Rheumatology

SECTION EDITOR

Nina T. Washington, MD, MPH
Cleveland, OH

MEDICAL EDITOR

Lynn Bullock, MD
Colorado Springs, CO

Table of Contents

JUVENILE IDIOPATHIC ARTHRITIS (JIA)

PREVIEW | REVIEW

- Which cytokines are believed to mediate juvenile idiopathic arthritis (JIA)?

- Name and describe the fever seen in systemic JIA (sJIA).

- Name 2 poor prognostic indicators for sJIA.

- Describe the rash of sJIA.

- What is macrophage activation syndrome (MAS)?

- Which cell type engulfs other cell types (hemophagocytosis) in MAS?

- Which joint is frequently involved in oligoarticular JIA (oJIA) but is often silent, requiring diagnosis by magnetic resonance imaging?

- When uveitis occurs with some of the subtypes of JIA, in which eye chamber is it found?

- Although the incidence of positive antinuclear antibody (ANA) is highest in oJIA, the presence of a positive ANA in some subtypes of JIA increases the risk of developing what eye finding?

- In polyarticular JIA, what does the presence of rheumatoid factor and anti-cyclic citrullinated peptide antibodies indicate?

- What criteria are required to make the diagnosis of psoriatic JIA (psJIA)?

- True or false? In psJIA, arthritis can precede the psoriasis by years.

- Arthritis of which joints is unique to psJIA?

- What is enthesitis-related arthropathy?

- Which biologics are used for JIA?

TERMINOLOGY / OCCURRENCE

JIA (formerly juvenile rheumatoid arthritis [JRA]) is the most common rheumatic disease diagnosed in children, affecting ~ 300,000 children in the U.S. Incidence (new cases) per year varies by location and is ~ 10/100,000. Prevalence of JIA in North America is ~ 1/1,000 children.

The International League of Associations for Rheumatology (ILAR) renamed and replaced the terms juvenile rheumatoid arthritis and juvenile chronic arthritis with the new nomenclature, juvenile idiopathic arthritis. The 2001 ILAR JIA criteria have been endorsed by the World Health Organization and are widely accepted in the U.S. and the international community.

JIA is defined as follows:

- Occurring before 16 years of age
- Persistent synovitis in ≥ 1 joints
- Synovitis for ≥ 6 weeks

All other potential diagnoses (e.g., infection, malignancy) must be excluded.

JIA TYPES

The ILAR classification system identifies 7 JIA categories:

1) **Systemic** (sJIA)—arthritis + fever + systemic findings, including rash, hepatomegaly, splenomegaly, lymphadenopathy, or serositis

2) **Oligoarticular** (oJIA; formerly pauciarticular-onset juvenile rheumatoid arthritis, pauciarthritis)—no > 4 joints affected during the first 6 months of disease; 2 subcategories:
   - Persistent oligoarthritis (affecting ≤ 4 joints for the duration of the disease)
   - Extended arthritis (affecting ≥ 5 joints after the first 6 months of disease)

3) **Polyarthritis rheumatoid factor (RF) negative** (poJIA RF–)—affecting ≥ 5 joints during the first 6 months of disease and RF–

4) **Polyarthritis RF positive** (poJIA RF+)—affecting ≥ 5 joints during the first 6 months of disease and RF+

5) **Psoriatic** arthritis (psJIA)

6) **Enthesitis-related arthropathies** (ERAs)

7) **Unclassified** (uJIA)

Keep going back to Table 20-1 on page 20-2 as you read through the topics that follow. The table puts it all together and makes it easy to compare and contrast findings of these different subtypes.

The etiologies of these autoimmune disorders differ based on the subtypes. Genetic predispositions and environmental exposures that increase an individual's risk also likely differ based on subtype. Some human leukocyte antigen (HLA) alleles appear to be important, and many believe that some microbial antigens are responsible as well.

JIA is thought to be initiated by presentation of antigens to T lymphocytes by antigen-presenting cells (e.g., macrophages, B cells, dendritic cells). This T-cell activation causes production of T and B lymphocytes. Cytokines are then released, including tumor necrosis factor (TNF; a.k.a. tumor necrosis factor-α [TNF-α]), interleukin-1 (IL-1), and interleukin-6 (IL-6), which cause release of other mediators, including prostaglandins, complement, and proteases.

Synovial fluid white blood cell (WBC) counts, composed mostly of lymphocytes, are usually between 2,000 and 30,000 cells/mL but can be as high as 100,000 cells/mL in some patients. The inflamed synovium is infiltrated with lymphocytes and plasma cells. Pannus formation occurs, which is an abnormal growth of the synovium into the articular cartilage.

Table 20-1: JIA Subtypes						
	Systemic JIA	**Oligoarticular JIA**	**Polyarticular RF− JIA**	**Polyarticular RF+ JIA**	**Juvenile Psoriatic JIA**	**Enthesitis-Related Arthropathies**
Peak age of onset	2 years	1–3 years	Dual peaks (1–3 years, then 9–14 years)	Teenage	Dual peaks (2–3 years, then mean age of 10 years)	Teenage
Sex	Equal	F > M	F > M	F > M	F > M*	M > F
ANA+	Rare	Majority	Majority	Rare	Majority of younger age	Rare
RF+	No	No	No	Yes	No	No
Anti-CCP+ (anti-cyclic citrullinated peptides)	No	No	No	Yes	No	No
HLA-B27+	No	No	No	No	Majority of older age	Majority
Anterior Uveitis	Rare	Silent	Silent	Rare	Silent	Typically, acute
Enthesitis	No	No	No	No	Older age	Yes
Dactylitis	No	Rare	No	No	Yes	Yes
Fevers	High-spiking	No	No	No	No	Rare

Adapted from: Stoll ML and Cron RQ. *Pediatric Rheumatology Online Journal* 2014 Apr 23;12:13.
By definition, children with unclassified JIA meet criteria for none of the categories listed in the table or for ≥ 2 of the categories.
*Among psoriatic individuals with an older age of onset, the male:female ratio is close to 1, and the incidence of positive antinuclear antibody (ANA+) is lower.

Clues for diagnosis of JIA:

- **Morning stiffness** that improves with movement later in the morning
- Changes in walking, running, climbing, or willingness to play, especially in the morning hours. These changes are sometimes described by the parents as the child "walking like an old man/woman."
- Voluntary guarding of an inflamed joint
- Leg-length discrepancies
- Child needs help with dressing, eating, bathing, and using the toilet.
- Loss of developmental milestones

Radiologic studies are nonspecific early in the course but can be helpful if you notice certain things. For example: If the JIA involves the fingers, it is characteristic to see widening of the midportion of the affected phalanges from periosteal new bone formation, although it takes months to years of active inflammation for these changes to appear. Bone erosions are rarely detected early in the course of most adult rheumatoid arthritis and JIA, with the occasional exception of the temporomandibular joint (TMJ), which can present with erosive changes.

Systemic JIA (sJIA)

sJIA (formerly Still disease) is a form of juvenile arthritis characterized by significantly high levels of systemic inflammation. By definition, sJIA requires the occurrence of daily fever (fevers of ≥ 102.2°F [39.0°C] must be present for ≥ 2 weeks with daily fevers for at least 3 days), arthritis, and other systemic findings (Table 20-1). sJIA occurs in ~ 10% of individuals with JIA. This type affects boys and girls equally. Whereas older children and adolescents may be diagnosed with sJIA, peak age of onset is between 1 and 5 years of age. The effects of the disease trail off into adulthood. The key to making the diagnosis is observing 1 or 2 fever spikes on a daily basis that return to normal without antipyretics; this is called a **quotidian fever**. Usually, the fever is in the evening and can be associated with severe malaise, myalgia, and arthralgia. However, the fever is present in this pattern in only 30% of children at disease onset. One Pennsylvania-based sJIA registry found 98% of patients had fever at the time of diagnosis, but patterns of fever were greatly varied. When the fever is gone, the child appears better and may have no significant symptoms. Poor prognostic indicators with sJIA include persistent fever, active disease 1 year after onset, steroid dependency, polyarthritis, and diagnosis before 4 years of age.

Clinical manifestations of sJIA:

- The sJIA rash is migratory with pink- to salmon-colored macules and discrete borders with or without central clearing, usually coinciding with the fever. You see the rash on the trunk, thighs, and axillae. Mild irritation, such as rubbing or scratching (**Koebner phenomenon**), may cause the rash to appear. Occasionally, the rash is very pruritic. Biopsy shows nonspecific lymphocytic infiltration, so this is not a recommended diagnostic test.

- Synovitis may or may not appear initially, but the diagnosis is more difficult until the joint involvement has declared itself. Arthritis can occur as oligoarticular (~ 25–30%) or polyarticular (70–75%) involvement. The amount of arthritis predicts the long-term outcome.
- Severe myalgias may be present. Creatine kinase (CK; a.k.a. creatine phosphokinase [CPK]) is usually normal, but the aldolase can be quite elevated.
- Pericarditis and myocarditis
- Pleuritis
- Lymphadenopathy
- Hepatosplenomegaly
- Abdominal pain
- Weight loss and fatigue

Laboratory findings in sJIA can be very abnormal, with occasional leukemoid reaction (> 40,000 WBC/μL), thrombocytosis (occasionally > 1 million cells/μL), microcytic anemia of chronic disease, and high C-reactive protein (CRP) and erythrocyte sedimentation rate (ESR) values. CRP and ESR are acute phase reactants commonly used to detect and follow the inflammatory state of rheumatologic diseases. Even though they are called acute phase reactants, they can be elevated in acute and chronic inflammatory conditions. Abnormal liver enzymes and bilirubin are not unusual. Ferritin, which typically is used to measure body iron stores, is also an acute phase reactant and levels are often elevated (normal < 200 ng/mL). Ferritin levels that are very elevated (e.g., > 5,000–10,000 ng/mL or higher) raise suspicion of macrophage activation syndrome (see Macrophage Activation Syndrome (MAS)). RF is usually negative, and the antinuclear antibody (ANA) is rarely positive. In contrast to oligoarticular JIA, uveitis is rare in the systemic form of JIA.

Macrophage Activation Syndrome (MAS)

Children severely affected by sJIA can develop a life-threatening condition called macrophage activation syndrome (MAS; a.k.a. acquired hemophagocytic syndrome). Although MAS can be caused by infections (e.g., Epstein-Barr virus [EBV], parvovirus B19, varicella) and drugs (e.g., sulfa drugs, nonsteroidal antiinflammatory drugs [NSAIDs]), the usual cause in these patients is uncontrolled sJIA.

Characteristics of MAS:

- Persistent fever
- Hepatosplenomegaly
- Markedly high ferritin
- Cytopenias (affecting at least 2 of the 3 cell lines)
- Liver dysfunction marked by elevated liver function tests (LFTs), coagulopathy, low fibrinogen, and/or elevated triglycerides
- Neurologic dysfunction

Prompt diagnosis is possible with frequent laboratory (1–2×/week) and clinical (every 1–2 weeks) monitoring during active systemic disease. ESR can drop precipitously

due to the low fibrinogen. Hemophagocytosis by macrophages/histiocytes is evident on bone marrow biopsy, although not always present.

Prompt treatment with high-dose corticosteroids, IL-1 or IL-6 inhibitors, and/or cyclosporine can prevent life-threatening complications in MAS.

Oligoarticular JIA (oJIA)

oJIA affects ≤ 4 joints during the first 6 months of disease. Note that the prefix oligo- means few (usually in contrast to poly-, meaning many). oJIA occurs in ~ 30% of individuals with JIA and usually presents between 1 and 5 years of age, with an average age of onset of 1–3 years. Females outnumber males 3:1 overall, but in those with uveitis, females outnumber males 6.5:1. These patients often present with few symptoms and slow onset. Approximately 25% do not have any pain but have incidental joint swelling. The joints most commonly involved (in most frequently seen order) are the knee, ankle, fingers/toes, elbows, and wrists, but rarely the hips. Asymptomatic TMJ involvement is typical in patients with oJIA and is best diagnosed by magnetic resonance imaging (MRI). Fever, rash, and night pain are not seen in oligoarticular disease.

The 2 subtypes of oJIA are defined by the course of the arthritis after 6 months of disease. **Persistent oligoarthritis** is when the child has ≤ 4 joints involved throughout the course of disease, and **extended oligoarthritis** (a worse prognosis) is when the child develops disease in ≥ 5 joints after the first 6 months. See Table 20-1.

Asymptomatic anterior uveitis occurs in ~ 30% of patients, usually with oJIA, and ANA positivity predicts higher risk of developing uveitis. Screening frequency is based on various risk factors. Uveitis presents most commonly within the first 5–7 years of initial JIA presentation. The 2019 American College of Rheumatology/Arthritis Foundation (ACR/AF) guidelines recommend performing ophthalmologic screening for uveitis with slitlamp exam every 3 months in all children and adolescents with oJIA who are also ANA positive, < 7 years old at disease onset, and have disease duration ≤ 4 years. Screening every 6–12 months is suggested for all other patients with JIA.

If uveitis is found, treat aggressively to prevent synechiae (i.e., iris adhesions; Figure 20-1), cataracts, glaucoma, and blindness. Uveitis and arthritis do not necessarily happen at the same time. Even a child with no active arthritis is at risk.

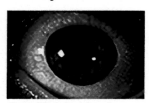

Figure 20-1: Peripheral anterior synechiae

Laboratory studies are nonspecific in oJIA. Approximately 70% of children with oJIA have a positive ANA in low titer (≤ 1:320). It is very important to know that a positive ANA is not a diagnostic tool for JIA. It is used as a prognostic indicator for risk of uveitis in children with JIA. Other laboratory tests—including RF and hemoglobin—are usually normal in patients with oJIA; inflammatory markers, including ESR and CRP, can be normal in many of these patients. An elevated platelet count, which is a nonspecific marker of inflammation, can be encountered in any patient with JIA and inflammation.

Polyarticular JIA (poJIA)

poJIA involves ≥ 5 joints during the first 6 months of the disease and is found in ~ 30–40% of individuals diagnosed with JIA. There is a higher prevalence in girls compared to boys (~ 3:1). poJIA affects large and small joints (metacarpophalangeals [MCPs] and proximal interphalangeals [PIPs]) and typically involves the cervical spine, hips, shoulders, and temporomandibular joints. Symmetrical joint involvement can occur, as in adult rheumatoid arthritis. Cervical spine fusion and micrognathia are typical late findings of polyarticular disease (for both polyarticular onset and systemic onset). Fatigue is a common presenting symptom; weight loss and rheumatoid nodules (usually RF+) also can occur. There are 2 distinct groups with polyarticular disease: those who are RF– and those who are RF+. See Table 20-1 on page 20-2.

RF– poJIA has 2 age peaks: the first occurs from 1 to 3 years of age and the second from 9 to 14 years of age. Most children with poJIA are RF–, are younger, and have a less aggressive course than RF+ poJIA. These children generally do not have anti-cyclic citrullinated peptide (anti-CCP) antibodies either.

RF+ poJIA represents only ~ 4–5% of all children with JIA. Think of this as being an early form of adult rheumatoid arthritis. RF+ disease occurs more frequently in older adolescents; the disease course corresponds to adult rheumatoid arthritis with a more aggressive course. RF positivity is a poor prognostic finding and mandates aggressive management of the patient. Anti-CCP antibodies, often seen in adult rheumatoid arthritis, are detectable in a significant proportion of RF+ JIA patients and are also associated with erosive arthritis in this group. Most, but not all, RF+ poJIA patients are anti-CCP antibody positive and vice versa.

Approximately 50–80% of children with RF– poJIA have a positive ANA. Uveitis is less common with polyarticular onset, compared to oligoarticular onset, affecting only 10–15% with a positive ANA. Uveitis is typically asymptomatic; children < 7 years of age with a positive ANA and poJIA have intermediate risk of uveitis and should be monitored more closely, as outlined under Oligoarticular JIA (oJIA) on page 20-3.

Juvenile Psoriatic Arthritis (psJIA)

psJIA is defined by:

- Arthritis and psoriasis, or
- Arthritis and at least 2 of the following:
  ○ Dactylitis
  ○ Nail findings (pitting [Figure 20-2], oil spots, or onycholysis)
  ○ Family history of psoriasis in at least one 1st degree relative

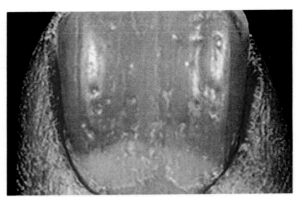

Figure 20-2: Pitted nail as seen in psoriatic arthritis

Arthritis can precede the psoriasis by many years. Arthritis develops in ~ 7% of patients with cutaneous psoriasis, but it is much more likely to develop (> 30%) in those with **psoriatic nail involvement**. Initially, the arthritis is an asymmetric oligoarthritis of small and large joints. **Distal interphalangeal (DIP) joint arthritis** is also typical, which makes psoriatic arthritis unique compared to the other JIA subtypes. Note: DIPs are the distal joints, PIPs are the middle joints (proximal interphalangeal joints), MCPs are the joints at the base of the fingers (metacarpophalangeal joints), and MTPs (metatarsophalangeals) are the joints at the base of the toes. In some, the arthritis can involve more joints, and they can have a polyarticular pattern. Some patients have a chronic oligoarthritis or DIP arthritis and never progress to polyarthritis. Some patients also present with back pain or spondyloarthropathy and appendicular arthritis. HLA-B7 antigen is positive in this group of adolescents. Acute or chronic anterior uveitis is common, as is ANA positivity (30–50% of patients). See Oligoarticular JIA (oJIA) on page 20-3 for uveitis screening guidelines.

Dactylitis can be present and looks like a sausage digit where there is inflammation at the joints and in the soft tissue—such as synovium, tendon sheath, and enthesis—of a finger or toe.

Younger patients with psJIA are more commonly girls, whereas children presenting during adolescence are more often boys. See Table 20-1 on page 20-2.

Enthesitis-Related Arthropathies (ERA)

An enthesis is the point where a tendon or ligament inserts into a bone. Enthesitis is inflammation and tenderness of this area. ERA is:

- Enthesitis and arthritis or
- Either enthesitis or arthritis with ≥ 2 of the following:
  ○ History or presence of sacroiliac (SI) joint tenderness and/or inflammatory lumbosacral pain
  ○ Presence of HLA-B27 antigen
  ○ Onset of arthritis in a male > 6 years of age
  ○ Acute symptomatic uveitis
  ○ A 1st degree relative with ankylosing spondylitis, ERA, sacroiliitis with inflammatory bowel disease (IBD), or reactive arthritis

You may be familiar with older terminology for 1 or more of the ERAs. In their 2001 guidelines, ILAR recommends that the following entities (some historical) be referred to as ERAs: juvenile spondyloarthropathy, SEA syndrome (syndrome of seronegativity, enthesopathy, and arthropathy), HLA-B27-associated arthropathy and enthesopathy syndrome, oligoarticular-onset JIA Type II, and juvenile ankylosing spondylitis.

ERA has different characteristics, compared to the other childhood inflammatory arthritides (Table 20-1 on page 20-2):

- Older children are affected more often.
- Males are more commonly affected.
- It is familial 10–20% of the time.
- Arthritis is typically peripheral, with lower limb involvement in an asymmetric manner.
- Enthesitis is a common finding.

Constitutional symptoms are less common, with fever and weight loss occurring in < 10% of children with ERA. Conduct a complete review of systems to be sure there is no growth delay, abdominal pain, or blood in the stools (as can be seen with IBD).

Clinically, these children (usually boys) present with morning pain and stiffness that is relieved by playing or other activity. The pain is predominantly in the joints of the lower extremities and is frequently in the lower back/buttocks and at the entheses of the heels, feet, and knees. The enthesitis at the patellar tendon can be misdiagnosed as Osgood-Schlatter disease, which is an overuse injury of the patellar ligament over the tibial tuberosity. The oligoarthritis of ERA is commonly asymmetric. The entheses that are affected can be exquisitely tender to palpation. You can elicit SI pain by direct palpation or pelvic manipulation. Lumbar flexion is often limited (i.e., the patient has a positive Schober test) and remains flat (no lumbar curvature) on exam.

Acute symptomatic iritis (i.e., an acutely painful, red eye) occurs in ~ 5–10% of children with ERA and requires referral to an ophthalmologist. See Oligoarticular JIA (oJIA) on page 20-3 for uveitis screening guidelines.

ESR is normal in 50% of patients, and HLA-B27 is positive in 50–90%.

Children with a chronic course are more likely to develop sacroiliitis with spondylitis and progress into adulthood with ankylosing disease of the back and SI joints.

DIFFERENTIAL DIAGNOSIS OF JIA

Joint inflammation, which manifests as heat, pain, and swelling, is required to make the JIA diagnosis. If pain occurs without evidence of inflammation, think of an orthopedic problem, such as avascular necrosis (AVN), slipped femoral epiphysis, or Osgood-Schlatter disease. Also consider other conditions, such as benign nocturnal limb pains of childhood (i.e., "growing pains"), benign hypermobility, and psychogenic/amplified pain syndrome. The differential diagnosis of sJIA includes various illnesses with fever, joint symptoms, rash, lymphadenopathy, and lab abnormalities such as:

- Malignancies (e.g., leukemia, lymphoma, neuroblastoma)
- Bone or joint infections
- Systemic lupus erythematosa (SLE)
- Acute rheumatic fever
- Serum sickness
- Kawasaki disease (KD)
- Sarcoidosis
- Sjögren syndrome (SS)

Figure 20-3 summarizes some emergent differential diagnoses of sJIA.

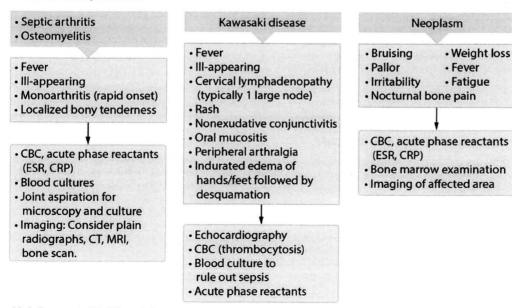

Figure 20-3: Emergent sJIA differential

TREATMENT OF JIA

NSAIDs are often used initially, typically with disease-modifying antirheumatic drugs (**DMARDs**). Try **steroid joint injections** if no improvement occurs with NSAIDs. Many pediatric rheumatologists start a DMARD immediately after ruling out other possible diagnoses. The DMARD most commonly used for JIA is methotrexate. It is administered 1×/week either as pills or injected subcutaneously. It is important that patients who take methotrexate be on folic acid supplementation to decrease risk for methotrexate side effects such as liver abnormalities, oral ulcers, and cytopenias.

Biologic therapies that target a specific cytokine are commonly used for children with aggressive disease or disease refractory to DMARDs, although not all are approved by the Food & Drug Administration (FDA) for treatment in children.

Biologic treatments for JIA include:

- Tumor necrosis factor inhibitors (e.g., etanercept, adalimumab, infliximab)
- T-cell modulators (abatacept)
- IL-6 receptor blockers (tocilizumab)
- IL-1 blockers (e.g., anakinra, canakinumab, rilonacept). A 2019 study has shown good results with using anakinra as a 1st line drug.

TNF inhibitors appear to work very well for poJIA but less so for sJIA patients (who respond well to IL-6 and IL-1 inhibition). **Abatacept**, a soluble fusion protein that inhibits the costimulation of T cells, is also useful for refractory cases of poJIA.

Test for latent tuberculosis infection, hepatitis B virus, and hepatitis C virus prior to initiating biologic therapy. Once a patient is on a biologic therapy, avoid live attenuated vaccines.

Generally, do not use oral corticosteroids except for very severe disease, flares of disease, or systemic manifestations. Try to use the lowest doses possible (< 0.25 mg/kg/day or < 10 mg/day) to minimize side effects, which include diabetes, stunted growth, osteoporosis, infection, cataracts, glaucoma, hypertension, hyperlipidemia, mood changes, and adrenal insufficiency.

Follow patients closely every 1–3 months; remission is the goal of therapy, and patients can then be seen every 4–5 months. Physical and occupational therapy, orthotics, and splinting can prevent deformities and help children maintain function.

OUTCOMES OF JIA

Long-term follow-up studies show that patients with JIA treated in the era before biologics had a higher rate of disability than previously thought, with 25–50% of them having functional limitations. Data shows steady improvement in functional capacity over the past 40 years due to better treatments, including medication and joint replacement. Up to 30–40% still have active synovitis as adults and require ongoing rheumatologic care. Mortality from JIA is rare; < 0.5% in the U.S. Deaths in children with sJIA related to amyloidosis, infections, and MAS have declined as a result of better disease recognition and control.

ARTHRITIS ASSOCIATED WITH INFLAMMATORY BOWEL DISEASE (IBD)

PREVIEW | REVIEW

- What percentage of patients with inflammatory bowel disease (IBD) have arthritis?
- In arthritis with IBD, how do the peripheral and axial forms of arthritis differ?
- What are the systemic symptoms of arthritis with IBD?

Arthritis occurs in ~ 25% of patients with IBD (i.e., Crohn disease, ulcerative colitis). Characteristics of IBD-associated arthritis depend on whether it is peripheral or axial:

- **Peripheral arthritis** (more commonly affected)
  - Incidence in girls = incidence in boys
  - Not associated with HLA-B27
  - Arthritis flares with gut flares
- **Axial arthritis** (e.g., spine, hips, SI joints)
  - Incidence in boys >> incidence in girls
  - Associated with HLA-B27
  - Not dependent on gut flares

Look for the following systemic symptoms and signs to help diagnose arthritis with IBD: fatigue, iron deficiency anemia, low albumin, persistently elevated inflammatory markers, weight loss, growth delay, fever, oral ulcers, abdominal pain/tenderness, diarrhea, erythema nodosum, pyoderma gangrenosum, and clubbing.

Arthritis coinciding with a gut flare, typically peripheral arthritis, usually responds to appropriate therapy for the gut disease such as corticosteroids or oral DMARDs (sulfasalazine, methotrexate, infliximab, and adalimumab). Spinal disease sometimes needs treatment even when gut disease is inactive. Typical agents used are NSAIDs and the monoclonal antibody TNF inhibitors (infliximab and adalimumab). Oral DMARDs do not help with spinal disease, they only help with peripheral disease. The FDA added label warnings of increased risk of hepatosplenic T-cell lymphoma (HSTCL) in children who receive TNF inhibitors, especially when used in combination with azathioprine or 6-mercaptopurine (6-MP); however, HSTCL has been described in patients receiving azathioprine and 6-MP alone. NSAIDs are used sparingly because of risk for IBD flares and gastrointestinal side effects.

INFECTION-RELATED ARTHRITIS

PREVIEW | REVIEW

- In infectious arthritis, what are the differing characteristics between bacterial and viral etiologies?
- Which gram-negative organism is usually the cause of infectious arthritis in neonates and infants?
- Infections of which 2 systems typically occur prior to reactive arthritis (ReA)?
- What is the typical triad of ReA?
- Can urethritis occur in ReA even if the organism is of gastrointestinal origin?

INFECTIOUS ARTHRITIS

Infectious arthritis is most frequently caused by the direct spread of bacteria into the joint space, but it can also be caused by viruses and fungi. Presenting symptoms include fever, substantial pain, and decreased range of motion of the affected, often erythematous joint. The arthritis can affect 1 joint or multiple joints, depending on the causative agent.

Bacteria tend to affect single, large joints, although certain pathogens (especially *Staphylococcus aureus* and *Neisseria gonorrhoeae*) can affect multiple joints. **Viral** etiologies cause a rash and commonly can have symmetric involvement of smaller joints. **Fungal** causes are rare and typically occur in the neonate or immunocompromised patient. Fungal causes have a more indolent course and occur with disseminated disease.

A good history and physical are important, with special attention given to location and number of joints affected. Diagnosis is made by isolation of the pathogen by culture or polymerase chain reaction (PCR) from synovial fluid or blood. The mainstay of treatment is drainage and lavage of the joint space and antimicrobial therapy (unless viral) targeted toward the inciting organism.

Some of the microbes that cause arthritis include:

- *S. aureus* (most common)
- *N. gonorrhoeae*
- Group B *Streptococcus*
- *Escherichia coli* (causes arthritis in neonates and infants)
- Viruses
  - Parvovirus B19
  - HBV

REACTIVE ARTHRITIS (ReA)

ReA (formerly postinfectious arthritis; Reiter syndrome) usually occurs 1–4 weeks after the following:

- Gastrointestinal (GI) infection with
  - *Yersinia enterocolitica*
  - *Shigella flexneri*
  - *Salmonella typhimurium*
  - *Campylobacter jejuni*
  - *Clostridioides* (formerly *Clostridium*) *difficile*
  - *Giardia lamblia*
- Genitourinary (GU) infection caused by *Chlamydia trachomatis* (usually lasts 3–6 weeks but occasionally remains chronic)
- Lyme disease
- Streptococcal infection

ReA is thought to occur due to molecular mimicry and cross-reactivity of T lymphocytes to bacterial antigens in the eyes, joints, genitals, and urinary tract. ReA typically manifests as a triad of **urethritis, conjunctivitis,** and **arthritis** (thus the catch phrase, "can't pee, can't see, can't climb a tree"). Not all symptoms necessarily occur, or they can occur at separate times. Urethritis can occur even if the infectious trigger is GI in origin; urinalysis may show a sterile pyuria. Males with ReA sometimes develop lesions on the end of the penis known as **circinate balanitis.** Mucocutaneous features, including oral ulcers, genital ulcers, balanitis, and papular skin lesions (e.g., **keratoderma blenorrhagicum** on the palms and soles), are common as well. Look for enthesitis (inflammation of the sites where tendons and ligaments connect to bones), dactylitis (sausage-like digits), and arthritis that affects the large weight-bearing joints. The sacroiliac joints, knees, and ankles are more commonly involved than are joints of the upper extremities. Aortic regurgitation, although rare, caused by inflammation of the aortic wall and valve may also occur. Due to the severity of the systemic symptoms, ReA can present like septic arthritis, requiring aspiration of joint fluid. In the acute phase, patients may experience symptoms such as fatigue, malaise, myalgia, weight loss, and fever. Conversely, it is not uncommon for patients to be afebrile with no constitutional symptoms. Initial laboratory findings are notable for an elevated erythrocyte sedimentation rate and elevated C-reactive protein. Patients with chronic arthritis may exhibit normocytic anemia.

A convincing history of infection occurring 2–4 weeks prior to onset of urethritis, conjunctivitis, and arthritis is usually sufficient to make the diagnosis; however, obtaining stool, urethral, conjunctival cultures, and/or blood serologies—looking for presence of current or recent infection—is recommended. Up to 50% of patients with ReA are HLA-B27 positive. Patients are seronegative for rheumatoid factor (RF) and antinuclear antibody (ANA). The arthritis usually lasts for 3–6 months but occasionally can remain chronic. Note that ocular findings of anterior uveitis and keratitis are also possible.

Treat with NSAIDs for at least 2–4 weeks. Resistant cases may benefit from sulfasalazine, methotrexate, and/or anti–tumor necrosis factor agents. Antibiotics are not required unless there is evidence of active infection.

VASCULITIDES

PREVIEW | REVIEW

- What is the most common vasculitis in childhood? Which antibody mediates it?

- What is a predisposing factor in 50% of immunoglobulin A vasculitis (IgAV) cases?

- What do you do if a child with IgAV has persistent, severe abdominal pain? What do you suspect as an etiology?

- What system are you concerned about for at least 3–6 months after diagnosis of IgAV?

- Are most cases of IgAV self-limited?

- How common are recurrences in IgAV during the first 2 years following the initial presentation?

- What is the nasal deformity seen in granulomatosis with polyangiitis (GPA)?

- What laboratory test is useful in diagnosing GPA?

- What is the main cause of death in Kawasaki disease (KD)? When does this usually occur?

- What are the diagnostic criteria for KD?

- What gallbladder abnormality is seen in KD?

- What are the cardiac manifestations of KD?

- What is the treatment for KD?

- What are potential therapies available for KD refractory to IV immunoglobulin?

- What is polyarteritis nodosa (PAN)?

- Which organ system is typically spared in PAN?

- What is Takayasu arteritis?

- What is the classic triad of Behçet disease?

- Which skin lesions are commonly seen in Behçet disease?

OVERVIEW

The vasculitic disorders are relatively uncommon in children. Severity and manifestations are dependent on the size of the vessels.

Small-vessel vasculitis, caused by immune complexes, presents with purpura. Examples of small-vessel vasculitis include:

- Drug reactions
- Serum sickness
- IgA vasculitis (IgAV; formerly Henoch-Schönlein purpura)
- Granulomatosis with polyangiitis (GPA)

Medium-vessel vasculitis causes organ system damage and includes:

- Polyarteritis nodosa (PAN)
- Kawasaki disease (KD)

Large-vessel vasculitis can cause claudication symptoms. Takayasu arteritis is the classic form of a large-vessel disorder.

SMALL-VESSEL VASCULITIDES

Immunoglobulin A Vasculitis (IgAV)

IgAV (formerly Henoch-Schönlein purpura) is a small-vessel vasculitis. It is the most common vasculitis of childhood, affecting ~ 1 in 5,000 children. It presents as a tetrad of **a**rthritis, **a**bdominal pain, **r**enal disease, and **p**alpable **p**urpura (mnemonic: **AARPP**). The mean age at diagnosis is 4 years, and > 75% of those affected are < 7 years of age. The age range is typically 3–15 years, but IgAV is seen in older adolescents and adults as well. IgAV affects boys more frequently than girls with a ratio of nearly 2:1. Seasonality is important, with more cases reported in the winter and spring. IgAV is an immune-mediated leukocytoclastic vasculitis with neutrophil infiltration and primarily IgA deposition in vessel walls, along with small amounts of IgG and C3.

The specific cause of IgAV is unknown. In ~ 50% of cases, an upper respiratory infection or gastroenteritis precedes the disease. The literature has listed a number of possible "triggers": bacteria (e.g., *Streptococcus pyogenes*, *Legionella*, *Mycoplasma*, *Yersinia*), viruses (e.g., Epstein-Barr virus [EBV], varicella, cytomegalovirus [CMV], parvovirus, hepatitis B virus), drugs (e.g., penicillin, cephalosporins, thiazide diuretics), vaccines (e.g., measles, yellow fever), food additives, and insect bites.

Skin lesions (Figure 20-4 and Figure 20-5) are present in all IgAV patients and are the presenting finding in ~ 50%. The rash begins as small wheals or red maculopapules that progress to petechial and palpable purpuric lesions. They are generally found on the dependent, pressure-bearing areas (i.e., lower extremities, buttocks). They can occur in other areas as well, particularly the face and ears in younger children. The skin lesions last from 4 days to 4 weeks. Angioedema sometimes precedes the rash.

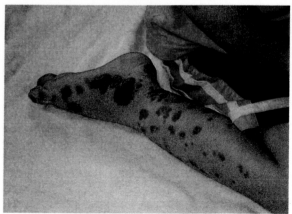

Figure 20-4: IgAV palpable purpuric skin lesions on the lower extremities

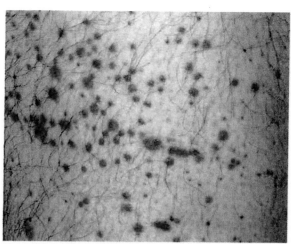

Figure 20-5: IgAV skin lesions; maculopapules and petechiae

The 2nd most common manifestation is **joint involvement,** occurring in 50–80% of patients. In ~ 25% of patients, arthritis is the initial manifestation and makes the diagnosis difficult until the rash appears. The arthritis/arthralgia is transient and mainly of the large joints, particularly the knees and ankles. Joint effusions do not usually occur. Periarthritis, with edema around the joints and inflammation involving the tendon sheaths, is the most common musculoskeletal manifestation. Chronic arthritis is not present.

The next most prevalent manifestations are the **GI manifestations.** The most typical GI manifestation is abdominal pain that is colicky in pattern and sometimes involves vomiting. The pain can precede the rash (in up to 20% of cases)—again, making the diagnosis more difficult until the rash appears. Occult bleeding is common in those with abdominal pain, and melena can occur. Hematemesis can occur but is less typical. Fortunately, only ~ 5% have a major GI bleeding episode. Ultrasound (U/S) may show increased echogenicity and/or thickening of the wall of the 2nd portion of the duodenum and hydrops of the gallbladder. These changes occur only if the patient has GI symptoms, which occur in ~ 50–75% of patients.

If abdominal pain is severe or persistent, perform U/S to evaluate for intussusception, which is the most common GI complication of IgAV (can occur in 5–10% of patients).

Renal manifestations affect between 30% and 50% of patients with IgAV and are usually mild and transient. Renal complications, however, are the most common overall long-term morbidity of IgAV. Look for isolated microscopic hematuria or hematuria and proteinuria at initial presentation. A renal biopsy (when performed in severe cases) shows IgA deposition just as with IgA nephropathy (a.k.a. Berger disease). Generally, < 1–2%

have residual renal disease and even fewer progress to end-stage renal disease. At greater risk for permanent renal damage are children:

- > 10 years of age
- with purpura that lasts > 1 month
- with severe, persistent GI symptoms (e.g., hemorrhage, pain)
- with arthritis/arthralgia
- with leukocytosis > 15, thrombocytosis > 500, decreased C3 levels, and elevated ASO titers

Other manifestations include orchitis and pulmonary hemorrhage. Acute appendicitis is often mistakenly suspected when severe GI symptoms precede the other classic manifestations.

IgAV is a clinical diagnosis without specific confirmatory laboratory tests. Nonspecific findings include high WBC counts, elevated ESR (increased in ~ 50% of patients), elevated serum IgA levels, and normal platelet and coagulation studies. Ultrasonography, as mentioned previously, can be helpful.

Order serial urinalysis for at least 3–6 months after diagnosis to monitor for renal involvement.

There is no specific or standardized therapy for IgAV. Supportive outpatient care is generally sufficient. Skin lesions do not need specific therapy unless they are severe and ulcerated. Use NSAIDs for pain control but avoid if renal disease and significant GI disease are present. Use of corticosteroids is not generally recommended but is reserved for those with severe abdominal pain, gastrointestinal hemorrhage, severe scrotal swelling/edema, or severe nephritis. No randomized controlled trials to date show the benefit of early corticosteroid therapy for treatment or prevention of IgAV nephritis. Most improve without specific therapy, although uncontrolled trials have used intravenous (IV) pulses of methylprednisolone, cyclophosphamide, and azathioprine for refractory cases.

Prognosis of IgAV is excellent. Most problems stem from acute GI bleeds early in the illness or from long-term renal involvement; otherwise, the disease tends to be self-limited and lasts 4 weeks in ~ 65% of children. IgAV recurs in up to 40% of patients from 6 weeks to 2 years after initial presentation.

Granulomatosis with Polyangiitis (GPA)

GPA is very rare in children and is characterized by necrotizing granulomatous vasculitis of small-sized vessels involving the upper and lower respiratory tracts and the kidney—**pulmonary-renal syndrome.** Other potentially confounding pulmonary-renal syndromes include microscopic polyangiitis (MPA), sarcoidosis, systemic lupus erythematosus (SLE), and Goodpasture syndrome. (Anti–glomerular basement membrane disease involving both the kidneys and lungs is termed Goodpasture syndrome; additional information on Goodpasture syndrome is available in the Nephrology & Urology section.) GPA can present in adolescence and affects males and females equally. Common symptoms are fever, weight loss, arthralgias or migratory large joint arthritis, cough, nasal stuffiness, epistaxis, resistant ear infections, and persistent sinusitis. Nasal deformity ("saddle nose"; Figure 20-6) and subglottic stenosis can also occur in children with GPA and, less commonly, in relapsing polychondritis.

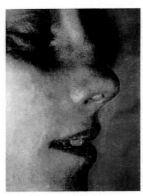

Figure 20-6: Saddle nose

Lung findings (nodules, infiltrates, hemoptysis, or pleuritis) are reported in 70% of children with GPA. **Ocular findings** (conjunctivitis, dacryocystitis, scleritis, and proptosis) occur in ~ 15–20% of these children. **Renal involvement** is uncommon in these children at presentation but eventually occurs in 60–70% of patients. Finding cytoplasmic antineutrophil cytoplasmic antibody (**c-ANCA** specific for proteinase 3 [PR3]) aids in the diagnosis. c-ANCA positivity is found in > 90% of patients with diffuse disease and only ~ 50% of those with limited (i.e., no renal involvement) disease. You must perform a biopsy to confirm the diagnosis.

Consider using steroids, methotrexate (especially for limited disease), rituximab, and cyclophosphamide. Chronic therapy with trimethoprim/sulfamethoxazole prevents relapses and decreases the risk for *Pneumocystis jiroveci* pneumonia. Relapses occur in 30–50% of patients. Long-term use of cyclophosphamide increases risk for infertility, lymphoma, hemorrhagic cystitis, and secondary cancers.

MEDIUM-VESSEL VASCULITIDES

Kawasaki Disease (KD)

KD (a.k.a. mucocutaneous lymph node syndrome), a medium-vessel vasculitis, is the 2nd most common vasculitis of childhood. It is the leading cause of acquired heart disease in children in the U.S. It generally occurs in children < 5 years of age, affects boys more than girls (1.5:1), and occurs year-round with clusters in the winter and spring. Incidence is highest in children of Asian descent. In Japan, the incidence is 90/100,000 in children < 5 years of age. The reported incidence in the U.S. is ~ 9/100,000 to 19/100,000. Nearly 1–3% of affected individuals have a recurrence. Recurrence is most likely in boys < 6 months of age or > 6 years of age. The etiology of this disorder is unknown. KD simulates an infectious disease, but no consistent organism can be identified. One theory points to staphylococcal and streptococcal superantigen stimulation of the immune system.

Myocardial infarction is the main cause of death in KD and most commonly occurs during the 1st year from the onset of illness. Fatality rates are 0.16% in infants < 1 year of age and 0.05% in children > 1 year of age.

A clinical diagnosis requires fever for at least 5 days and a minimum of 4 of the following 5 findings (Table 20-2):

1) Bilateral conjunctival injection without exudate (occurs in 80–90% of KD patients)

2) Rash (occurs in > 90%) is typically macular and polymorphous in character with no vesicles, scaling, or crusting; it is found on the trunk and frequently more prominent in the perineal area later in the course; desquamation of the area follows.

3) Changes in lips and oral cavity (occurs in 80–90%) present with red pharynx; dry, fissured lips; and/or an injected, strawberry tongue (Figure 20-7).

4) Changes in the peripheral extremities (occurs in ~ 80%) present with redness and swelling of the hands/feet (Figure 20-8) and, later, desquamation of the fingers/toes (Figure 20-9).

5) Cervical lymphadenopathy (occurs in ~ 50%) is typically nonfluctuant with 1 node required to be at least 1.5 cm in diameter.

Table 20-2: Classic Clinical Criteria for Kawasaki Disease	
Criteria	**Frequency (%)**
Fever persisting at least 5 days	100
Polymorphous exanthem	> 90
Changes in lips and oral cavity: erythema, lips cracking, strawberry tongue, diffuse injection of oral and pharyngeal mucosae	80–90
Bilateral bulbar conjunctival injection without exudate	80–90
Changes in extremities Acute: Erythema of palms, soles; edema of hands, feet Subacute: Periungual peeling of fingers, toes in weeks 2 and 3	~ 80
Cervical lymphadenopathy (> 1.5-cm diameter), usually unilateral	~ 50

Adapted from: Newburger JW, et al. AHA Scientific Statement 2004. *Textbook of Pediatric Rheumatology*, 7th ed. Ross E. Petty, et al. (eds.) Elsevier, 2015.

Diagnosis with < 4 of the 5 criteria is possible if coronary aneurysm is demonstrated on echocardiogram or angiography. Fever is an absolute requirement. Baseline lab tests such as complete blood count (CBC), LFTs, ESR/CRP, and urinalysis are generally done. Serologies such as ANA, RF, and ANCA are not necessary and are usually negative.

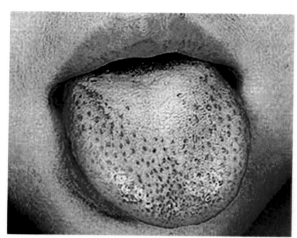

Figure 20-7: Strawberry tongue

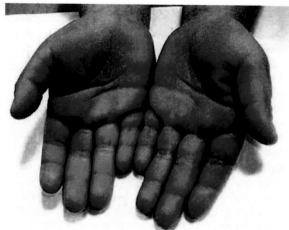

Figure 20-8: Kawasaki disease with redness and swelling of hands

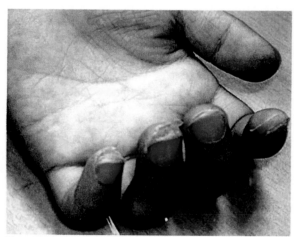

Figure 20-9: Kawasaki disease with desquamation of fingers

There is a syndrome known as **atypical** or **incomplete KD**, which is seen in patients who have fewer than the required 4 of 5 clinical findings needed for diagnosis. Usually missing is cervical lymphadenopathy and rash. It more often occurs in younger patients, especially infants < 1 year of age.

Think of KD in **3 stages**:

The **1st stage**, the acute phase, is the initial febrile period, usually lasting 1–2 weeks with temperatures of ≥ 104.0°F (40.0°C) and with at least 4 of the 5 findings. Irritability is a hallmark in this stage. Additional clinical findings may include aseptic meningitis, acute uveitis, diarrhea, mild obstructive jaundice with elevated transaminases, hydrops of the gallbladder, and sterile pyuria. Nearly 33% have polyarthritis or polyarthralgia, typically of the knees, ankles, and hands. Edema of the hands and feet is more common than localized inflammatory arthritis. Fluid aspirated from the joint shows polymorphonuclear leukocytes (PMNs), simulating septic arthritis but with a negative culture.

Be particularly aware of cardiac manifestations. Nearly 33% have pericardial effusions, and myocarditis is also common. Several coronary artery abnormalities—aneurysms are the main worry—may occur as early as day 3 of illness but are more typically seen 10 days to 4 weeks after onset. Even with treatment, they are found in 5–9% of patients. Increased risks of coronary aneurysm include male gender, age < 1 year or > 8 years, fever > 10 days, thrombocytopenia, hyponatremia, hypoalbuminemia, WBC > 15, and a recurrence of fever 36 hours after IVIG administration. See more about Kawasaki disease in the Cardiology section.

The **2nd stage**, the subacute phase, starts ~ 10–25 days after the initial fever presentation and persists until all clinical signs of inflammatory activity subside. The fever, rash, and lymph nodes usually resolve early in this phase, but irritability and conjunctival injection can persist. Skin changes occur during this stage, most commonly desquamation. Thrombocytosis generally occurs after day 7 of the illness. Coronary artery aneurysms occur in 25% of untreated individuals and in 5–9% of those who are treated. Oligoarticular disease can occur in 25% during the 2nd and 3rd weeks but is self-limited.

The **3rd stage**, the convalescent phase, occurs approximately the 3rd or 4th week, when clinical signs disappear, and usually lasts 3–4 weeks. Although less likely, coronary artery aneurysms may occur in the convalescent phase.

KD is mostly a clinical diagnosis. Use laboratory tests to exclude strep or staph infection and serum sickness. Laboratory findings include leukocytosis with a left shift, platelet counts commonly > 1 million during the subacute phase of the illness, and typically, the ESR and/or CRP are significantly elevated. Elevation of the gamma-glutamyl transferase (GGT) can help differentiate KD from other fever and rash syndromes that do not have gallbladder involvement. Be cognizant of possible multiorgan dysfunction. Approximately 1% of these patients can develop overt macrophage activation syndrome (MAS).

Treatment for KD is well established. Traditional recommendations are to give aspirin at a dosage of 80–100 mg/kg/day initially and IV immunoglobulin (IVIG) at a dosage of 2 g/kg as a single infusion over 12–14 hours. The IVIG typically causes a rapid improvement in fever and clinical symptoms. If the condition relapses or the patient does not respond well to treatment, repeat the dose of IVIG. Retreatment is needed in < 5–10% of cases. IVIG side effects are uncommon, but look for anaphylaxis and aseptic meningitis, which can occur 1–2 days after treatment. Corticosteroid therapy is controversial. Recent studies suggest the benefit of corticosteroid use as adjunctive therapy to ASA and IVIG (versus corticosteroid use in cases refractory to IVIG) when used in patients at high risk for developing coronary artery aneurysms. Infliximab, anakinra, and cyclosporine have also been used safely and successfully in patients who are IVIG failures. Continue high-dose aspirin until IVIG response is achieved and fever resolves. Reduce the aspirin dosage to 3–5 mg/kg/day for platelet inhibition. Discontinue when you are assured there is no cardiac involvement. Follow up with a cardiologist can be helpful in making this determination.

Every child with KD should have an initial echocardiogram at the time of diagnosis and a 2nd echocardiogram performed 6–8 weeks later. Myocardial infarction, if it occurs, usually does so during the 1st year after the onset of illness. Fatality rates are 0.16% in infants < 1 year of age and 0.05% in children > 1 year of age.

Polyarteritis Nodosa (PAN)

PAN is characterized by inflammation of medium-sized arteries and results in a focal segmental necrotizing vasculitis. PAN is rare in children. When it does appear, it occurs at a mean age of ~ 9 years, with males more frequently affected (~ 2:1). The exact etiology is unknown, although documented cases have occurred after hepatitis B or strep infection, or the use of certain drugs, all of which seem to implicate immune complexes.

PAN in childhood typically presents with constitutional symptoms (e.g., fever, fatigue, anorexia), musculoskeletal findings, and renal disease. The following may be observed: red rashes, IgAV-like lesions (i.e., maculopapular, purpuric), painful skin nodules (erythema nodosum), livedo reticularis (a persistent, purplish, network-patterned discoloration of the skin caused by dilation of capillaries), cutaneous ulcers, and, very rarely, infarction of digits. Musculoskeletal findings can include arthralgia, arthritis, and myositis. Renal arterial involvement occurs in ~ 50–60% of patients and can present as hematuria, proteinuria, or hypertension (HTN). There is an absence of lung involvement.

GI bleeding and ulcers as well as neurologic disease (mononeuritis multiplex, hemiparesis, or stroke) are seen much less often. One other thing to look for—orchitis! It occurs most commonly in those with concomitant hepatitis B infection.

Cutaneous PAN, a subset of PAN, has just the skin manifestations without the systemic findings. It responds well to oral prednisone; however, expect relapses. Occasionally, peripheral neuropathy develops in these patients. Diagnosis of PAN is difficult because there is no specific PAN test and the ANCA is negative. Diagnosis is usually based on criteria from the ACR, which includes:

- Skin lesions (e.g., purpura, livedo)
- Testicular pain/orchitis
- Mononeuritis multiplex (presenting as a foot drop)
- Renal involvement
- HTN
- Evidence of hepatitis B
- Weight loss
- Biopsy or angiographic findings

You can confirm diagnosis with biopsy of affected tissue (e.g., skin, kidney, muscle, sural nerve) or angiograph showing stenosis and aneurysm formation.

Treat with steroids and immunosuppressive agents. Daily steroids are most effective, and IV pulse cyclophosphamide is effective in some. Prognosis is poor without aggressive treatment.

PAN is a separate condition from microscopic polyangiitis (MPA). PAN is a medium-vessel vasculitis that causes aneurysms and stenosis, resulting in hematuria and renovascular HTN. PAN does not cause glomerulonephritis. MPA does.

MPA is a p-ANCA-associated (perinuclear antibodies to MPO [myeloperoxidase]), small-vessel vasculitis without granuloma formation. Glomerular involvement is extensive, causing rapidly progressive glomerulonephritis and a pulmonary-renal syndrome (resulting in pulmonary hemorrhage) similar to GPA.

LARGE-VESSEL VASCULITIS

Takayasu Arteritis (TA)

TA is a granulomatous vasculitis of large vessels that leads to arteritis of the aorta and its major branches, resulting in weak or absent pulses in the upper extremities. TA is very rare in children in the U.S. It is the 3rd most common childhood vasculitis in Japan after IgAV and Kawasaki disease.

Look for coarctation of the aorta and/or HTN with systemic findings of fever, arthritis, and myalgia. A simple, yet very useful, test to help identify TA as a possible diagnosis is to perform 4-extremity blood pressures. The proposed criteria for the diagnosis of TA in children are in Table 20-3. Unlike in adults, ischemic findings in children are infrequent.

Think of TA as occurring in phases: the inflammatory prepulseless stage and the noninflammatory occlusive stage. During the inflammatory stage, patients can have fever, fatigue, weight loss, arthritis, and elevated markers of inflammation. During the noninflammatory stage, patients can have symptoms that are secondary to vessel

Table 20-3: Proposed Criteria for the Diagnosis of Takayasu Arteritis in Children
Angiographic abnormalities (as demonstrated by CT or MRA) of the aorta or main branches, plus at least 1 of the following:
1) Decreased peripheral pulses and/or claudication of the extremities
2) Blood pressure difference of > 10 mmHg between arms
3) Audible bruits over aorta and/or major branches
4) Hypertension
Adapted from: Tann OR, et al. Takayasu's disease: A review. *Cardiology in the Young.* June 2008;18(3):250–259.

involvement, such as claudication, dizziness, headaches, and vision problems. During this stage, markers of inflammation can be normal. These stages can overlap or be separated by ≥ 10 years.

Glucocorticoids and cyclophosphamide are the mainstays of therapy. Consider surgery for stenotic lesions that do not respond to immunotherapy. Also consider antiplatelet agents or anticoagulation for patients with nonsurgical but stenotic lesions. Some studies suggest patients with refractory TA benefit from TNF or IL-6 blockade with biologic agents.

VASCULITIDES OF > 1 VESSEL SIZE

Behçet Disease

Behçet disease is unlike any other vasculitis in that it can involve blood vessels of any size and type including arteries or veins. Look for the classic triad:

1) Oral ulcers (painful, recurrent)
2) Genital ulcers (painful, recurrent)
3) Inflammatory eye disease

Behçet disease occurs sporadically in children in the U.S. It is much more common in children from the Mediterranean and the Far East. The key finding is **recurrent buccal aphthous ulcers,** which are found in nearly 100% of patients. Behçet disease can present as a periodic fever syndrome in younger children before the typical manifestations occur. Skin lesions (including erythema nodosum and necrotic folliculitis) are common. You occasionally see a positive pathergy test—prick the skin with a needle, and after 48 hours you see a pustule or papule surrounded by redness. Pathergy is found most often in individuals of Middle Eastern origin. Genital ulcers occur in ~ 75% of patients. Eye lesions also occur and can include both anterior and posterior uveitis, retinal vasculitis, and papilledema. Arthralgias or arthritis can also be seen.

Rarely, GI involvement mimics Crohn disease or ulcerative colitis. When this happens, it typically presents with diarrhea and GI bleeding from ulcerations within the GI tract. It can be very difficult to distinguish between Behçet disease and Crohn disease, which may represent a spectrum of disease with different modes of inheritance.

The diagnosis is clinical and requires observation of recurrent oral ulceration at least 3× over a 1-year period plus at least 2 of the following: recurrent genital ulceration, eye lesions, skin lesions, or positive pathergy test. Pathology shows a neutrophilic infiltrate in affected blood vessels.

Initially, treat with corticosteroids (oral or topical) for skin manifestations. Some patients with ulcerative manifestations benefit from colchicine and pentoxifylline. Use azathioprine for severe complications, such as pulmonary aneurysmal vasculitis, and central nervous system or eye involvement. Infliximab helps treat the colitis.

Childhood Primary Angiitis of the CNS (cPACNS)

CNS vasculitis is an inflammatory disease affecting the blood vessels of the brain. It can be primary or secondary (e.g., another autoimmune disease, infection, drugs).

cPACNS is a primary form of this vasculitis. This disease can present with arterial stroke in children. The etiology of this disorder is unknown, and the histopathology is nonspecific.

cPACNS is defined by the size of the artery/arteries involved and whether or not it is progressive over time. **Small-vessel cPACNS** has a normal angiography, and **medium- and large-vessel cPACNS** have abnormal angiography. Medium- and large-vessel disease are further identified by exhibiting evidence of ongoing inflammatory disease (i.e., new stenosis on angiography) after 3 months from onset.

Clinical presentations vary depending on the arteries involved. In medium- and large-vessel cPACNS, patients present with headaches, focal deficits, movement disorders, arterial ischemic strokes, and cranial neuropathies. Small-vessel cPACNS patients usually have seizures, psychiatric manifestations, and/or diffuse neurological deficits.

Laboratory abnormalities vary with the type of vasculitis. Small-vessel cPACNS often has abnormal blood tests, including high ESR, CRP, thrombocytosis, anemia, elevated C3, and an elevated von Willebrand factor. Normal inflammatory markers (ESR and CRP) do not rule out medium- or large-vessel cPACNS. Elevated opening pressures on lumbar puncture, abnormally high WBC counts, and high protein on cerebrospinal fluid analysis are not uncommon in small-vessel cPACNS. Angiography is considered the gold standard for diagnosis but is rather invasive. Magnetic resonance angiography (MRA) can miss smaller lesions, and findings can mimic benign conditions, such as reversible vasoconstriction syndromes. When available, high-resolution MRA with special attention to the cross section of the wall of the affected vessel can provide information about vessel wall inflammation without an angiogram. A leptomeningeal and brain biopsy is sometimes necessary to establish the diagnosis of small-vessel cPACNS. Histology of the tissue in this group is usually one of nongranulomatous inflammation with a lymphocytic infiltration.

Treatment for small-vessel and medium-to-large vessel progressive cPACNS typically consists of high-dose steroids and cyclophosphamide. Treatment for nonprogressive disease is controversial. Children with stroke are usually given heparin, and those with small-vessel disease are treated with antiplatelet agents. Supportive treatment with typical agents used for seizures, movement disorders, and psychosis are appropriate as adjunctive therapy.

SYSTEMIC LUPUS ERYTHEMATOSUS (SLE)

PREVIEW | REVIEW

- Which ethnic groups have higher rates of systemic lupus erythematosus (SLE)?
- What antibodies increase the risk for neonatal lupus?
- Which cardiac complication is seen in neonatal lupus?
- Which cardiac tests are indicated in newborns of mothers with anti-SSA and/or anti-SSB?
- Is a positive ANA common in pediatric SLE?
- With what are antiphospholipid antibodies associated?
- What is the most common cause of chorea in the U.S.?
- Which 2 autoimmune diseases are signified by the finding of a malar rash?
- Which hair finding is common in SLE?
- Where are the painless ulcerations typically located in patients with lupus?
- Which bone abnormality is common in SLE and is due to the SLE itself, antiphospholipid antibodies, and/or prolonged or high-dose steroid use?
- Which type of endocarditis is associated with SLE and antiphospholipid antibodies?
- Which drug class reduces lupus mortality and improves prognosis?
- What are the clinical side effects of long-term corticosteroid use in children with SLE?

OVERVIEW

Worldwide, the prevalence of SLE in children < 18 years of age varies from ~ 3 to 10 per 100,000, depending on the population being studied. Incidence is higher in females, especially those of childbearing age, and in Americans of African, Asian, and Hispanic descents.

Note: Pediatric SLE is different from neonatal lupus erythematosus. Neonatal lupus develops as a result of transplacental passage of maternal autoantibodies—typically anti-SSA (anti-Sjögren syndrome A; a.k.a. anti-Ro),

anti-SSB (anti-Sjögren syndrome B; a.k.a. anti-La), and, more rarely, U1 RNP antibodies. 50% of these mothers are healthy and asymptomatic and do not know they have these autoantibodies. For this reason, screen all mothers with SLE and pregnant women with a history of autoimmune disease for these antibodies. The risk of neonatal lupus in infants exposed to anti-SSA and anti-SSB antibodies is 2%, but substantially increases in cases where the mother had a previous pregnancy complicated by neonatal lupus. Common features of neonatal lupus erythematosus include an erythematous annular or discoid rash (usually on the scalp and face), periorbital erythema (resembling a raccoon-like appearance), cytopenias, elevated transaminases, and, most importantly, bradycardia from various forms of congenital heart block. Congenital complete heart block with severe bradycardia, which occurs in 1–3% of patients, requires the insertion of a pacemaker. In pregnant women with known positive anti-SSA and/or anti-SSB antibodies, initiate prenatal screening with fetal echocardiogram starting at week 16 of pregnancy, then every 2 weeks thereafter. If heart block is discovered on the fetal echocardiogram of a healthy pregnant woman, screen for anti-SSA, anti-SSB, and anti-U1 RNP antibodies. If there is evidence for cardiac conduction abnormalities, dexamethasone is often given in utero to decrease the risk for complete heart block and pacemaker dependency. In mothers with a known history of SLE or positive anti-SSA, anti-SSB, or anti-U1 RNP antibodies, recent studies have shown the benefit of 400 mg of hydroxychloroquine daily, starting at 6–10 weeks gestation, in reducing the risk or recurrence of neonatal cardiac lupus.

Most noncardiac features, such as the rash, resolve within 6 months as maternal antibodies disappear.

Remember: All infants born to mothers with anti-SSA and/or anti-SSB require a baseline electrocardiogram (ECG), followed by an echocardiogram if ECG abnormalities such as heart block and bradycardia are detected. Prolonged QTc syndrome can develop in children up to 12 months of age; because of this, an ECG should be repeated at least once by 12 months of age.

DIAGNOSIS

Patients with SLE often present with malaise, fever, and/or weight loss. Common manifestations in pediatric SLE are arthritis (80–90%), rash (70–80%), and nephritis (50–60%). Other clinical manifestations include hematologic, pulmonary, and neuropsychiatric abnormalities. Table 20-4 lists the American College of Rheumatology (ACR) 11 criteria for SLE. Patients must fulfill 4 of the 11 criteria for a diagnosis of lupus. Most clinical manifestations, if they are going to occur, do so in the first 4–5 years of diagnosis. The one exception to this is CNS disease, which may not develop for many years. There are 2 sets of SLE diagnostic criteria: ACR and Systemic Lupus International Collaborating Clinics (SLICC). Note that biopsy-proven lupus nephritis plus ANA and/or anti-double-stranded (anti-ds) DNA antibodies also support the diagnosis of SLE according to the SLICC.

Table 20-4: ACR Criteria for Diagnosis of Systemic Lupus Erythematosus (must have at least 4 of 11)

Clinical Criteria

1) Neurologic disorder (e.g., seizures, psychosis, chorea)
2) Malar rash
3) Discoid rash
4) Photosensitive rash
5) Oral ulcers and/or nasal ulcers
6) Serositis (e.g., pleuritis, pericarditis, peritonitis)
7) Renal disorder (e.g., proteinuria, hematuria, cellular casts)
8) Arthritis

Laboratory Criteria

9) Hematologic disorder (e.g., hemolytic anemia, leukopenia, lymphopenia, thrombocytopenia)
10) Immunologic disorder (e.g., positive antiphospholipid ab, anti-dsDNA, anti-Smith, false-positive syphilis test—rapid plasma reagin [RPR] or Venereal Disease Research Laboratory [VDRL])
11) Positive antinuclear antibody (ANA)

In 2012, new criteria for the diagnosis of pediatric SLE were proposed by the SLICC to provide more inclusive diagnostic criteria. Changes include the following:

- Recognizing other cutaneous features such as acute and chronic cutaneous lupus and alopecia
- Allowing biopsy-proven lupus nephritis with positive ANA/anti-dsDNA as an isolated diagnostic criterion
- Including a greater number of neurologic manifestations
- Including low complement measurements
- Counting autoantibodies as separate criterion
- Counting cytopenias as separate criterion

The SLICC criteria for SLE classification requires fulfillment of at least 4 criteria, with at least 1 clinical criterion AND 1 immunologic criterion OR lupus nephritis as the sole clinical criterion in the presence of ANA or anti-dsDNA antibodies (Table 20-5).

Laboratory Findings

Common laboratory findings in patients with SLE include the presence of autoantibodies.

A positive antinuclear antibody (**ANA+**) occurs in almost all pediatric patients with SLE (98–99% sensitivity).

Anti-dsDNA antibodies are the 2nd most common (found in 60–70% of pediatric patients with SLE at some point during the disease course); these antibodies fluctuate with disease activity and are typical with renal disease. **Anti-Smith** antibodies are found in ~ 33% of SLE patients. The presence of anti-dsDNA and/or anti-Smith antibodies has high specificity (97–99%) for SLE; anti-dsDNA strongly correlates with renal involvement in SLE.

Table 20-5: Full SLICC Criteria for Diagnosis of Systemic Lupus Erythematosus

Clinical Criteria

1) Acute cutaneous lupus
2) Chronic cutaneous lupus
3) Oral ulcers (painless and localized to the hard palate)
4) Nonscarring alopecia (diffuse thinning or hair fragility with visible broken hairs)
5) Synovitis involving ≥ 2 joints, characterized by swelling or effusion OR tenderness in ≥ 2 joints and ≥ 30 minutes of morning stiffness
6) Serositis
7) Renal
8) Neurologic
9) Hemolytic anemia
10) Leukopenia (< 4000/mm^3 at least once)
11) Thrombocytopenia (<100,000/mm^3) at least once

Immunologic Criteria

12) ANA above laboratory reference range
13) Anti-dsDNA above laboratory reference range, except ELISA: twice above laboratory
14) Anti-Smith
15) Antiphospholipid antibody (Any of the following: lupus anticoagulant, beta 2 glycoprotein, and/or anti-cardiolipin)
16) Low complement
17) Direct Coombs test in the absence of hemolytic anemia

Antiphospholipid antibodies (lupus anticoagulant, anti-cardiolipin, and β_2-glycoprotein-1 antibodies) are found in up to 50% of lupus patients. These antibodies affect pathways of coagulation and increase the risk of miscarriages, thrombocytopenia, livedo reticularis, and/or blood clots in ~ 25% of patients.

Anti-U1 RNP (anti-U1 ribonucleoprotein) antibodies are the least produced of the antibodies listed here. They are, however, also seen in high titers in the related condition—mixed connective tissue disease.

Hypocomplementemia is another finding seen in SLE. Complement proteins are consumed during immune complex formation in active SLE, particularly with nephritis. C3 and C4 often decline with active disease and may normalize with successful treatment. Inherited C4, C2, or other complement deficiencies correlate with more severe SLE.

Renal Manifestations

Renal involvement in SLE is very common and directly affects both morbidity and mortality. SLE with no renal involvement, or with nephritis requiring a short course of steroids, has a better outcome. SLE with nephritis requiring immunosuppressive therapy has a poorer outcome.

Lupus nephritis can be classified into 6 classes, shown in Table 20-6.

Infectious complications from immunosuppression are a major cause of morbidity and mortality in lupus nephritis. For more information on lupus nephritis, see the Nephrology & Urology section.

CNS Manifestations

CNS disease occurs in 10–30% of children with SLE. Headache is a frequent complaint in these patients. Psychiatric and mood disorders occur in ~ 10–20%. You must rule out psychosis or organic brain syndrome—usually by lumbar puncture—because infection or hemorrhage is possible. Seizures are also a common presentation for CNS disease. SLE is the most common cause of chorea in the U.S.! Chorea in SLE is often associated with antiphospholipid antibodies. Cranial nerve involvement is more common than peripheral nerve disease. Autonomic dysfunction is common but typically mild—changes in heart rate can be the only change you observe. Cognitive difficulties are common in patients with SLE. Neurocognitive testing is helpful in evaluating whether this is secondary to SLE. Order serum antiribosomal P antibodies and antineuronal antibodies (from cerebrospinal fluid) to help diagnose lupus psychosis or lupus cerebritis.

Skin Manifestations

Characteristic skin manifestations of SLE include butterfly rash (a.k.a. malar rash; Figure 20-10); discoid rash (uncommon in childhood SLE; Figure 20-11); and/or photosensitivity. A malar rash is usually due to either SLE or dermatomyositis; the rash involves the malar eminence and spares the nasolabial folds (unlike rosacea and psoriasis, which can involve the nasolabial folds). Fifth disease (parvovirus) can also present with a facial rash and is part of the differential diagnosis. Alopecia is fairly common. This can be diffuse, and generally mild, because of disease activity, scarring discoid lesions, and/or steroid use. Oral and nasal erosions can occur, as well as ulcerative lesions of the arms, legs, or ears. Oral lesions/ulcerations are usually painless and located on the hard palate or in the nares. A less common vesicular or bullous rash can develop and is associated with anti-SSA and anti-SSB antibodies. This condition is termed **subacute cutaneous lupus erythematosus (SCLE)** and has the same rash and antibodies as seen in neonatal lupus.

Table 20-6: Guidelines for Management of Lupus Nephritis

Class 1: Minimal Mesangial Lupus Nephritis
- Good prognosis; no immunosuppressive therapy required; short duration of steroids if needed

Class 2: Mesangial Proliferative Lupus Nephritis
- Fair prognosis; no immunosuppressive therapy required; short duration of steroids if needed

Class 3: Focal Lupus Nephritis (< 50% of glomeruli)
- 3(A): Active lesions
- 3(A/C): Active and chronic lesions
- 3(C): Chronic lesions
- Treat with steroids plus either CYP or MMF for induction therapy; use MMF or AZP for maintenance therapy.

Class 4: Diffuse Segmental or Global Lupus Nephritis (> 50% of glomeruli)
- Diffuse segmental (4-S) or global (4-G)
- 4(A): Active lesions
- 4(A/C): Active and chronic lesions
- 4(C): Chronic lesions
- Treat with steroids plus CYP or MMF for induction therapy; use MMF or AZP for maintenance therapy.

Class 5: Membranous Lupus Nephritis
- Associated with nephrotic range proteinuria
- Treat with steroids and MMF (if MMF ineffective, switch to CYP) for induction therapy; use MMF or AZP for maintenance therapy.

Class 6: Advanced Sclerosing Lupus Nephritis
- > 90% of glomeruli are globally sclerosed with no residual activity.
- Prepare for renal replacement therapy (hemodialysis/kidney transplant).

Notes:
- Classes 3 and 4 nephritis are associated with HTN, and risk for renal failure is high if not treated.
- Class 5 can occur in combination with Class 3 or 4.
- Monitor blood pressure, lipids.
- Use ACE inhibitors or ARBs to decrease proteinuria and preserve renal function.

References:
Weening JJ, et al. International Society of Nephrology Working Group on the Classification of Lupus Nephritis; Renal Pathology Society Working Group on the Classification of Lupus Nephritis. The classification of glomerulonephritis in systemic lupus erythematosus revisited. *Kidney Int.* 2004;65:521–530.
Hahn BH, et al. American College of Rheumatology Guidelines for Screening, Case Definition, Treatment and Management of Lupus Nephritis. *Arthritis Care Res* (Hoboken). Jun 2012;64(6):797–808.

ACE = angiotensin-converting enzyme
ARB = angiotensin II receptor blocker
AZP = azathioprine

CYP = cyclophosphamide
HTN = hypertension
MMF = mycophenolate mofetil

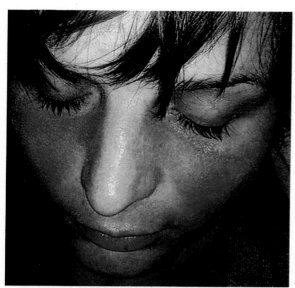

Figure 20-10: SLE with malar rash

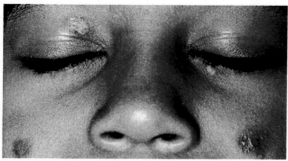

Figure 20-11: SLE with discoid rash

Musculoskeletal Manifestations

In SLE patients, look for nondeforming polyarticular arthritis, especially of small and large joints, with morning stiffness. You might find it difficult to distinguish poJIA from early-stage SLE arthritis. Over time, poJIA can show juxta-articular osteopenia and joint damage, such as erosions, on radiography. In SLE, the radiographs show nonerosive results even after years of arthritis. (SLE can cause **Jaccoud arthropathy,** a nonerosive arthritis with reversible subluxation at the MCPs of the hands.) **Avascular necrosis** (AVN), bony destruction and pain due to interruption of blood flow to the bone, is fairly common and is due to the disease itself, antiphospholipid antibodies, and/or prolonged or high-dose steroid use. AVN can be either symptomatic or asymptomatic. A nuclear bone scan reveals the sites of asymptomatic AVN; MRI confirms the diagnosis. Symptomatic AVN presents with nighttime pain, limp (often associated with progressively worsening groin, thigh, and/or knee pain and further exacerbated by weight-bearing), joint or bone tenderness, and a non-inflammatory effusion. Hips, knees, and shoulders are common sites of involvement. AVN is a common cause of morbidity in SLE.

Cardiopulmonary Manifestations

The most common cardiac abnormality in children with SLE is pericarditis. It occurs in 25–35% of patients and is associated with pleuritic disease as well. Tamponade is very rare in these patients. Myocarditis and endocarditis occur in < 10%. Valvular disease is common but is usually clinically insignificant. **Libman-Sacks endocarditis** (nonbacterial endocarditis with verrucous vegetations) is associated with SLE and antiphospholipid antibodies.

Pulmonary manifestations can vary from something as severe as pulmonary hemorrhage or infection to a more benign, indolent, decreased diffusion capacity. Pleural disease is very common and can present as pleuritis or pleural effusion. The pain is usually sharp/stabbing and worsens with deep inspiration.

Gastrointestinal Manifestations

Gastrointestinal manifestations occur in ~ 33% of patients with SLE. Abdominal pain is the most common presenting symptom. It can be due to serositis, autoimmune hepatitis, vasculitis, pancreatitis, or enteritis. Hepatomegaly is common; jaundice is rare.

Hematologic Manifestations

Cytopenias are common. Up to 75% of patients are found to have 1 or more cytopenias, including leukopenia (WBC < 4,000 cells/μL), lymphopenia (total lymphocyte count < 1,500 cells/μL), hemolytic anemia, or thrombocytopenia (platelet count < 150,000 cells/μL).

Normochromic normocytic anemia and hypochromic microcytic anemia are more common than Coombs-positive hemolytic anemia.

Lupus anticoagulant causes an in vitro prolongation of partial thromboplastin time (PTT) but not prothrombin time (PT). These patients do not bleed excessively; instead, they have an increased risk of arterial thrombosis, deep vein thrombosis, and thromboembolism.

Endocrine Manifestations

Antithyroid antibodies occur in nearly 50% of patients, and clinical hypothyroidism occurs in 10–20% of patients. Graves disease can occur, but it is much less common than hypothyroidism.

TREATMENT

Only 4 drug therapies are approved by the FDA to be used in SLE:

1) Low-dose aspirin
2) Glucocorticosteroids (e.g., prednisone)
3) Hydroxychloroquine
4) Belimumab

However, rheumatologists use multiple DMARDs and immunomodulators that are not approved by the FDA to manage their patients:

- Mycophenolate mofetil (MMF)
- Methotrexate (MTX)
- Azathioprine (AZP)
- Cyclophosphamide (CYP)
- Cyclosporine
- Leflunomide
- Rituximab

The reasons for lack of approval of these agents to treat lupus are multiple and include heterogeneity of the disease, inadequate outcome tools to assess disease activity and treatment response, and variable background medications that patients are taking during the trials—so gauging treatment response is difficult.

The treatment mainstay for lupus is antimalarial drugs. **Hydroxychloroquine** is helpful with skin and joint manifestations and can improve fatigue in many patients. Data shows that continued use of antimalarial therapy prevents disease flares (a 3× reduction in the rate of flares when compared to management that discontinues hydroxychloroquine), decreases mortality in patients, lowers serum cholesterol levels, and decreases the risk for neonatal lupus in mothers who take the drug. The risk of ophthalmic complications (retinal toxicity) is very low, but screen for this 1–2×/year with eye examinations performed by an ophthalmologist. Hydroxychloroquine is safe to use in pregnant patients with SLE.

Corticosteroids are used for many aspects of disease therapy. Use a low dosage (< 0.1–0.25 mg/kg/day or < 10–15 mg/day) for joint complaints and fatigue. Serositis responds to 20–30 mg/day, but nephritis and CNS disease often require high-dose steroids (2 mg/kg/day or pulse therapy 30 mg/kg/day of methylprednisolone).

Know the common side effects from long-term use of steroids:

- AVN
- Osteoporosis with fracture or vertebral collapse
- Growth failure
- Glaucoma and cataracts
- Diabetes mellitus
- HTN
- Accelerated atherosclerosis
- Infection

Cyclophosphamide (CYP) carries a lot of toxicity and is used mainly for initial control of aggressive disease. CYP increases the risk of infertility (10–20% risk in 25-year-old women and up to 50% risk in women > 32 years of age). The risk of malignancy, especially lymphoma, is an accumulated dose-related side effect. Minimize this risk by reducing the total dose of CYP, using monthly IV pulse therapy, and switching to a potentially less toxic agent after the first 6–12 months. The risk of bladder carcinoma is directly related to the development of hemorrhagic cystitis that is a result of bladder wall toxicity from this agent.

Other drugs effective for managing severe disease include:

- **Immunosuppressants**—MMF and AZP
- **Monoclonal antibodies**—belimumab and **rituximab**

Table 20-6 on page 20-16 reviews the management of lupus nephritis.

PROGNOSIS

Morbidity in SLE is due to disease manifestations (renal and CNS manifestations) and to medication toxicity (steroid side effects and infections from immunosuppression). Late morbidity and early mortality are due to premature atherosclerotic disease > 10–20 years after onset. SLE is an independent risk factor for coronary artery disease. Risk for atherosclerosis is multifactorial and includes endothelial damage secondary to chronic inflammation and immune dysregulation.

MIXED CONNECTIVE TISSUE DISEASE (MCTD)

PREVIEW | REVIEW

- What is the autoantibody affiliated with mixed connective tissue disease (MCTD)?
- What is the main cause of mortality in MCTD?

MCTD used to be referred to as an overlap syndrome with features of dermatomyositis, JIA, lupus, and/or scleroderma disorders, but it is now characterized as its own entity due to the presence of a distinctive autoantibody, anti-U1 RNP. Girls account for 80% of cases, and they characteristically present with Raynaud phenomenon, low-grade fever, arthritis, dorsal hand edema, rash, and myositis. Joint abnormalities are seen in 60–90% of children.

Over time, MCTD progresses like systemic sclerosis, and many patients develop:

- Restrictive lung disease
- GI disease—usually esophageal disease with dysphagia and abnormal esophageal function
- Cardiac problems—especially acute pericarditis with pericardial effusion and mitral valve prolapse
- Renal disease occurs in ~ 25% of pediatric patients, and the nephritis can be membranous, membranoproliferative, or mesangioproliferative.

Erosive arthritis is rarely seen except in those who are RF+. CNS disease and eye disease are also rare with this syndrome.

Mortality most often occurs due to chronic interstitial lung disease or pulmonary HTN. Mortality also results from severe thrombocytopenia and infectious complications of immunosuppression. The prognosis is generally better than in SLE or systemic sclerosis.

Labs in MCTD show a high-titer speckled ANA, anti-U1 RNP antibodies, RF, and hypergammaglobulinemia. Diagnosis requires high-titer antibodies against U1 RNP autoantigen.

As in SLE, use antimalarials to treat MCTD. Also, corticosteroids can be used with patients with severe disease. Many patients require more intensive immunosuppression, such as MTX for arthropathy or CYP for severe organ system involvement.

SJÖGREN SYNDROME (SS)

PREVIEW | REVIEW

- Name the diagnostic criteria for Sjögren syndrome (SS).
- Which antibodies are frequently present in pediatric SS?
- How do most pediatric cases of SS present?
- Patients with SS are at increased risk for which malignancies?

SS is a rare autoimmune exocrinopathy that causes a combination of signs/symptoms, of which dry eyes and dry mouth are the most notable. In pediatric cases, consider the following for diagnosis:

- Inflamed and dry eyes (keratoconjunctivitis sicca)
- Dryness of the mouth (xerostomia)
- Lymphocytic infiltrate on minor salivary gland biopsy
- Laboratory evidence of the following: RF+, ANA+, or Ro+ (SSA; 70%) or La+ (SSB; 50%) antibodies

Suspect SS in a child with recurrent parotitis in whom infection has been excluded. Girls outnumber boys 3:1. Most cases present with the recurrent parotitis and keratoconjunctivitis sicca. CNS (e.g., transverse myelitis) and renal (including renal tubular acidosis) manifestations are uncommon but do occur in children. Remember: Particularly young children may not yet be symptomatic with dry eyes and dry mouth. However, excessive dental caries can represent poor saliva production. One extraglandular manifestation to look for is hypergammaglobulinemic purpura—2- to 3-mm, palpable or nonpalpable purpura that can ulcerate on the lower extremities. Annular erythema, usually seen with anti-SSA (anti-Ro) or anti-SSB (anti-La), is also sometimes observed.

Primary SS is defined as an isolated disorder, whereas **secondary SS** is defined as being associated with another autoimmune disease. Some children with a diagnosis of primary SS go on to develop another autoimmune disorder, most commonly SLE.

Treat symptomatic patients with agents that increase moisture: artificial tears for the eyes, artificial saliva, and pilocarpine to stimulate exocrine secretions. Antimalarial agents can be used for skin rashes and joint symptoms. Suggest dental visits at least 2–3×/year due to marked increase in caries. Chewing sugarless gum can help stimulate salivary flow. Cyclosporine ophthalmic suspension and cevimeline are approved treatments for adults with SS but are not approved for children.

Children generally do well, but patients with SS are at increased risk for lymphoma, especially mucosa-associated lymphoid tissue (MALT) lymphoma and non-Hodgkin B-cell lymphomas.

Note: Children born to mothers with SS who have Ro (SSA) and/or La (SSB) antibodies are also at risk for developing neonatal lupus. See more about neonatal lupus under Systemic Lupus Erythematosus (SLE) on page 20-14.

AUTOIMMUNE MYOPATHIES

PREVIEW | REVIEW

- Describe the classic rashes of juvenile dermatomyositis (JDM).
- Does the muscle weakness of JDM mainly affect proximal or distal muscle groups?
- What is the primary therapy for JDM?

OVERVIEW

Juvenile dermatomyositis (JDM) is a systemic connective tissue disorder with chronic skeletal muscle and skin inflammation. Its etiology is unknown, but its pathogenesis is one of autoimmune angiopathy. Polymyositis is a much less common inflammatory myositis in children (< 10% of cases) that has no skin involvement. These diseases are very rare and occur at a rate of ~ 1.5–5/1,000,000. They affect girls more often than boys and have a bimodal pattern of incidence, peaking first at 3–7 years of age and again in the early teenage years.

JUVENILE DERMATOMYOSITIS (JDM)

There is a seasonal clustering of the onset of JDM, suggesting a viral or bacterial trigger for this illness.

Patients present with a rash and with muscle weakness. The symptoms develop gradually over a period of weeks to months. Rashes can be quite varied. Some children have only subtle skin lesions; others have severe, vasculitic, ulcerative rashes. The typical rashes include the classic heliotrope rash (faint purple-to-red discoloration of the eyelids, with or without periorbital edema; Figure 20-12) and Gottron papules (red plaques over the extensor surfaces—most often occurring on the small joints of the hands; Figure 20-13). Periungual changes, such as cuticular overgrowth and dilated tortuous capillaries (visualized by nailfold capillaroscopy), can occur. You might also observe SLE-like malar and facial redness and red rashes on sun-exposed areas. Photosensitivity is common and can precipitate flares.

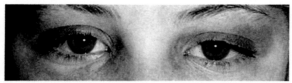

Figure 20-12: Heliotrope rash

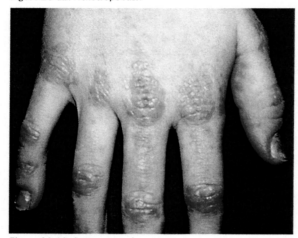

Figure 20-13: Gottron papules

The muscle weakness is always proximal and symmetric in nature. This presents with difficulty in grooming hair, getting up off the floor, and climbing stairs. Some distal weakness occurs in severe cases. When distal weakness is present early on, consider a different form of muscle disease, such as muscular dystrophy, congenital myopathies, and CNS denervation. Children with JDM can also develop muscle involvement of the GI tract, resulting in difficulty swallowing or hoarseness/dysphonia. Dysfunctional swallowing can be asymptomatic and may only be detectable with barium swallow testing. Dysphonia and dysphagia are very serious manifestations, requiring aggressive, prompt treatment.

Nearly 70% of patients have arthralgias. When true arthritis occurs, oligoarthritis (affecting ~ 65%) is more common than polyarthritis (30–35%). Contractures of large joints can occur after prolonged muscle weakness. You see fever and Raynaud phenomenon in ~ 25% at the onset of disease.

Be aware of the potential complications of JDM. Ulcerations are rare but can be severe if they occur. Ulcerative skin disease is a poor prognostic sign and can portend GI vasculitis—one of the most serious, life-threatening complications of JDM. Dystrophic calcification (calcinosis cutis universalis) of the skin, subcutaneous

tissue, and fascia occurs in ~ 33% of affected patients. Calcinosis is much less common today because of better recognition of the complication and prompt treatment. Risk factors for complications are inadequate steroid therapy and delay of therapy for > 4 months from onset of myositis. Another late complication of JDM is lipodystrophy. This is characterized by insulin resistance, hyperlipidemia, and asthenic body habitus. Muscle strength can be completely normal, or the patient can still have active myositis.

Diagnostic criteria are defined in Table 20-7. MRI (T2 or short TI inversion recovery [STIR] imaging) of the thigh muscles, demonstrating inflammation as symmetrical muscle edema, has become the preferred modality over electromyography (EMG) since EMG is invasive and uncomfortable. Be aware that edema on MRI is not specific to inflammatory myopathies. A diagnosis of juvenile polymyositis is based on similar criteria, except that the rashes are absent.

Table 20-7: Diagnosis of Juvenile Dermatomyositis
Presence of heliotrope rash or Gottron papules is required   Plus at least 3 of the following 4 findings = Definite Dx   Plus at least 2 of the following 4 findings = Probable Dx
1) Symmetric proximal muscle weakness
2) Elevated CK, aldolase, LDH, or transaminases
3) EMG abnormalities   • Small amplitude, short duration, polyphasic motor-unit potentials   • Fibrillations, positive sharp waves, increased insertional irritability   • Spontaneous, bizarre, high-frequency discharges
4) Muscle biopsy abnormalities of   • Degeneration   • Regeneration   • Necrosis   • Phagocytosis   • Interstitial mononuclear cell infiltrate
CK = creatine kinase (a.k.a. creatine phosphokinase [CPK])   LDH = lactate dehydrogenase

Begin primary therapy with prednisone 2–3 mg/kg/day. In more severe cases of myositis, many rheumatologists give IV pulse methylprednisolone at 30 mg/kg/dose for ≥ 3 doses. Sunscreens, sun avoidance, and hydroxychloroquine are important adjunctive therapies for rashes. Additionally, prescribe physical and occupational therapy. The 2nd line therapies—and therapies for severe exacerbations—include IV methylprednisolone, IVIG, MTX, cyclosporine, and AZP. Utilizing these adjunctive therapies frequently allows for successful tapering of steroids and avoidance of steroid-induced morbidities. If patients do not respond, try 3rd line therapy—a combination of 2nd line therapies plus 1 of the following:

• Other immunomodulators (anti-TNF agents and rituximab)
• IV cyclophosphamide

Prednisone and other immune modulators have reduced mortality from 40% to < 3%. Approximately 60–80% of patients recover after their initial episode (uniphasic disease course) or after 1 or more recurrences. Fewer than 20% have difficult-to-control disease with persistent myositis over a long period of time. Unlike adult dermatomyositis, in which the dermatomyositis is often a paraneoplastic syndrome, childhood dermatomyositis rarely predisposes to malignancy. Therefore, screening for malignancy is not routinely indicated in children with this disease.

JUVENILE POLYMYOSITIS

Juvenile polymyositis is extremely rare and generally has a chronic course. It has the same clinical features as JDM except there is no rash. Patients can present with proximal girdle weakness. Labs indicate elevated CPK and aldolase, EMG indicates muscle irritability, and MRI shows muscle edema. Differential diagnoses include muscular dystrophy. Frequently, biopsy is indicated to clarify the diagnosis. Treatment is the same as for JDM.

SCLERODERMA

PREVIEW | REVIEW

- What is the most common form of localized scleroderma seen in children?

- In what disorder is en coupe de sabre seen?

- Explain how localized scleroderma can affect soft tissue and bone.

- What are the common antiinflammatory treatments used for linear scleroderma?

- What are the 2 broad subtypes of juvenile systemic sclerosis (JSS)?

- Which part of the GI tract is most commonly affected in JSS?

- Which class of antihypertensive do you use to reduce the incidence of scleroderma renal crisis?

- Which laboratory findings are helpful in diagnosing JSS?

- Why are corticosteroids typically not used in JSS?

SCLERODERMA DISORDERS

Scleroderma means "hard skin." Recognize that when you read the term scleroderma, usually systemic sclerosis is what is being discussed. Tip: Only when you see the words "localized" or "linear" before "scleroderma" is the discussion not talking about systemic sclerosis. This is confusing; so, in this topic, we use "systemic sclerosis" when discussing the systemic form and "localized scleroderma" when discussing the localized form. Nice and simple.

There are 2 major categories of scleroderma disorders:

1) **Localized scleroderma** (linear scleroderma and morphea) is found much more often in children than in adults and is the most common category found in children.
2) **Systemic sclerosis** (diffuse and limited cutaneous sclerodermas) is rare.

The etiology of scleroderma is unknown. Both localized and systemic types involve an abnormality in the regulation of fibroblasts and collagen production along with an endothelial vasculopathy. Endothelin, an endothelial cell-dependent vasoconstrictor, is increased in scleroderma disorders.

LOCALIZED SCLERODERMA

Localized scleroderma is the most common form of scleroderma in children with an incidence of ~ 50/100,000. Examples of localized scleroderma are morphea, plaque morphea, generalized morphea, linear scleroderma (Figure 20-14), and deep morphea (Figure 20-15).

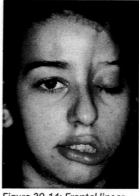
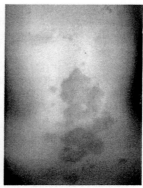

Figure 20-14: Frontal linear (localized) scleroderma

Figure 20-15: Deep morphea (localized scleroderma)

Plaque morphea occurs gradually and is characterized by an oval or circular area of cutaneous induration with a central ivory color surrounded by a purplish halo. If the plaques become more extensive and involve 3 separate anatomic sites, it is called **generalized morphea**. If generalized full-thickness skin involvement occurs, it is called **deep morphea**. Typically, this involves the scalp, face, trunk, and extremities.

Linear scleroderma (formerly linear morphea) is the most common localized scleroderma seen in children. It is characterized by linear streaks of the upper or lower extremity that usually are dermatomal. If the streaks cross a joint, flexion contractures can develop. The streaks become more indurated and gradually extend deeper into underlying muscle and bone (melorheostosis). Streaks involving the face are known as "en coupe de sabre" because they resemble a depression due to a dueling stroke from a sword. These patients can have associated ipsilateral CNS findings, seizures, uveitis, dental defects, and facial abnormalities, including Parry-Romberg syndrome.

Base your diagnosis of these forms of localized scleroderma on clinical findings of the skin lesions; some cases require biopsy. Depth of disease determines the subtypes. Plaque morphea is confined to the dermis, while linear scleroderma can go to muscle and bone. Laboratory testing is not helpful; antibodies to centromere, SCL-70 (topoisomerase 1), nuclear RNP, Smith, and SSA are not present. Occasionally, antibodies to single-stranded DNA are present in linear scleroderma.

Although localized scleroderma is generally a benign condition that resolves in 3–5 years, all pediatric patients suspected of having this disorder should be referred to a specialized pediatric rheumatology center. Localized scleroderma can lead to significant limb growth abnormalities when there is extensive subdermal involvement; this sometimes requires systemic therapy including steroids and/or methotrexate. If a joint is involved, prescribe physical therapy to prevent contractures.

JUVENILE SYSTEMIC SCLEROSIS (JSS)

JSS can be divided into 2 subtypes:

1) **Diffuse cutaneous scleroderma:** proximal and distal skin involvement with internal organ dysfunction of the GI tract, lung, heart, and kidney

2) **Limited cutaneous scleroderma:** mostly distal skin involvement. This was formerly **CREST** syndrome: **c**alcinosis, **R**aynaud phenomenon (Figure 20-16), **e**sophageal dysmotility, **s**clerodactyly, and **t**elangiectasia (Figure 20-17).

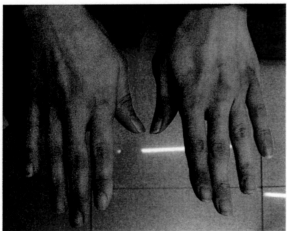

Figure 20-16: Skin changes in Raynaud phenomenon

Although both of these subtypes are rare disorders in childhood, anti-SCL-70 + diffuse scleroderma is seen more than anticentromere + limited scleroderma.

Children with either form of JSS usually present with **Raynaud phenomenon** (spasm of the digital arteries with blanching and numbness or pain of the fingers and toes, often precipitated by cold). Classic signs of Raynaud phenomenon are triphasic color changes of the digits: white, blue, and red on rewarming. Fingertip ulcerations

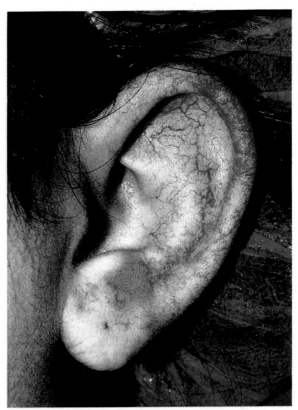

Figure 20-17: Telangiectasias

occur frequently in children. Gradual thickening of the skin of the distal extremities occurs and slowly progresses, eventually involving the face and trunk.

The **GI tract** is commonly affected—particularly the distal esophagus, where both systemic forms of scleroderma affect distal smooth muscle, resulting in dysphagia. Gastroesophageal (GE) reflux is common.

Lung involvement is initially asymptomatic but gradually manifests in a dry cough. Alveolitis develops first; then pulmonary interstitial fibrosis worsens, most often in patients with diffuse cutaneous scleroderma. Pulmonary HTN occurs, which leads to right heart failure. This is found more frequently in those with limited cutaneous scleroderma.

Renal crisis occurs only in ~10% of patients and, for the most part, only in diffuse cutaneous scleroderma patients. Managing HTN with angiotensin-converting enzyme (ACE) inhibitors decreases the incidence of renal crisis.

Clinical diagnosis is dependent on findings of sclerodactyly (stiffness and tightness of the skin of the fingers), nail bed capillary findings showing periungual tortuous dilated loops (visualized by nailfold capillaroscopy), and internal organ involvement.

Laboratory testing shows that 80% of patients have a nucleolar or speckled ANA, and 50% have antibodies to SCL-70 in diffuse cutaneous scleroderma. Anticentromere antibodies, if they occur, are seen with limited cutaneous scleroderma and primary biliary cirrhosis. Which test is used to determine esophageal abnormalities? Esophageal manometry is the most sensitive test. Use barium swallow to show severe motor dysfunction and/or reflux.

High-resolution CT scan is a sensitive test for lung abnormalities such as fibrosis or alveolitis. Monitor patients for carbon monoxide diffusion capacity (DLCO) using pulmonary function tests (PFTs), which are highly sensitive in detecting pulmonary HTN. It is essential to monitor patients at risk for pulmonary HTN with echocardiography to assess right-side heart pressures and pulmonary pressures. Consider right heart catheterization in such patients.

Treatment is mainly supportive. Order aggressive physical and occupational therapy to prevent progression to flexion contractures. Raynaud phenomenon responds to calcium channel blockers (nifedipine) and α-blockers (doxazosin). Corticosteroids are relatively contraindicated due to an increased risk of renal crisis. ACE inhibitors to prevent (and treat) renal crisis, and anti-GE reflux agents are important adjunctive therapies. If it is necessary to use corticosteroids, as in myositis, try to use dosages ≤ 10 mg/day. You can use MTX, although avoid it in patients with significant interstitial lung disease. CYP reverses alveolitis and stabilizes, if not reverses, severe scleroderma lung disease; MMF may have a role as well. Systemic vasodilators, such as sildenafil and iloprost, are used for pulmonary HTN, as well as endothelin receptor antagonists. Prognosis is poor for individuals with internal organ involvement; those with limited cutaneous scleroderma generally do better.

SARCOIDOSIS

PREVIEW | REVIEW

- List the most common systems affected in sarcoidosis.
- What is the triad of clinical manifestations typically seen in Blau syndrome?
- Describe the skin findings in sarcoidosis.

Sarcoidosis is an uncommon multisystem granulomatous disease (with increased relative prevalence in the southeastern U.S.) that mainly affects the lungs, lymph nodes, eyes, and skin. The etiology is unknown but results from an immunologic response that causes accumulation of inflammatory cells (granulomas). Symptoms vary depending on the system affected. However, most present with fatigue, fever, and weight loss. **Blau syndrome**, a familial form of sarcoidosis, typically presents with uveitis, rash, and "boggy" arthritis.

Lung involvement is common and presents with a persistent dry cough. Chest x-ray reveals hilar infiltrates and sometimes parenchymal infiltrates. PFTs demonstrate restrictive changes. See more on sarcoidosis in the Pulmonary Medicine section.

Granulomatous infiltration of the liver, spleen, and lymph nodes is typical and presents as hepatomegaly, splenomegaly, and lymphadenopathy (peripheral but especially hilar/mediastinal), respectively. Most are asymptomatic, but monitoring liver functions is warranted.

The most common skin findings are nodules on the face, neck, back, and extremities (e.g., erythema nodosum). The lesions are red-brown, maculopapular, and < 1 cm in diameter.

Eye involvement includes uveitis and conjunctival granulomas. All patients with sarcoidosis require complete ophthalmological examination.

Diagnosis is made by biopsy of the affected tissue demonstrating noncaseating granulomatous lesions. A patient with sarcoidosis must be monitored with serial testing, including chest x-ray, PFTs, LFTs, renal function tests, and ophthalmologic slit-lamp examination. Serum angiotensin-converting enzyme and lysozyme levels are often elevated during active disease.

Corticosteroids are the mainstay of treatment. Duration is 8–12 weeks, followed by a 6–12-month wean. Immunosuppressive drugs, such as methotrexate, are also used. Monoclonal antibodies to TNF are also effective.

PAIN SYNDROMES

PREVIEW | REVIEW

- Is morning pain a common finding with growing pains?
- Are unilateral findings common in growing pains?
- Describe some of the tasks that can be attempted to determine if a child has hypermobility syndrome.
- If you find hypermobility syndrome, which traits do you look for to determine if a hereditary syndrome might be present?
- What are recommended exercise activities for hypermobility syndrome?
- What are the clinical findings in patients with amplified musculoskeletal pain syndromes (AMPS)?
- What is common regarding school attendance in patients with AMPS?

GROWING PAINS

Growing pains are the most common cause of recurrent limb pain in children. Rheumatologists refer to this as "benign nocturnal limb pains of childhood." Actually, the pain is not due to growing. The name was probably coined because the pain occurs in children (who are growing).

We do not know what causes growing pains. Musculoskeletal symptoms may be prevalent in the families of these children, but a true familial tendency has not been proven. These symptoms may also be associated with emotional disturbances.

So then, what are they? Classically, growing pains are characterized as a deep aching located in nonarticular areas, generally within muscle groups, especially thighs and calves, but rarely back or forearms. Pain is bilateral, typically occurs late in the day or evening, and commonly awakens a child from sleep. Limping and mobility problems do not occur. Usually, there are no objective findings. Unilateral symptoms require further evaluation.

Remember: The other diagnosis that causes nighttime bone pain, since it is difficult for most patients to differentiate between bone and muscle pain, is malignancy. Perform a thorough review of systems, including whether the child is experiencing weight loss, night sweats, or daytime pain as well. Bone pain from metastases is usually unilateral and can manifest in other areas (e.g., spine, ribs, skull) that are not typical for growing pains.

Laboratory testing is not indicated in situations where the clinical picture is compatible with growing pains, except to rule out other etiologies. WBC, ESR, CK, and all serologic tests are normal.

Treat symptomatic patients with heat, massage, and acetaminophen or ibuprofen for pain. Sometimes, a dose of these medications before bed for children with frequent episodes can decrease the severity of the spells. Normally, it just takes time. If the pain is persistent, explore psychological stressors and family dynamics. Growing pains occur most commonly in preschool and elementary-age children. Growing pains generally disappear by 12–13 years of age.

HYPERMOBILITY SYNDROME

Benign hypermobility joint syndrome is fairly common and is seen in 4–13% of children, with girls more commonly affected. Most of these children are asymptomatic. You can demonstrate hypermobility by having the child attempt 5 tasks:

1) Extend the wrist and metacarpophalangeal joints so that the fingers are parallel to the dorsum of the forearm (bilateral).

2) Passively oppose the thumb to the flexor aspect of the forearm (bilateral).

3) Hyperextend the elbows 10° or more (bilateral).

4) Hyperextend the knees 10° or more (bilateral).

5) Flex the trunk with the knees fully extended so the palms rest on the floor.

The ability to perform these tasks in ≥ 5 locations (a point for each side of the body plus flexing the trunk) indicates hypermobility on the Beighton scale. If found, look for other signs of inherited diseases of connective tissue, such as high-arched palate, ocular/cardiac lesions, skin hyperelasticity, arachnodactyly, and velvety skin texture. Variants of **Ehlers-Danlos syndrome** or **Marfan syndrome** are most common.

Joint and muscular pain, as well as transient joint effusions, can occur in those with benign hypermobility syndrome. The knees and the hands are most commonly affected.

Treat pain with NSAIDs or acetaminophen. Swimming and other low- to no-impact sports are good exercise recommendations. Psychological factors seem to exacerbate or prolong the course. Premature osteoarthritic changes can occur in some of these children, but generally, the prognosis is good. If Marfan syndrome (i.e., tall stature, high-arched palate, lens dislocation) or Ehlers-Danlos syndrome (i.e., velvety, loose skin with thin, widened scars) is suspected, perform cardiac screening with echocardiography, and consider the involvement of a genetics specialist.

AMPLIFIED MUSCULOSKELETAL PAIN SYNDROMES (AMPS)

In general, AMPS are the result of an amplified pain signal. The 3 primary causes are injury, illness, and psychological stressors. The most common psychological stressors include family or school issues, but AMPS can be complicated from the stress of having chronic pain and not having an accurate diagnosis and/or appropriate plan for improvement.

AMPS can present with pain in 1 affected limb (e.g., a distal lower extremity) or with diffuse pain throughout the body. Most children describe the pain as constant; however, it can be intermittent in some. The pain that patients experience is real.

Juvenile (primary) fibromyalgia is a subset of AMPS. Typical features include widespread musculoskeletal aches and pain and any combination of poor sleep, fatigue, headache, cognitive complaints, and anxiety. Diagnosis requires the presence of symptoms daily or every other day for the past 3 months. Although children often fail to fulfill the diagnostic criteria for fibromyalgia outlined for adults, they may have tender points. Figure 20-18 shows the 18 total trigger points that can be found by digital palpation (as previously used for the adult criteria). For adults, newer diagnostic criteria have been developed that do not involve determining the total number of tender points. These new criteria were validated in girls 11–17 years of age but not the general pediatric population. Juvenile fibromyalgia has a high familial association.

It is important to remember that patients with fibromyalgia do not have evidence of articular swelling, loss of joint motion, or muscle weakness. If these are present, consider another diagnosis. However, keep in mind that secondary fibromyalgia can develop in individuals with JIA or SLE.

Complex regional pain syndrome (CRPS; formerly reflex sympathetic dystrophy [RSD]) is another subtype of AMPS. The characteristic features of CRPS include allodynia (pain aggravated by light touch) and/or hyperalgesia of the involved extremity. Patients have localized autonomic dysfunction with edema, coolness or excess warmth,

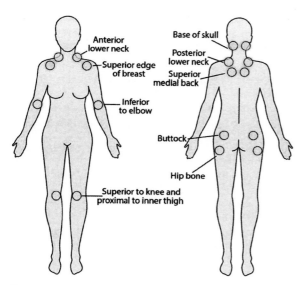

Figure 20-18: Tender points common in juvenile fibromyalgia

mottling, and/or sweatiness. CRPS may be preceded by a soft-tissue injury, such as a sprain, but often there is no identifiable preceding trauma. Plain radiographs of the involved region are obtained to rule out fractures or tumors and may reveal osteoporosis in late stages.

Appropriate therapy for AMPS includes aggressive physical and occupational therapy, preferably by a therapist with experience in treating this diagnosis. In many cases, physical therapy includes desensitization to textures, pressure, and temperatures (particularly in those with allodynia). Focus should also be placed on improvement of sleep hygiene. Treatment results are often better when professional psychological support, such as cognitive-behavioral therapy, is provided. Improvement, and resolution of symptoms, is better in children than in adults and is particularly good in children who partake in an aggressive treatment program with a multidisciplinary approach.

School absenteeism can be a big problem in patients with AMPS. Be sure to ask about school attendance as you are exploring if a patient has AMPS.

Because fatigue and pain can be seen in some patients with an autoimmune disorder (e.g., SLE, juvenile dermatomyositis, JIA, Hashimoto thyroiditis), be sure to check appropriate laboratory tests (e.g., CBC, ESR, CRP, CMP, ANA, CK, and thyroid function tests) to rule out these conditions. Laboratory tests are normal in patients with AMPS.

AMYLOIDOSIS

PREVIEW | REVIEW
- What are some diseases that cause amyloid deposition?
- What is the most serious manifestation of amyloid deposition?

Amyloidosis is the extracellular accumulation of protein fibrils that then interfere with specific organ functions. You can see amyloid by staining with Congo red then looking for green-yellow birefringence under polarized light.

Amyloid accumulation occurs with many diseases, including infectious diseases (tuberculosis, leprosy, and chronic osteomyelitis), familial Mediterranean fever, inflammatory bowel disease, Behçet disease, and SLE. In the past, amyloidosis was found in children with long-standing JIA (typically systemic disease), particularly in Europe. This complication has virtually disappeared with the advent of better, aggressive therapies.

Renal disease is the most prevalent and serious manifestation of amyloid deposition. Patients present with proteinuria, with rapid progression to nephrotic-range proteinuria, and then eventually renal failure. Renal vein thrombosis due to proteinuria is also common. Hepatosplenomegaly can occur but usually does not cause abnormalities.

There is no specific "amyloidosis blood test," but look for markedly increased ESR, CRP, and serum amyloid A levels if active inflammation, proteinuria, and hypoalbuminemia are present. The key is to find amyloid deposition in tissue. Rectal biopsy, gingival biopsy, or aspiration of subcutaneous abdominal fat are potential sites for tissue acquisition.

Prevention is much more effective than treatment. As such, aggressive therapy for diseases that predispose to amyloidosis is important. For example, the use of colchicine is effective in treating familial Mediterranean fever and preventing amyloidosis. Renal transplant is successful in some patients, but there is recurrence in some individuals who have had transplants.

PERIODIC FEVER SYNDROMES

PREVIEW | REVIEW
- What is periodic fever, aphthous stomatitis, pharyngitis, and cervical adenitis syndrome?
- Which periodic fever syndrome does not have a known genetic abnormality?
- Where is the gene responsible for familial Mediterranean fever (FMF)?
- What is the product of the FMF gene?
- How do you treat FMF?
- Define the genetic defect in hyper-IgD syndrome.
- What are cryopyrin-associated periodic syndromes?
- Name the 3 periodic fever syndromes due to cryopyrin abnormalities.
- What is the neutrophilic pattern in cyclic neutropenia?

OVERVIEW

Fever is a common cause of presentation to the pediatrician. Recurrent fevers are most often due to repeated infections, frequently viral. Fever of unknown origin (FUO), documented fever for > 1 week with no etiology identified on initial evaluation, is often due to infections but can also be due to malignancies and rheumatic diseases, such as systemic JIA or SLE.

Periodic fever syndromes are defined as ≥ 3 episodes of unexplained fever in a 6-month period. This group of disorders can follow a definitive periodic pattern or can have variable intervals between attacks. Initially, you may think these children have recurrent infections. The periodicity is ultimately recognized before these diagnoses are considered. Specific genetic abnormalities have been identified for many of these disorders.

PERIODIC FEVER, APHTHOUS STOMATITIS, PHARYNGITIS, AND CERVICAL ADENITIS (PFAPA) SYNDROME

PFAPA is a benign syndrome that typically begins in children ≤ 5 years old (the mean age is ~ 3 years old). It is a relatively common disorder with no known genetic cause.

PFAPA has no recognizable Mendelian inheritance pattern. It is not prominent in any ethnic group and is not associated with amyloid deposition. Children with PFAPA have normal growth parameters and are in good health between episodes.

There are no laboratory tests to diagnose PFAPA. The diagnosis is based on the fever pattern and physical exam. In contrast to familial Mediterranean fever (FMF; see Familial Mediterranean Fever (FMF)), the fever generally lasts longer in PFAPA (~ 3–7 days with an average of 5 days). It should be considered in patients with at least 3 similar recurrent episodes lasting no longer than 5–7 days and who are well between episodes. Some children can manifest joint pain, abdominal pain, rash, headache, vomiting, or diarrhea. The flares respond quickly to prednisone. Prompt resolution of symptoms following a single dose of prednisone (1 mg/kg; maximum 60 mg) is typical. Some patients may experience recurrence of symptoms within 2–3 days of treatment. In such cases, a repeat dose of prednisone at 1 mg/kg may be administered. If there is incomplete response, subsequent PFAPA episodes may be treated with a single dose of prednisone 2 mg/kg. If fevers persist or recur in ≤ 21 days, prophylactic therapy should be considered. The periodicity of febrile episodes ranges from 3–6 weeks with an average interval of 4 weeks. Febrile episodes are unaccompanied by any sign of infection.

Although episodes are typically very responsive to steroids, the interval to the next episode can decrease with steroid use. The decision to treat often depends on whether the symptoms interfere with the family's work or school routines. In children who do not respond to the short course of steroids, consider cimetidine, colchicine, and/or tonsillectomy. There is anecdotal evidence for the use of IL-1 blockade such as anakinra. However, additional trials are needed before this is considered standard of care.

The fever cycles of PFAPA generally stop recurring by ~ 10 years of age.

FAMILIAL MEDITERRANEAN FEVER (FMF)

FMF (a.k.a. familial paroxysmal polyserositis, familial recurrent polyserositis) is an autosomal recessive disorder mainly seen in Armenians, Turks, Levantine Arabs, and Sephardic Jews. The responsible gene (*MEFV*) is localized to chromosome 16. The product of this gene is a protein called pyrin (a.k.a. marenostrin), which is responsible for the regulation of PMN inflammatory response and biochemically interacts with TNF, IL-1, and other cytokines. Patients have benefited from therapy with newer anticytokine biologic agents (specifically IL-1 inhibition). Curiously, some patients with documented FMF have only 1 *MEFV* gene or even none, prompting researchers to investigate other possible loci or mediators for this disease.

Children usually present with symptoms before 10 years of age. Most children have attacks of fever that can last from several hours to 5 days. The fever typically recurs in predictable cycles (e.g., 3–5 days every month for one patient, several times a year for another patient). Severe abdominal pain occurs with the fever. Pleuritis, pericarditis, and scrotal swelling also can occur. An erysipelas-like rash can appear around the ankles. Arthritis, arthralgia, and myalgia are common.

Make your diagnosis based on the clinical pattern, family history, and response to colchicine. Laboratory results are nonspecific, but ESR, CRP, fibrinogen, and WBC counts are usually quite high during the episodes and can normalize between flares. Genetic testing is diagnostic in > 50% of patients, but not all gene defects have been identified.

Treat FMF with daily colchicine, which treats acute attacks, prevents future attacks, and prevents development of amyloidosis. The most common side effects are diarrhea and bone marrow suppression (particularly if renal disease is present). Colchicine prevents amyloidosis in all patients and prevents attacks in ~ 65% of patients with FMF. Increasing the dosage to 2 mg/day in 2 divided doses prevents attacks in 95% of patients. Amyloidosis is of high concern in untreated individuals. Drugs that target IL-1 are being used to treat patients with disease refractory to colchicine.

HYPER-IgD SYNDROME (HIDS)

HIDS is an autosomal recessive disorder that affects mainly individuals of Dutch or French descent. It is due to a mutation in the *MVK* gene that encodes mevalonate kinase, which likely results in excess production of IL-1. A majority of patients present by 1 year of age, and the fevers generally last 3–7 days. Fever episodes usually occur every 1–2 months. Clinically, these patients can have abdominal pain, nausea/vomiting, and nondestructive large-joint arthritis. They can also have a diffuse nonmigratory erythematous macular rash. Lymphadenopathy, headaches, oral/vaginal ulcers, and splenomegaly also can occur during febrile episodes. Characteristically, as expected, IgD is often elevated (> 100 IU/mL) but not always, and IgA is also elevated in most cases. This helps differentiate this disease from other periodic fever syndromes. Amyloidosis is rare in this disorder.

Treatment can include colchicine, prednisone, NSAIDs, etanercept, and anakinra.

CRYOPYRIN-ASSOCIATED PERIODIC SYNDROMES (CAPS)

CAPS are a group of autoinflammatory diseases with autosomal dominant inheritance and variable expression.

There are 3 periodic fever syndromes resulting from inheritable abnormalities in cryopyrin (due to mutations in the *NLRP3* gene). These are familial cold autoinflammatory syndrome (**FCAS**), Muckle-Wells syndrome, and neonatal-onset multisystem inflammatory disease (**NOMID**). These disorders have overlapping clinical presentations, including fever, acute-phase inflammation, a neutrophilic urticarial skin rash, and joint involvement. There are distinguishing features as well, including sensorineural hearing loss in Muckle-Wells syndrome and CNS involvement in NOMID.

The diagnosis is made by genetic testing. Other tests include skin biopsy of the rash, an eye examination, hearing tests, lumbar puncture, and imaging of the brain and inner ears with MRI.

Cryopyrin is involved with the activation of IL-1β. Targeted inhibition of the IL-1 pathway has resulted in new treatments for these diseases. Approved drugs include rilonacept, anakinra, and canakinumab.

OTHER CAUSES OF PERIODIC FEVERS

Consider **cyclic neutropenia** (really an immunodeficiency syndrome) in your evaluation of recurrent fevers. This can be autosomal dominant or sporadic in inheritance. It usually presents in early childhood. Absolute neutrophil counts of < 200 cells/μL occur every 21 days (with a range of 14–36 days) like clockwork, with each episode lasting 3–10 days. Clinical symptoms include fever, malaise, lymphadenopathy, and mouth sores. Blood counts 3×/week every 6–8 weeks are sometimes necessary to make the diagnosis. Treatment with granulocyte colony-stimulating factor (G-CSF) is effective in raising blood neutrophil counts.

THE MEDSTUDY HUB: YOUR GUIDELINES AND REVIEW ARTICLES RESOURCE

For both review articles and current pediatrics practice guidelines, visit the MedStudy Hub at

medstudy.com/hub

The Hub contains the only online consolidated list of all current guidelines focused on pediatrics. Guidelines on the Hub are easy to find, continually updated, and linked to the published source. MedStudy maintains the Hub as a service to the medical community and makes it available to anyone and everyone at no cost to users.

FIGURE SOURCES

Figure 20-1: Jonathan Trobe, M.D., CC BY 3.0
Figure 20-2: Nailsjournal.com
Figure 20-3: MedStudy illustration
Figure 20-4: Okwikikim
Figure 20-5: Hektor, CC BY-SA 3.0
Figure 20-6: Frederick Stucker, MD
Figure 20-7: Afag Azizova, CC BY-SA 3.0
Figure 20-8: Dong Soo Kim, CC BY 2.0
Figure 20-9: Dong Soo Kim, CC BY 2.0
Figure 20-10: Doktorinternet, CC BY-SA 4.0
Figure 20-13: Elizabeth M. Dugan, Adam M. Huber, Frederick W. Miller, Lisa G. Rider, CC BY-SA 3.0
Figure 20-14: Gambichler et al., CC BY-SA 2.0
Figure 20-15: Leith C Jones, CC BY 3.0
Figure 20-16: Intermedichbo, CC BY-SA 3.0
Figure 20-17: Klaus D. Peter
Figure 20-18: MedStudy illustration
The remaining figures are from the MedStudy archives.

Ophthalmology &ENT

SECTION EDITORS

Erik Langenau, DO, MS
Professor, Pediatrics
Chief Academic Technology Officer,
Department of Professional Development and Online Learning
Philadelphia College of Osteopathic Medicine
Philadelphia, PA

Victoria Wurster Ovalle, MD, MEd
Pediatric Emergency Medicine Physician
Osceola Regional Medical Center
Kissimmee, FL

MEDICAL EDITOR

Lynn Bullock, MD
Colorado Springs, CO

Table of Contents

NORMAL VISUAL DEVELOPMENT

PREVIEW | REVIEW

- At what age does visual fixation achieve accuracy?
- Are most infants nearsighted or farsighted at birth?

ANATOMY OF THE EYE

To understand vision, visual development, and pathology, it is helpful to refamiliarize yourself with the anatomy of the eye. In Figure 21-1, you will find the important structures of the eye. Processing visual input is complex. Light first enters through the cornea and travels through the anterior chamber, lens, and posterior chamber. Light sensors within the retina (cones and rods) then process electrical stimuli to the optic nerve, tracts, and visual cortex. For vision to occur, each of these structures must function properly.

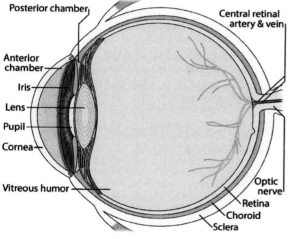

Figure 21-1: Structures of the eye

SOME IMPORTANT BASICS

As newborns grow, we see changes in the maturation of vision, eye movements, and depth perception. It is helpful to review some key concepts:

- Visual fixation can be demonstrated soon after birth and achieves accuracy by 6–8 weeks.
- By 2 months of age, infants should track across midline. Object tracking to 180° and conjugate gaze should be present by 4 months of age.
- Normal involuntary eye movements that provide stability of visual images are:
  - optokinetic nystagmus (tested by inducing nystagmus when looking at a series of vertical lines moving across the visual field), and
  - vestibulo-ocular reflex (tested by moving the infant's head back and forth horizontally and vertically and finding that the eyes remain fixed looking in the forward direction).

- Stereopsis (a.k.a. binocular depth perception) is when 2 separate images from both eyes are combined into 1 image in the brain. Stereopsis and binocular visual function develop between 3 and 7 months of age.
- Accommodation is the ability to focus the intraocular lens for near-viewing and is present at birth; however, it is not accurate until 2–3 months of age.
- Due to its size and shape, the normal eye at birth is often hyperopic (i.e., typically, infants are farsighted at birth). As the visual system matures, the eye elongates and becomes less hyperopic. Although most newborn full-term infants are normally mildly farsighted, premature infants and infants with low birth weights tend to be either less hyperopic or even myopic (nearsighted) and often also have some degree of astigmatism (misshapen cornea resulting in improperly refracted light and blurred vision).
- Color discrimination occurs by 2 weeks of age and improves over the next 3 months.

Vision Screening Guidelines

Evaluation of the eyes and visual system should begin in the newborn period and continue through adolescence during routine well-child visits. Evaluation for all ages should include ocular history, pupillary and red reflex exams, eye alignment assessment, and external inspection of the eyes and lids. Evaluating the ability to fixate on objects should begin at 2 months of age. Instrument-based screening (e.g., photoscreening) may be used to assess risk factors for amblyopia beginning at 12 months of age until the child can cooperate with visual acuity testing. Visual acuity testing may begin as early as 3 years of age; it should be started with formal vision testing at 4 years of age, using age-appropriate assessments (i.e., eye charts with figures, letters, or numbers).

Referral criteria to an ophthalmologist include:

- Physical abnormalities of the eyes or lids
- Abnormal red reflex
- Inability to fixate by 3–4 months of age
- Malalignment of eyes (strabismus) after 4 months of age
- Inability to perform visual acuity testing by 4 years of age (e.g., uncooperative child)
- Abnormal visual acuity
  - Vision worse than 20/50 in children 3–4 years of age
  - Vision worse than 20/40 in children 4–5 years of age
  - Vision worse than 20/30 in children > 5 years of age
  - More than a 2-line difference between eyes at any age

Early detection of eye abnormalities leads to earlier treatment and a greater chance of maintaining ocular health.

Refer to Vision and Hearing Screening in the Preventive Pediatrics section for more information.

EYE DISORDERS

PREVIEW | REVIEW

- What are some abnormalities that can cause an abnormal red reflex?
- What are the most common risk factors for retinopathy of prematurity?
- What is strabismus?
- What are the causes of amblyopia?
- What is the incidence of color vision abnormalities in boys compared with girls?
- Which brain lesion is suggested by upbeating jerk nystagmus? Downbeating jerk nystagmus?
- What are the symptoms of a corneal abrasion?
- How do you diagnose corneal abrasion?
- What is the most prevalent malignant ocular tumor in childhood?
- How does retinoblastoma usually present?
- What is a hyphema?

OVERVIEW

Common visual disorders include amblyopia, strabismus, significant refractive error, color vision defects, and ocular disease. In the U.S., the leading causes of blindness in children are cortical visual impairment, retinopathy of prematurity, and optic nerve hypoplasia. The leading cause of "acquired" blindness in children is ocular trauma, most often following a sports-related injury or an accidental or intentional injury by another child.

An abnormal red reflex can be caused by a number of abnormalities (e.g., strabismus, cataracts, glaucoma, retinoblastoma, high refractory error); refer immediately.

CATARACTS

A cataract is an opacification of the lens. Early detection and treatment are imperative for a good outcome.

Congenital cataracts are caused by abnormal lens development in utero and are present at birth, although they sometimes go undetected for a period of time. A unilateral cataract is usually sporadic and not associated with a systemic disease. Bilateral cataracts, however, can be caused by autosomal dominant inheritance, trisomy syndromes (i.e., 13, 18, 21), metabolic disorders (e.g., galactosemia), and intrauterine infections (i.e., **TORCH** [**t**oxoplasmosis, **o**ther, **r**ubella, **c**ytomegalovirus, and **h**erpes simplex]). See the Infectious Disease section for more on TORCH. Cataracts in older children can occur following ocular trauma, glucocorticoid treatment, and ionizing radiation.

The simultaneous red reflex test is the most useful assessment to detect lens opacity. If abnormal, a complete eye examination must be done by an ophthalmologist. Not all cataracts are visually significant. However, cataracts

that are centrally located and are > 3 mm require immediate removal to prevent vision loss. Smaller ones can be observed for a period of time but must be removed at the first indication of visual interference.

RETINOPATHY OF PREMATURITY (ROP)

ROP is caused by abnormal development of blood vessels in the retina of preterm infants. Prematurity is the most important risk factor for ROP, followed by low birth weight. Other risk factors include prolonged exposure to high levels of supplemental oxygen, assisted ventilation for > 7 days, surfactant therapy, hyperglycemia, insulin therapy, and cumulative illness severity.

Severe ROP occurs mainly in infants born at < 28 weeks of gestation and with a birth weight of < 1,250 g.

Indications for screening remain controversial and vary among institutions. In general, screen all infants weighing ≤ 1,500 g at birth or with a gestational age of < 30 weeks. Also, screen those with a birth weight between 1,500 g and 2,000 g or a gestational age ≥ 30 weeks whose unstable clinical course places them at increased risk for ROP. The ROP screening should be performed with a dilated eye exam by a pediatric ophthalmologist.

Treatment is by the ophthalmologist and varies depending on severity of the ROP. Options include surveillance, laser photocoagulation, and intravitreal injection of monoclonal antibodies.

DACRYOSTENOSIS (NASOLACRIMAL DUCT OBSTRUCTION)

Dacryostenosis is caused by obstruction of the nasolacrimal duct and is very common in newborns. The main symptom is persistent tearing in the affected eye. Treatment consists of lacrimal sac massage. Most cases resolve by 6 months of age. Refer to an ophthalmologist for possible duct probing if the condition persists after 6–7 months of age.

STYE / CHALAZION

A **stye (hordeolum)** is a small, painful, localized, erythematous, infectious abscess of the eyelid (Figure 21-2). External styes, on the visible part of the eyelid, arise from a blocked and then infected eyelash follicle gland or meibomian gland. Internal styes, on the inside of the eyelid, arise

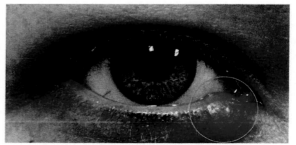

Figure 21-2: Stye (hordeolum)—infectious

only from meibomian gland obstruction and infection. (Meibomian glands secrete a vital oil that stabilizes the tear film and keeps it from quickly evaporating.) Most styes resolve spontaneously within 3–5 days. Warm compresses and regular cleaning of the lid margins often decrease the duration of illness. Antibiotics are not usually required.

A **chalazion** is a noninfectious, localized, painless, rubbery eyelid swelling, caused by obstruction of a meibomian gland with subsequent granulomatous inflammation (but again, no infection; Figure 21-3). It typically resolves without treatment within a few months. Antibiotics are not indicated. Protracted cases, or those with increasing pain or obstructed vision, warrant referral to an ophthalmologist.

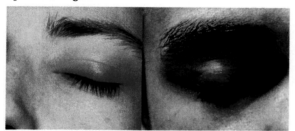

Figure 21-3: Chalazion, mild (L) and moderate (R)--noninfectious

STRABISMUS

Strabismus is the continuous or intermittent malalignment of one or both eyes, in which one or both eyes are turned in (esotropia), out (exotropia), up (hypertropia), or down (hypotropia). In childhood, the most common forms are infantile and accommodative esotropia. Physical exam reveals an asymmetric corneal light reflex and abnormal cover/uncover test (i.e., movement of the uncovered eye that is fixated on a target when the other eye is covered). While ocular instability of infancy is frequently present in normal newborns during the first few months of life, refer to an ophthalmologist for possible pathologic strabismus if it persists past 4 months of age. Treatment may involve a combination of corrective lenses, patching, cycloplegics, and/or surgery.

Pseudoesotropia (pseudostrabismus) is the result of a wide nasal bridge and/or epicanthal folds, which obscure the nasal sclera, particularly when the child looks to the right or left. On formal testing, symmetric light reflex is demonstrated on both examination of the corneal light reflex and the cover/uncover test, thereby confirming that the child has pseudostrabismus.

AMBLYOPIA

Amblyopia, a functional reduction in visual acuity caused by disuse or misuse of visual pathways, occurs in 1–4% of 3-year-old children. It also affects depth perception and binocularity. Amblyopia is the most common cause of visual loss in individuals < 45 years of age. Amblyopia can result from early childhood refractive disorders, strabismus, cataracts, corneal opacities, or anisometropia (an

unequal refractive error between the eyes). Treatment often involves encouraging use of the amblyopic eye by obscuring vision in the better-seeing eye with a patch or cycloplegic eye drops.

COLOR VISION DEFECTS

Color differentiation is present by 2 years of age. Abnormal color vision occurs in ~ 8–10% of boys and < 0.5% of girls; it is due to X-linked protan and deutan deficits (red–green color blindness). While most color vision defects are congenital, rare acquired color vision abnormalities are usually caused by retinal and optic nerve abnormalities.

CORTICAL VISUAL IMPAIRMENT

Damage to the geniculostriate pathway (composed of the visual cortex and optic radiations) causes cortical visual impairment. There is reduced vision and absence of optokinetic nystagmus, but pupillary light reflexes are intact. Hypoxia is the most common cause. Other etiologies include meningitis, encephalitis, metabolic disease, head trauma, and hydrocephalus. Generally, children with cortical visual impairment have other associated abnormalities such as cerebral palsy, seizures, or paralysis.

NYSTAGMUS

As we track objects across the visual field, eye movement is usually smooth ("smooth pursuit"). Nystagmus is an involuntary oscillation of the eyes. The movements can be pendular (like a pendulum) or jerk.

Optokinetic nystagmus is nystagmus while tracking objects across the visual field. This is an attempt to stabilize the visual image during tracking and is considered part of normal development for early infants.

Pendular nystagmus has a sinusoidal oscillation. It is typically acquired, and it is due to visual loss or can be a late unremitting sign of multiple sclerosis. The sinusoidal oscillation can occur in any direction; however, it is usually horizontal.

Jerk nystagmus has 2 components: slow and fast. The eyes "drift" (slow component) and try to quickly recover (fast component). The fast direction defines the direction of the nystagmus. The nystagmus is sometimes—but not always—associated with vertigo. Jerk nystagmus is most common in vestibular disorders but does not indicate whether the lesion is within the central nervous system or if it involves the cranial nerve itself. **Upbeating jerk nystagmus** usually indicates a brain lesion in the pons; however, it can be seen in brain lesions of the medulla or cerebellum (i.e., infratentorial). **Downbeating jerk nystagmus** indicates a brain lesion at the cervicomedullary junction.

Spasmus nutans is an acquired nystagmus of unknown etiology, presenting within the first 6–24 months of life. In contrast to congenital nystagmus, this nystagmus is often intermittent, asymmetrical, and either bilateral or unilateral. It is characterized by a fine, horizontal, rapid pendular nystagmus. In its complete form, spasmus nutans is also associated with torticollis and slow head nodding. All symptoms may present at varying intervals or simultaneously. At presentation, complete evaluation for evidence of a space-occupying lesion, drug ingestion, and/or central nervous system infection is indicated prior to confirming the diagnosis of spasmus nutans. Affected individuals require continued evaluation by an ophthalmologist to monitor for, and to treat, strabismus and amblyopia. Spontaneous resolution usually occurs within several months to several years.

Most congenital nystagmus is horizontal and conjugate. It is often associated with visual loss. This type usually has a blending of jerk and pendular waveforms.

Gazing in particular directions precipitates the abnormal eye movements in certain types of nystagmus. For instance, drugs (e.g., antiseizure medications) can cause horizontal and vertical gaze-evoked nystagmus (occurring when the person looks right, left, or up). In other words, it is present "in all directions." Isolated vertical gaze-evoked nystagmus typically indicates disease in the posterior fossa.

OPTIC NERVE HYPOPLASIA

Optic nerve hypoplasia is a nonspecific finding due to damage of the visual system prior to full development. It is characterized by pallor of the disc, loss of substance of the nerve head, and enlargement of the disc cup.

Intracranial tumors and hydrocephalus are the most common causes of optic atrophy in children. Other causes are hypopituitarism, hypothyroidism, growth hormone deficiency, and/or neonatal hypoglycemia.

Maternal risk factors are diabetes, alcohol abuse, and exposure to toxins.

Optic nerve hypoplasia is an example of a midline facial defect. Other defects include neural tube defects, single central incisor, cleft lip/palate, tracheoesophageal fistula, conotruncal heart defects, diaphragmatic hernia, omphalocele, imperforated anus, and microphalus or undescended testicle.

GLAUCOMA

Glaucoma refers to increased ocular pressure, often leading to damage of the optic nerve. Although common in older adults, it is rare in children. Many cases of pediatric glaucoma have no specific identifiable cause and are referred to as primary glaucoma. A variety of causes can result in secondary glaucoma. Some examples include trauma, intraocular hemorrhage, surgical complications (e.g., after cataract removal), chronic steroid use, and Sturge-Weber syndrome. Surgery, especially in infants, is often required to relieve intraocular pressure.

PAINFUL ERYTHEMATOUS EYE

The painful red eye is a typical primary care complaint. Although conjunctivitis is the usual cause, consider also corneal abrasion, foreign body, subconjunctival hemorrhage, glaucoma, iritis, keratitis, and scleritis. Evaluate with history, visual acuity testing, and penlight examination. If there is moderate-to-severe pain with vision abnormalities, distorted pupil, or corneal involvement, refer urgently to an ophthalmologist for further evaluation, as there is likely to be a serious underlying cause.

Conjunctivitis

Conjunctivitis is inflammation of the conjunctiva. It can be either infectious (bacterial or viral) or noninfectious (typically allergic). Allergic conjunctivitis is covered in the Allergy & Immunology section, so we will concentrate on infectious etiologies here. Both viral and bacterial conjunctivitis are very contagious and spread by direct contact.

Viruses are the most frequent cause of conjunctivitis. The most common etiology is **adenovirus**. The patient with viral conjunctivitis presents with red conjunctiva and a gritty sensation in the eye, which often accompanies an upper respiratory infection. Viral conjunctivitis usually produces a watery discharge, starts in one eye, and spreads to the other eye within 24–48 hours. Although there is no specific treatment for viral conjunctivitis, many patients receive some relief with lubricant drops.

Bacterial conjunctivitis is often caused by *Streptococcus pneumoniae*, *Haemophilus influenzae*, or *Moraxella catarrhalis*. Bacterial conjunctivitis produces a purulent discharge and tends to be unilateral, although it can be in both eyes. Treatment for bacterial conjunctivitis often includes erythromycin ophthalmic ointment or trimethoprim–polymyxin ophthalmic drops 4×/day for 5–7 days. Use fluoroquinolone drops in contact lens wearers due to the increased incidence of *Pseudomonas* in these patients.

Corneal Abrasion

Corneal abrasions are very common; fortunately, most superficial abrasions heal quickly without sequelae. Symptoms of a corneal abrasion include pain, tearing, photophobia, and blurry vision. Infants can present with inconsolable crying. Corneal ulcers are uncommon but potentially much more serious. Contact lens wearers are at increased risk.

Diagnosis of corneal abrasion is best made with fluorescein dye and either a Wood lamp or the blue light of a slitlamp (Figure 21-4). An abrasion is transparent on gross examination without fluorescein. An ulcer is opaque. Both illuminate with fluorescein.

Treat corneal abrasions with a topical antibiotic ointment and oral analgesia. Topical anesthetics are helpful in the emergency department or office to provide temporary pain relief and allow examination, but do not send the patient home with anesthetic drops—they can be toxic to the cornea with repeated use, and the child may retraumatize the eye. Topical cycloplegic drops have traditionally

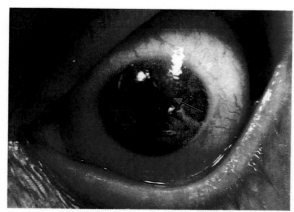

Figure 21-4: Corneal abrasion with fluorescein staining

been used to control pain, but recent research shows little clinical benefit. Semipressure patches are no longer recommended and have not been found to reduce pain or improve healing.

Multiple vertical abrasions suggest a foreign body retained in the upper eyelid; the lid must be everted to find and remove the object. Remove superficial foreign bodies with a cotton swab (after topical anesthesia, of course). Refer to an ophthalmologist for removal of deeper foreign bodies.

Recheck corneal abrasions for resolution in 24–48 hours. Corneal ulcers should be treated by an ophthalmologist.

PRESEPTAL AND ORBITAL CELLULITIS

Preseptal cellulitis is an infection of the eye involving tissues anterior to the orbital septum (i.e., anterior to the orbital contents). **Orbital cellulitis** is an infection involving structures behind the orbital septum. It is imperative to distinguish between preseptal cellulitis, which is typically mild, and orbital cellulitis, which is far more serious. Although both present with eye pain and a red swollen eyelid, only orbital cellulitis causes pain with eye movement, ophthalmoplegia, chemosis, and/or proptosis.

Diagnose preseptal cellulitis by history and physical exam. Preseptal cellulitis is typically caused by contiguous spread of infection from surrounding soft tissue due to trauma or from sinusitis. The usual pathogens are *Staphylococcus aureus* and *Streptococcus pyogenes* when the infection originates from local trauma and *Streptococcus pneumoniae* when it originates from sinusitis. Antibiotic selection will depend on local surveillance of sensitivities and resistance patterns. Treatment is usually outpatient and consists of 7–10 days of:

- clindamycin, or
- combination therapy of trimethoprim/sulfamethoxazole (TMP/SMX) plus 1 of the following—amoxicillin, amoxicillin/clavulanic acid, cefpodoxime, or cefdinir.

Patients < 1 year of age are usually hospitalized for treatment.

Orbital cellulitis is a serious infection and, if suspected clinically, requires a CT scan for diagnosis. It typically originates from sinusitis, particularly ethmoidal. Orbital cellulitis is usually caused by multiple organisms, but the most commonly identified pathogens are *S. aureus* and streptococci. Admit the patient for parenteral antibiotic therapy with vancomycin plus ampicillin–sulbactam, ceftriaxone, or cefotaxime. Metronidazole may be needed for anaerobic coverage as well, especially if you suspect a dental or sinus source. Once the patient improves, typically within 3–5 days, switch treatment to the same oral drug regimen used for preseptal cellulitis for a total duration of combined antibiotic therapy (both IV and oral) of at least 2–3 weeks. Surgery is sometimes required if the patient does not respond to antibiotic therapy. Possible complications include orbital abscess, subperiosteal abscess, and intracranial extension.

PAPILLEDEMA

Papilledema is optic nerve swelling due to increased intracranial pressure (Figure 21-5). It is imperative to urgently recognize and evaluate papilledema. Underlying causes include a mass lesion, brain abscess, cerebral edema, obstructive hydrocephalus, and pseudotumor cerebri. Symptoms can include headache, nausea and vomiting, and pulsatile tinnitus. Visual symptoms are often absent. If they occur, they include diplopia and brief visual obscurations that are often unilateral.

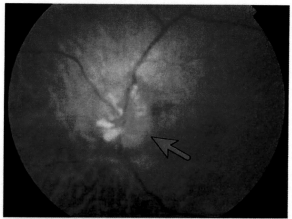

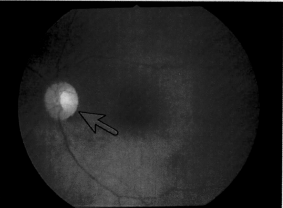

Figure 21-5: Papilledema (top) with arrow showing obscured disc margin. Normal fundus (bottom).

Diagnosis is made by funduscopic examination, and findings can range from loss of spontaneous venous pulsations to obscured disc margins (Figure 21-5 on page 21-5), venous congestion, and papillary hemorrhages. Once the diagnosis of papilledema is made, neuroimaging is required. An MRI may be indicated for a complete tumor or vascular evaluation. Often, a CT is preferred because it is more available, performed quickly, and typically does not require sedation. If neuroimaging is normal, evaluate the opening pressure and spinal fluid with a lumbar puncture. A result of > 27 cm H_2O is considered an elevated opening pressure. Treatment varies and depends upon the underlying etiology.

RETINOBLASTOMA

Retinoblastoma is the leading malignant ocular tumor of childhood, with an incidence of 3.7 cases per million. The tumor arises from the primitive retinal cells—most present at < 4 years of age. It can be genetic or sporadic. Approximately 60% of cases are unilateral and nonhereditary; the remaining 40% are hereditary, with ~ 1/3 of these bilateral. Bilateral involvement is most common in those < 1 year of age. Germinal retinoblastoma is the result of inactivation of the *RB1* gene on chromosome 13q14 and is inherited in an autosomal dominant pattern.

Retinoblastoma typically presents with a white pupillary reflex—leukocoria; however, strabismus can also be the initial presenting sign.

Treatment depends on the size and location of the tumor. Options include enucleation, chemotherapy, radiation therapy, laser therapy, and cryotherapy.

There is a significant risk of secondary malignancies, especially osteosarcoma, soft tissue sarcomas, and malignant melanoma.

SUBCONJUNCTIVAL HEMORRHAGE

A subconjunctival hemorrhage presents as a painless red discrete discoloration on the sclera. It is caused by rupture of small scleral capillaries beneath the bulbar conjunctiva, and results from mild trauma or increased capillary pressure. It is commonly seen in infants after vaginal delivery and in older children after forceful vomiting when increased pressure results in rupture of the capillaries. Most spontaneously resolve over 2–3 weeks without treatment.

HYPHEMA

A hyphema is the presence of blood in the anterior chamber of the eye. It usually occurs after blunt or penetrating injury. It appears as a bright or dark red fluid level between the cornea and iris (Figure 21-6); early injuries sometimes show diffuse murkiness before the blood settles. Complete opacification of the anterior chamber ("8-ball hyphema") can occur in more severe injuries. Consultation with an ophthalmologist is required. Consider ruptured globe and intraocular foreign body if the history or physical exam is concerning—such as struck by a sharp object (e.g., knife, scissors) or shot with a BB gun. A clue to a ruptured globe is a teardrop-shaped or eccentric pupil. Protect any serious eye injury from further trauma with a rigid shield, and consult an ophthalmologist.

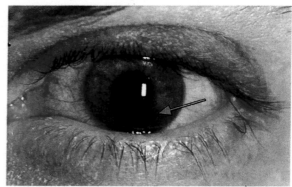

Figure 21-6: Hyphema

Treatment includes topical steroid and cycloplegic drops. Use ondansetron and analgesics to alleviate vomiting and/or pain, which can otherwise further elevate intraocular pressure. Although most children with minor hyphemas do well, they are at risk of rebleeding (usually in the 1st week after initial injury); this increases the risk for long-term complications such as glaucoma. Prevent secondary bleeding with antifibrinolytic therapy (e.g., aminocaproic acid). Closely monitor intraocular pressures.

ORBITAL BLOWOUT FRACTURE

Blunt trauma to the eye, such as being punched or struck by a baseball, can cause fracture of the orbital walls or floor. Herniation of orbital contents into a paranasal sinus can entrap extraocular muscles and other structures. Orbital floor fractures are the most common. Symptoms can include vertical diplopia and limited vertical gaze (due to entrapment of the inferior rectus muscle). Other findings can include circumferential ecchymosis, subconjunctival hemorrhage, hyphema, and enophthalmos (eye appears sunken in).

Consult an ophthalmologist and obtain a CT scan of the orbits (Figure 21-7). Advise these patients to avoid blowing their nose and prescribe antibiotics to prevent infection. Refer early to a maxillofacial surgeon, as operative treatment will likely be needed. Exact timing depends on the severity of entrapment and other findings.

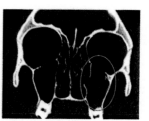

Figure 21-7: Orbital blowout fracture

EAR DISORDERS

PREVIEW | REVIEW

- A child with a preauricular pit is at increased risk for what kind of impairment?
- What are the most common bacterial pathogens of acute otitis media?
- What is the pattern of inheritance for the majority of inherited deafness cases?
- What are the most common causes of conductive hearing loss in children?
- What is the most likely type of hearing loss for those with severe and profound hearing loss?
- What is the most common infectious cause of congenital deafness?
- Interpret common tympanogram results.

ANATOMY OF THE EAR

Reviewing the anatomy of the ear is helpful to understanding audio processing, normal hearing, and hearing pathology (Figure 21-8). Sound travels through the outer ear, striking the tympanic membrane. The membrane transfers sound into mechanical stimuli, using the ossicles of the middle ear. Sound is then transmitted to the inner ear where the cochlea is important for audio processing by providing input to the audio cortex via the auditory nerve. The semicircular canals are important for balance and spacial orientation.

PREAURICULAR SINUSES AND PITS

A preauricular sinus/pit is a common congenital abnormality. There is an increased risk of hearing impairment in children with a preauricular pit, so all affected patients need an audiologic examination. There is no increased risk of renal abnormalities with isolated preauricular sinus/pit. However, if there are other dysmorphic features or malformations or hearing loss, order a renal ultrasound to rule out associated syndromes. See the Genetics section for more on associated syndromes with preauricular sinus/pit.

EXTERNAL EAR

Otitis Externa

Otitis externa (a.k.a. swimmer's ear) is inflammation of the outer ear canal. It is common in swimmers, because water remaining in the ear canal provides a favorable environment for bacterial overgrowth. The most common etiologies are *Pseudomonas aeruginosa* and *Staphylococcus aureus*, although cultures are typically not done. Although bacterial infection, including aerobic and anaerobic infections, is the most common cause of otitis externa, it can also be caused by allergic reactions and fungal infections.

Symptoms include pruritus, pain, drainage, redness, and muffled hearing. On physical exam, the ear canal is red, swollen, and often scaly. A key finding is worsening pain with manipulation of the pinna, which does not occur with otitis media.

Treatment escalates with severity. Mild infection treatment is usually topical with a combination preparation of an acidic solution (e.g., acetic acid) plus hydrocortisone.

Moderate infection treatment is the same as mild disease with the addition of a topic antibiotic that covers both *S. aureus* and *P. aeruginosa* (e.g., aminoglycosides, polymyxin B, quinolones). Note: Never give topical aminoglycosides unless you can confirm the tympanic membrane is intact.

Severe infection treatment is the same as moderate disease with the addition of an ear wick if the canal is getting occluded and the addition of oral antibiotics if the

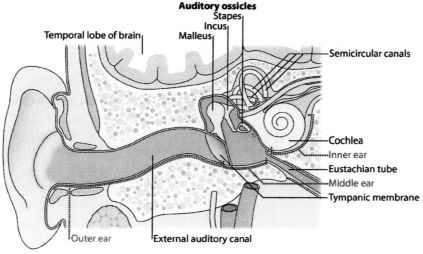

Figure 21-8: Ear anatomy

infection spreads outside of the ear canal. Oral antibiotics are typically reserved only for patients with infection spread and complications. Oral antibiotics must also cover *S. aureus* and *P. aeruginosa*.

Duration of treatment is typically 5–7 days; however, it may be as long as 2 weeks depending on severity and response to treatment.

Foreign Body

Most foreign bodies of the external ear canal occur in children ≤ 6 years of age and can include beads, food, toys, rocks, and insects. Although foreign bodies can cause pain and/or decreased hearing, many are asymptomatic and are found incidentally on exam or are brought to medical attention by a caregiver who saw the patient place an object into the ear. Diagnosis is made by otoscopy. Removal techniques include irrigation and instrumentation under direct visualization. Mineral oil or lidocaine can be placed in the ear canal to kill live insects prior to removal. Referral to an ENT specialist is necessary if proper instruments are unavailable or if removal is difficult.

External Ear Injury

Any external ear injury, including **laceration**, should trigger the physician to perform a complete HEENT examination, looking for other coexisting injuries such as perforation of the tympanic membrane, skull fracture, or a C-spine injury. Such injuries may present with signs and symptoms that include bleeding from the ear, hearing loss, loss of consciousness, or obvious head trauma.

Typically, a laceration of the ear should be sutured. Healing by secondary intention carries a greater risk of ear deformities/poor cosmesis and chondritis. When repairing ear lacerations, an auricular field block is generally superior to local infiltration because it provides better analgesia without distorting important landmarks.

Auricular hematoma is caused by blunt trauma to the auricle. Accumulation of blood between the cartilage and the perichondrium interrupts the blood supply to the cartilage. It commonly occurs in the anterior superior portion of the auricle. Drain as soon as possible to prevent necrosis and "cauliflower ear," followed by pressure bandaging to reduce the risk for reaccumulation of the hematoma. Prophylactic oral antibiotics with good cartilage penetration against skin flora are often recommended. Common choices are fluoroquinolones or amoxicillin/clavulanic in younger children. Refer to an ENT specialist if drainage is delayed > 7 days.

MIDDLE EAR

Acute Otitis Media (AOM)

AOM is an acute inflammation of the middle ear caused by infection. Most episodes of AOM are triggered by an upper respiratory infection causing blockage of the eustachian tube. The typical pathogens of AOM are viruses: *Streptococcus pneumoniae*, nontypeable *Haemophilus influenzae*, and *Moraxella catarrhalis*. Risk factors include young age (6–18 months), family history, day care attendance, lack of breastfeeding, and tobacco smoke exposure. The most common symptom is ear pain, but in younger children, the symptoms are nonspecific and can include fever, anorexia, and irritability. Tugging at the ears is nonspecific and is an unreliable sign for diagnosis. (Tugging at the ears may be a sign of pain or simply a soothing technique.) According to the American Academy of Pediatrics (AAP) guidelines, diagnosis of AOM is made by pneumatic otoscopy when the following criteria are met: bulging tympanic membrane (or new-onset otorrhea not due to otitis externa), middle ear effusion, and signs of acute inflammation such as pain, erythema, or opaque tympanic membrane.

High-dose amoxicillin (80–90 mg/kg/day) is the drug of choice for AOM. If patients fail to respond within 48 hours, broaden coverage to include penicillin-resistant *S. pneumoniae*, β-lactamase-producing *H. influenzae*, and *M. catarrhalis*, by switching to amoxicillin/clavulanate or a 2nd or 3rd generation cephalosporin.

In 2013, the AAP published updated guidelines for the diagnosis and management of uncomplicated AOM in children 6 months to 12 years of age. The guidelines base initial antibiotic treatment on age (6 months to 2 years of age vs. > 2 years of age), severity of symptoms, laterality of disease (unilateral vs. bilateral), and presence of otorrhea.

Antibiotics should be initiated for all children who have AOM with otorrhea, severe symptoms (e.g., fever > 102.2°F [39.0°C], toxic appearance, otalgia for > 48 hours), or poor follow up. Antibiotics should also be started for children 6 months through 23 months of age with bilateral AOM, even if not severe.

Treat all infants < 6 months of age who have AOM with antibiotic therapy.

Observation without antibiotics can be considered for children 6 months to 2 years of age with unilateral AOM without otorrhea, and for children ≥ 2 years of age with unilateral or bilateral otitis without otorrhea. Monitor for resolution of symptoms and follow up closely. Start antibiotics if the child worsens or fails to improve within 48–72 hours from onset.

Recurrent Acute Otitis Media (AOM)

Recurrent AOM is defined as ≥ 3 episodes within a period of 6 months or ≥ 4 episodes within a period of 12 months. Treatment remains controversial and may include a combination of the following: avoidance of second-hand smoke (parental smoking), vaccination with pneumococcal conjugate vaccine, breastfeeding, prophylactic antibiotics, and adenoidectomy with or without tympanostomy tube placement.

Otitis Media with Effusion (OME)

OME is a middle ear effusion without clinical signs of infection. It is typically seen during the resolution of AOM or with eustachian tube dysfunction. OME is often asymptomatic but can present with some hearing loss. Spontaneous resolution usually occurs within 6 weeks. Tympanostomy tube placement is recommended for patients with persistent OME.

Chronic Suppurative Otitis Media

Chronic suppurative otitis media refers to a perforated tympanic membrane with chronic drainage lasting > 6 weeks. Typical causes include recurrent AOM, injury, or tympanostomy tube placement. The patient presents with painless drainage and possibly decreased hearing. The most common pathogens are *Pseudomonas* and *Proteus*. Treatment consists of ototopical therapy with a quinolone (5 drops 3×/day for 2 weeks). This can be combined with ear wicking, suctioning of the otorrhea, or using gauze to absorb the drainage.

Complications of Otitis Media

Tympanosclerosis is scarring of the tympanic membrane. Tympanosclerosis can be caused by recurrent AOM, chronic OME, trauma, or congenital anomalies. It can be asymptomatic; however, it is often associated with conductive hearing loss due to limited mobility of the tympanic membrane.

Cholesteatoma is an abnormal growth of squamous epithelium in the middle ear; progressive enlargement can destroy the nearby ossicles, thus causing hearing loss. It can also cause cranial nerve palsies and vertigo. Rarely, it can cause intracranial abscess, meningitis, and venous thrombosis. Cholesteatoma occurs most commonly in children with recurrent or chronic otitis media, extruded tympanostomy tubes, cleft palate, craniofacial abnormalities, trisomy 21 (a.k.a. Down syndrome), and 45,X (a.k.a. Turner syndrome). Diagnosis is made on otoscopy exam when a white mass is seen behind an intact eardrum. Surgical removal is required. There is a > 50% recurrence rate within 5 years of surgery.

Mastoiditis occurs when the mastoid air cells of the temporal bone, which are contiguous with the middle ear cavity, become infected. The most common pathogens include *S. pneumoniae*, *S. pyogenes*, nontypeable *H. influenzae*, *S. aureus*, and *P. aeruginosa*. Physical features include fever; postauricular erythema, tenderness, and swelling; and protrusion of the auricle.

Immediate diagnosis and treatment can prevent serious complications (e.g., meningitis, osteomyelitis). Confirmatory CT may reveal opacification of the middle ear and mastoid, coalescence of the mastoid air cells, and/or irregularity of the mastoid cortex and bony septae contours.

Treat uncomplicated cases with IV vancomycin +/– ceftazidime or cefepime, until culture results from tympanocentesis are available. Switch to oral antibiotics once improvement is seen and sensitivities are known. If needed, additional drainage of the middle ear can be achieved with myringotomy. Complicated cases may also require a mastoidectomy to remove the infected mastoid cortical bone.

Middle Ear Trauma

Trauma to the middle ear can result in tympanic membrane perforation, temporal bone fracture, or hearing loss, among other injuries.

Causes of traumatic tympanic membrane perforations include direct trauma, head trauma, barotrauma, and blast injury. Symptoms include pain, bleeding, hearing loss, and tinnitus. Small perforations are typically managed conservatively, with close follow up with an ENT specialist along with initiation of prophylactic antibiotic ear drops for 1–2 weeks. Those with suspected hearing loss should also be referred for formal audiometry testing.

Indications for surgical management of a tympanic membrane perforation include:

- Large perforations unlikely to heal spontaneously
- Hearing loss
- Chronic perforations
- Perforations of the posterior region of the tympanic membrane

In cases of severe head injury, look for signs or symptoms of a temporal bone fracture—hearing loss, dizziness, vertigo, hemotympanum, otorrhea, or Battle sign (retroauricular hematoma). Along with a noncontrast head CT, these patients require a dedicated noncontrast temporal bone CT. Patients with a temporal bone fracture require evaluation by a pediatric ENT specialist.

HEARING PROBLEMS

Deafness is defined as hearing loss at > 90 dB, which results in the inability to distinguish between elements of spoken language. "Mild" hearing loss is defined as a 25-dB loss; even a 15-dB loss can result in problems with speech perception, especially during early childhood.

Deafness is inherited in ~ 50% of cases. Of these, 80% are inherited as autosomal recessive, 18% as autosomal dominant, and 2% as X-linked recessive. Deafness can be due to either an isolated event or associated with a syndrome (e.g., Treacher-Collins, Alport, Crouzon, Waardenburg, trisomy 21). One form of the prolonged QT syndrome, Jervell and Lange-Nielsen syndrome, is associated with sensorineural hearing loss—**syncope** and a history of **hearing loss** are important clues to this diagnosis!

According to the CDC, 1–3/1,000 children have hearing loss. Hearing loss is generally classified into 1 of 3 categories: conductive, sensorineural, or cortical.

Conductive hearing loss (more common) is due to disruption of mechanical components required for the transduction of sound wave energy. Cerumen impaction, ossicular chain fixation, and fluid in the middle ear—due either to acute otitis media or otitis media with effusion—are the most common causes of conductive hearing loss. With prolonged middle ear effusion, sounds are distorted by the fluid, leading to problems in early language discrimination. In children with persistent middle ear effusions, closely monitor language development for any delay because prolonged hearing loss during the critical period of speech acquisition can lead to significant impediments.

Most children have, at various points in time, some degree of intermittent conductive hearing loss, usually limited to sounds at 50 dB or lower; sounds louder than this can be conducted directly by bone to the cochlea.

Sensorineural hearing loss (less common) is caused by dysfunction of the sensory epithelium, cochlea, or neural pathways leading to the auditory cortex via cranial nerve 8 and other connections. Severe and profound hearing loss is always sensorineural and most often affects higher frequencies.

The most common infectious cause of congenital deafness is cytomegalovirus (**CMV**), which causes sensorineural hearing loss in 30–50% of symptomatic infants and 8–12% of asymptomatic infants. Other congenital infections that can cause sensorineural hearing loss include toxoplasmosis, rubella, and syphilis. Routine immunization with *H. influenzae* Type b and pneumococcal vaccines has decreased the rate of bacterial meningitis and the resulting hearing loss. Other causes of acquired sensorineural hearing loss include prolonged exposure to loud noise—a typical cause of high-pitched hearing loss in adolescents—ototoxic drugs (e.g., aminoglycosides, salicylates, loop diuretics), and trauma.

Cortical dysfunction can also cause hearing loss with impaired ability to perceive or process sounds.

Table 21-1 lists risk factors for neonatal hearing loss as identified by the Joint Committee on Infant Hearing. Approximately 50% of infants with sensorineural hearing loss have ≥ 1 risk factor. Universal screening is recommended for all infants, whether they are at increased risk or not. See the Preventive Pediatrics section for more information.

Screening is performed with either otoacoustic emissions or an automated auditory brainstem response test. The key to success in treating hearing loss is early diagnosis and intervention (e.g., hearing aids, implants).

TYMPANOGRAMS

Tympanometry objectively tests middle ear function by determining the compliance of the eardrum in response to a range of air pressures in the external canal. The tympanometer is inserted into the external canal, forming a seal from outside air pressure. Air pressure is then changed in the canal from a negative pressure, through atmospheric pressure ("0"), to a positive pressure, measured in decaPascals (daPa). During this process, a low frequency sound is injected into the external canal and a little microphone on the tympanometer measures how much of that sound is reflected back—the more reflected back, the less compliant the eardrum. The resulting tympanogram plots the induced pressure on the *x* axis and resulting compliance on the *y* axis.

Findings on tympanograms are classified as Types A (Figure 21-9 through Figure 21-11), B (Figure 21-12), and C (Figure 21-13).

Type A, normal middle ear pressure peak (Figure 21-9):

- These values form the dimensions of the "normal box" shown in this and the other tympanograms.
  - Peak –150 to +50 daPa
  - Peak compliance (*y* axis) between 0.2 and 1.8 cc
- There is absence of middle ear pathology.
- Tympanic membrane (TM) is mobile and intact.
- Eustachian tube function is normal.
- If the patient has hearing loss, it is likely sensorineural.

Table 21-1: Risk Factors for Hearing Loss in Neonates
Family history of sensorineural hearing loss
Congenital infection—especially cytomegalovirus
Presence of craniofacial anomalies
Birth weight < 1,500 g
Neonatal jaundice resulting in exchange transfusion
Ototoxic medications (e.g., furosemide, aminoglycosides)
Bacterial meningitis
Apgar scores of ≤ 3 at 5 minutes
Physical findings consistent with a syndrome associated with hearing loss

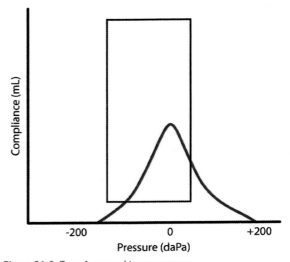

Figure 21-9: Type A, normal tympanogram

Type A(s), shallow; poorly compliant middle ear system (Figure 21-10):

- Compliance curve is in the normal position.
- Peak compliance is very low (below 0.2 cc).
- Think ossicular fixation, TM scarring, or otosclerosis for Type A(s).
- Not due to middle ear effusion
- Conductive hearing loss

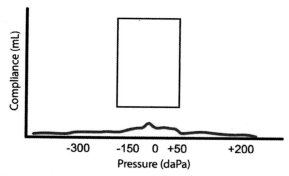

Figure 21-10: Type A(s), shallow

Type A(d), highly compliant middle ear system (Figure 21-11):

- Peak compliance occurs between –150 and +50 daPa (i.e., normal).
- Peak compliance is very high.
- Think ossicular disarticulation or hypermobile TM with Type A(d).
- Conductive hearing loss is possible.

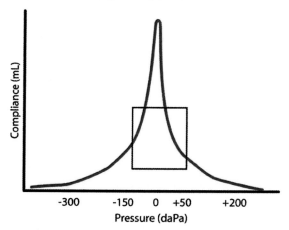

Figure 21-11: Type A(d), disarticulation

Type B, retracted, poorly mobile (Figure 21-12):

- Compliance curve is nearly flat to completely flat and always below normal.
- Negative middle ear pressure (Peak compliance is shifted left.)
- Think middle ear effusion or perforated eardrum with Type B.
- Conductive hearing loss

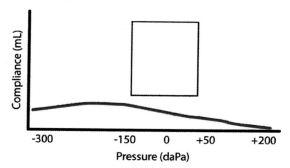

Figure 21-12: Type B, retracted, poorly mobile

Type C, normal compliance but negative pressure in the middle ear (Figure 21-13):

- Clear peak
- Peak compliance has normal amplitude.
- Peak compliance is shifted to the left (negative middle ear pressure).
- Think eustachian tube blockage with Type C.
- Conductive hearing loss is likely.

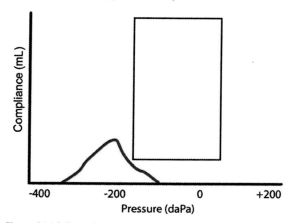

Figure 21-13: Type C, negative pressure

CONGENITAL DISORDERS OF THE NOSE

PREVIEW | REVIEW

- What is the most common congenital anomaly of the nose?
- What is CHARGE syndrome?

CHOANAL ATRESIA

Choanal atresia is the most common congenital anomaly of the nose and occurs in ~ 1/7,000 newborns. It is characterized by a bony (90%) or membranous (10%) septum between the nose and the pharynx, unilaterally or bilaterally. Nearly half of these infants have other associated congenital anomalies. Look for **CHARGE** syndrome (coloboma, **h**eart disease, **a**tresia of the choanae, **r**estricted growth and development, **g**enital anomalies, and **e**ar anomalies/deafness) with choanal atresia.

Symptoms vary, depending upon the infant's ability to breathe through the mouth and the severity of the atresia. These infants often appear normal initially but present early, because infants are primarily nose breathers. Infants with bilateral atresia frequently have respiratory distress and cyanosis. Even infants who are able to adequately breathe through their mouths still have difficulty breathing while feeding. Symptoms often improve with crying. Infants with unilateral choanal atresia are often asymptomatic until blockage (e.g., secretions) of the nonaffected side occurs.

Diagnosis is suggested by the inability to pass a firm catheter through each nostril past a depth of ~ 3–4 cm. Confirm with CT scan. Due to the high association of other anomalies, consultations with a cardiologist and ophthalmologist are warranted.

Treat initially by providing an adequate oral airway, which also allows the infant to feed. Usually, an orogastric tube is sufficient for infants who can breathe by mouth. Consider performing corrective neonatal surgery if the infant does not have other associated defects. Infants with severe bilateral involvement, who cannot breathe effectively by mouth, require a tracheotomy until reconstructive surgery can be safely performed. Unilateral correction can usually be delayed for several years. Restenosis after surgery is not uncommon.

ACQUIRED DISORDERS OF THE NOSE

PREVIEW | REVIEW

- What is the most common etiology for epistaxis (nose bleed)?

- When an adolescent presents with epistaxis, which type of illicit drug usage should you ask about?

- Which studies do you do for a child with recurrent or severe epistaxis?

- If you find nasal polyps in a child < 12 years of age, what diagnosis do you consider first?

- What is an effective treatment of nasal polyps?

NASAL FOREIGN BODY

A nasal foreign body is typically associated with fetid breath and foul-smelling, thick, purulent, copious nasal discharge. Sometimes, the discharge is bloody. Although more often unilateral, bilateral discharge with similar characteristics may occur after insertion of a foreign body into both nares. Common nasal foreign bodies include beads, small toys, wads of paper, corn, peas, and beans.

Alkaline button batteries are of specific concern because they may cause liquefaction necrosis and perforation of the septum.

A foreign body may be removed with forceps, suction, or curette. Topical anesthetics can reduce pain. Avoid pushing the foreign body further into the nasal cavity. If left undiagnosed, a foreign body may lead to sinusitis or cause damage to the nasal septum; however, these sequelae are uncommon because the foul odor of the discharge generally prompts the child's caregiver to seek medical attention.

EPISTAXIS

Epistaxis (nose bleed) is common in children. It usually occurs during the dry, winter months. The most frequent cause of epistaxis is "nose picking." Besides nose picking, other causes include trauma (particularly playing sports), foreign bodies, and neoplasms (nasopharyngeal carcinomata, rhabdomyosarcomas, and lymphomata) of the nose. Question any adolescent with epistaxis regarding drug use. Mucosal irritation is often seen in those who inhale cocaine or other substances (e.g., glue, cinnamon), resulting in epistaxis. Coagulopathies can predispose to prolonged epistaxis. Hereditary hemorrhagic telangiectasia can also present with recurrent epistaxis.

Most bleeding originates from the Kiesselbach plexus (anterior portion of the nasal septum). Treat by pinching the nose for 5–10 minutes to compress the nasal alae, putting pressure on this area. If bleeding does not stop, try other therapies, including vasoconstrictor nose sprays or cautery of the bleeding site with silver nitrate. If bleeding still persists, refer the patient to the emergency department or an ENT specialist for nasal packing and further monitoring.

Search for other underlying conditions if epistaxis continues to recur or is difficult to correct. In children with recurrent or severe epistaxis, order coagulation and hematologic studies. Also, fully evaluate the nasal passages and look for nasal masses or other causes of epistaxis.

NASAL POLYPS

Nasal polyps are benign tumors that form in the nasal passages and are usually due to chronically inflamed nasal mucosa. One of the most common causes of nasal polyps in children is **cystic fibrosis** (CF). Evaluate for CF in any child < 12 years of age who has nasal polyps—even in the absence of other findings for CF. Other predisposing conditions for nasal polyps include chronic sinusitis and allergic rhinitis.

Children with nasal polyps present with mouth breathing and a nasal-sounding voice. Polyps are sometimes visible using an otoscope or nasal speculum (Figure 21-14). However, diagnosis of smaller polyps requires nasal endoscopy

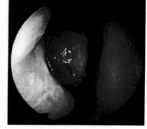

Figure 21-14: Nasal polyps

or CT scan. The polyps may appear as gray, grapelike masses found between the nasal turbinates and septum.

Nasal steroids are quite effective for many polyps, especially in children with CF. Surgically remove polyps if they do not respond to steroids and cause symptomatic obstruction, recurrent sinus infection, or nasal deformity. Nasal polyps can recur after surgery. Nasal decongestants are not effective in decreasing polyp size.

NASAL FRACTURES

Nasal fractures are rare in children < 5 years of age. Incidence of fractures increases after this and peaks in the later teen years. Nasal fractures usually result from trauma sustained during sports and play. Most of these injuries are minor, but check all patients for associated injury of the cervical spine, orbit, maxilla, and teeth. Order x-rays as needed.

If the patient has diplopia, decreased visual acuity, or any sensory or motor defects, immediately consult an ophthalmologist or neurologist.

Do a thorough palpation of the nasal bones and facial bones, especially the maxilla and orbital rim. Check for broken teeth and malocclusion. Palpate the mandible.

Specialized training is needed to perform closed reduction of a nasal fracture. Usually it is done in the emergency department. Follow up after closed reduction in 3–5 days.

NASAL SEPTAL HEMATOMA

Nasal septal hematoma, caused by nasal trauma, can potentially compromise the blood supply to the septum, resulting in septal perforation, saddle nose deformity, or abscess. Diagnose by physical examination findings of a swollen, fluctuant, and tender septum. Immediately drain the septal hematoma and pack the nasal cavity to prevent bleeding or recurrence of the hematoma. While packing is in place, broad-spectrum antibiotics should be given, including coverage for staph infections. Follow up closely with an ENT specialist.

CONGENITAL DISORDERS OF THE MOUTH AND PHARYNX

PREVIEW | REVIEW

- True or false? Cleft palate is typically associated with a genetic disorder.
- How is lingual ankyloglossia (tongue-tie) surgically managed?
- What is the most common location for an ectopic thyroid?
- What are some characteristics of a thyroglossal duct cyst?

CLEFT LIP AND PALATE

A cleft lip is caused by the incomplete fusion of embryonic structures that surround the primitive oral cavity (Figure 21-15). It can be unilateral or bilateral. Cleft palate involves the soft palate, sometimes the hard palate (Figure 21-16), and may extend to a cleft lip. A cleft lip or palate can run in families; however, the majority of cases are spontaneous and not associated with any genetic syndrome.

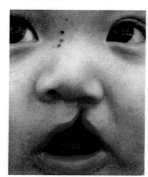

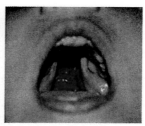

Figure 21-16: Cleft palate

Figure 21-15: Cleft lip

Submucosal cleft palate is often not obvious until several years of age. The uvula is usually bifid. Occasionally, a blue line is visible in the midline of the soft palate due to a lack of midline musculature. This is known as a **zona pellucida**. A notch of the posterior hard palate can sometimes be palpated.

Treatment requires a multifaceted approach and includes craniofacial teams, speech pathologists, and occupational therapists. Address feeding issues first. In general, cleft lip repair is done between 2 and 6 months of age. Repair of cleft palate is generally done between 9 and 18 months of age.

LINGUAL ANKYLOGLOSSIA (TONGUE-TIE)

Lingual ankyloglossia (Figure 21-17) is a common disorder in which the lingual frenulum limits the movement of the anterior tongue tip. Infants have difficulty extending the tongue past the alveolar ridge, which can make breastfeeding difficult.

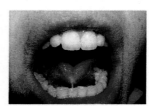

Figure 21-17: Lingual ankyloglossia (tongue-tie)

Most newborns can adjust and do well without operative intervention. Speech difficulties, especially with the English language, are rare.

Some infants and children with lingual ankyloglossia require frenulectomy, which is often performed by a dentist or oral surgeon in the outpatient office setting.

OPHTHALMOLOGY / ENT

LINGUAL THYROID

A lingual thyroid is the most common location for an ectopic thyroid (90% of cases). Thyroid tissue fails to descend into the neck from its site of origin in the tongue base. Usually, the lingual thyroid appears as a raised, violaceous mass visible at the base of the tongue. The lingual thyroid can enlarge with upper respiratory infections, puberty, or pregnancy, causing dysphagia or airway obstruction. Thyroid hormone may be used to reduce the size of the thyroid remnant, particularly for those who are hypothyroid. Because the ectopic thyroid may be the patient's only thyroid tissue, a thorough endocrine evaluation is required prior to surgical excision.

THYROGLOSSAL DUCT CYSTS

Thyroglossal duct cysts, often seen with ectopic thyroid glands, are cystic masses in the midline of the neck. The cysts typically move with swallowing or movement of the tongue. Generally, these cysts are asymptomatic unless they become infected. If infection occurs, a cyst can rapidly increase in size and cause respiratory compromise. Treatment consists of surgical removal of thyroglossal duct cysts. If infection is involved, treat with antibiotics first; perform surgery once the infection is resolved.

TEETH

See the Preventive Pediatrics section for information on teeth.

INFECTIONS OF THE MOUTH, NOSE, PHARYNX, AND UPPER RESPIRATORY TRACT

PREVIEW | REVIEW

- Does secondhand smoke increase the risk of developing an upper respiratory infection (URI)?
- Which viruses typically cause most URIs?
- Is routine viral testing appropriate in children with URIs?
- Does green nasal discharge in the first few days of a URI indicate that bacterial sinusitis is likely?
- If a child presents at Day 9 of a URI with new fever, worsening nighttime cough, and increased sinus drainage, what do you suspect?
- A child with severe immunosuppression presents with a suspected sinus infection. What is the best way to diagnose the infection and treat appropriately?
- What is Pott's puffy tumor?

- In a diabetic adolescent with uncontrolled serum glucose and the finding of a black eschar in the nose, what infection do you suspect?
- What is the most common cause of acute pharyngitis in children?
- Is the older child who has a sore throat, conjunctivitis, runny nose, and hoarseness likely to have *S. pyogenes*?
- In a 1-year-old with sore throat accompanied by runny nose, hoarseness, cervical lymphadenitis and poor appetite, is *S. pyogenes* the likely etiology?
- Does treatment with penicillin shorten the disease course in acute pharyngitis?
- How soon can a child return to school after being treated for acute pharyngitis?
- In a retropharyngeal abscess, what does the lateral x-ray show?
- How is the voice described in peritonsillar abscess?
- What are the indications for tonsillectomy?
- Does tonsillectomy help with chronic otitis media?
- Does adenoidectomy help with chronic otitis media?

THE COMMON COLD

Viral upper respiratory infections (URIs), usually called common colds, are the most frequently occurring illnesses in children. Most children have between 3 and 8 "colds" a year, most often in the fall and winter months. Certain factors increase a child's risk for developing a URI. They include young age, lack of breastfeeding, attending day care, inhaling secondhand smoke (or actively smoking), lower socioeconomic status, and overcrowding.

The majority of URIs are viral. **Rhinoviruses** cause nearly 33% of cases, followed by **coronaviruses, adenoviruses,** and **coxsackieviruses.** After each viral infection, the child develops lifelong immunity to that serotype. The problem is that each virus has potentially hundreds of other serotypes to which immunity is not conferred. Some viruses that cause URIs can spread to the lower respiratory tract, most notably the **parainfluenza** viruses, human **metapneumovirus,** and respiratory syncytial virus (**RSV**). Viruses that cause URIs rarely cause acute bloodstream infection or viremia.

URIs clinically present with low-grade fever, malaise, and upper respiratory symptoms of runny nose, cough, and congestion. Viral shedding peaks at 2–7 days after initial symptoms and can last as long as 2 weeks.

Viruses that cause URIs are transmitted in 1 of 3 ways:

1) Large-particle droplets, which can travel through coughing or sneezing and spread to another person
2) Small-particle aerosols, which travel longer distances and can directly enter the alveoli

3) Secretions that get on hands or other surfaces (fomites), which can transmit the virus by direct physical contact (The recipients inoculate themselves by touching their nose or other mucous membranes with their contaminated hands and/or fingers.)

Do not order laboratory tests in children with URIs unless the diagnosis is unclear or if the history/physical is incompatible with a diagnosis of URI.

Treat symptoms as needed. Acetaminophen is used most often for fever and pain management. It is generally regarded as safe for infants and children with proper dosing. No pharmacologic therapy has been shown to reduce the duration of a URI, and most have been shown to be ineffective for children < 6 years of age. Over-the-counter medications for cough and cold (e.g., antihistamines, antitussives, decongestants, expectorants, mucolytics) should be avoided in all children < 4 years of age. Many of these over-the-counter medications have resulted in the death of children, especially for children < 2–4 years of age. Alternative symptomatic treatments for young children include nasal saline with bulb suction, humidified air, honey (if > 1 year of age), and mentholated rubs.

Complications of the common cold may include acute otitis media, sinusitis, asthma exacerbation, bronchiolitis, and pneumonia. Thick, "green" nasal discharge by itself in the first few days of a URI does not mean the patient has bacterial sinusitis. It usually signifies an increase in the number of inflammatory cells.

ACUTE SINUSITIS

Almost all cases of sinusitis are viral in origin. The common bacterial causes of acute sinusitis are *Streptococcus pneumoniae*, *Moraxella catarrhalis*, and nontypeable *Haemophilus influenzae*.

Children with sinusitis usually present clinically with cough, nasal discharge, and halitosis. The more "adult-like" presentation is seen in adolescents and includes facial pain, tenderness, and facial edema. In children, the cough is bad in the daytime and worsens with supine position. Nasal discharge can be clear or green. Sore throat is common from postnasal drainage. Fever occurs more typically in older children.

Clinically, viral sinusitis is almost indistinguishable from bacterial sinusitis. Most URIs improve in 7–10 days. A clinical diagnosis of acute bacterial sinusitis can be made when there is (1) nasal discharge or nighttime cough that lasts longer than 10 days without improvement, (2) worsening of symptoms such as nasal discharge, cough, and fever after initial improvement, or (3) severe symptoms with rapid onset (e.g., fever > 102.2°F [39.0°C], purulent discharge for at least 3 consecutive days). Sinus x-rays and CT scans are usually not reliable and are not recommended for uncomplicated sinusitis.

For children with immunocompromise, a life-threatening illness, or an illness that is unresponsive to empiric therapy, referral to an ENT specialist to obtain valid bacterial cultures by aspirating the sinus by direct maxillary antral puncture or endoscopic middle meatal aspiration may be required.

Antibiotic treatment is aimed at the most common bacterial etiologies. Amoxicillin with or without clavulanic acid is the 1st line treatment for acute bacterial sinusitis. Clavulanic acid is often added because of the increasing rate of β-lactamase production by *H. influenzae* and *M. catarrhalis*. High-dose amoxicillin (80–90 mg/kg/day) therapy is often used, due to a dramatic rise in *S. pneumoniae* resistance to amoxicillin and TMP/SMX. Treatment duration is 10–21 days. Potential adjunct therapies may include nasal saline irrigation, decongestants, antihistamines, mucolytics, or intranasal corticosteroids. However, these adjunct treatments have not been shown to be effective in reducing duration or severity of symptoms; therefore, they are not routinely recommended.

Complications of sinusitis are relatively rare but are very important to consider. These include:

- Preseptal (periorbital) cellulitis—mild complication characterized by swelling and erythema of the lids and periorbital area; no proptosis or limitation of eye movement
- Orbital cellulitis—pain with eye movement, conjunctival swelling (chemosis), proptosis, limitation of eye movements (ophthalmoplegia), diplopia, vision loss
- Septic cavernous sinus thrombosis—bilateral ptosis, proptosis, ophthalmoplegia, periorbital edema, headache, change in mental status
- Meningitis—fever, headache, nuchal rigidity, change in mental status
- Osteomyelitis of the frontal bone with a subperiosteal abscess (**Pott's puffy tumor**)—forehead or scalp swelling and tenderness, headache, photophobia, fever, vomiting, lethargy
- Epidural abscess—papilledema, focal neurologic signs, headache, lethargy, nausea, vomiting
- Subdural abscess—fever, severe headache, meningeal irritation, progressive neurologic deficits, seizures, signs of increased intracranial pressure (e.g., papilledema, vomiting)
- Brain abscess—headache, neck stiffness, changes in mental status, vomiting, focal neurologic deficits, seizures, deficits in cranial nerves 3 and 6, papilledema

For any of these complications, order a CT scan and hospital admission for IV antibiotics. The exception to treating with IV antibiotics is preseptal cellulitis in a child > 1 year of age who shows no signs of systemic toxicity.

Unusual organisms can also cause sinusitis, depending on underlying conditions. For instance, in children with prolonged neutropenia due to chemotherapy, the risk of *Aspergillus* or *Candida* sinusitis is increased. Mucormycosis, potentially seen in patients with uncontrolled diabetes, is another serious fungal disease that can be life-threatening. It can present as a black eschar on the nasal turbinate and may lead to osteomyelitis or intracranial abscess.

CHRONIC RHINOSINUSITIS

Chronic sinusitis is defined as an inflammatory process affecting the paranasal sinuses that lasts at least 12 weeks despite medical therapy. It is often a continuation of acute sinusitis; however, it can also be caused by mechanical obstruction or allergic edema. Risk factors include immunodeficiency, nasal polyposis, anatomic abnormalities, URIs, allergic rhinitis, asthma, inhaled irritants, and exposure to cigarette smoke.

Staphylococcus aureus (including methicillin-resistant *S. aureus* [MRSA]), fungi, aerobic gram-negative bacilli, and anaerobes are the most common causes of chronic rhinosinusitis. Pathogens responsible for acute sinusitis (e.g., *S. pneumoniae*, nontypeable *H. influenzae*, *M. catarrhalis*) do not typically cause chronic rhinosinusitis.

Common symptoms include chronic cough, intermittent fever, mucopurulent discharge (anterior and/or posterior nasal), congestion, facial pain/pressure, halitosis, and decreased sense of smell. These patients often have received multiple short courses (5–7 days) of oral antibiotics that improve symptoms, but the symptoms return upon discontinuation. A clue to diagnosis is cough that worsens upon lying down and awakening due to postnasal drainage of secretions.

Diagnose with history, physical exam, and objective evidence of inflammation.

Documentation of sinus mucosal disease on CT imaging (i.e., sinus opacification, mucosal thickening) or by direct endoscopic examination is required to confirm the diagnosis of chronic rhinosinusitis and to rule out associated anatomical abnormalities.

Treatment of chronic sinusitis is controversial and may include broad-spectrum long-term antibiotics, oral or intranasal steroids, nasal irrigation, or a variety of surgical procedures. Treatment is often complex and requires referral to an ENT specialist.

LUDWIG ANGINA

Ludwig angina is an aggressive, rapidly spreading, bilateral polymicrobial (oral flora including anaerobes) cellulitis of the submandibular and sublingual spaces. It is most often a complication of an infection of the 2nd and/or 3rd mandibular molar roots. Patients appear very ill, with fever, severe dysphagia, and stiff neck. They have difficulty opening the mouth (trismus). As the infection progresses, patients often purposely lean forward in an attempt to maximize airway space and improve, at least temporarily, their respiratory status. The cellulitis has a characteristic "brawny" or woody texture and is often associated with palpable crepitus within the submandibular and sublingual spaces. The floor of the oropharynx is usually inflamed and tender to palpation.

CT is the imaging modality of choice in patients with deep neck-space infections such as Ludwig angina. Monitor closely for evidence of airway compromise such as cyanosis and increasing stridor.

Treat immunocompetent patients with intravenous ampicillin–sulbactam, a combination of penicillin G plus metronidazole, or clindamycin. Additional coverage may be needed for immunocompromised patients or those where MRSA is a concern. Patients who do not improve with appropriate antimicrobial therapy, or in whom fluctuance is identified, require surgical intervention and drainage. Additionally, extract any tooth implicated as the source of infection.

ACUTE PHARYNGITIS

Acute pharyngitis is most commonly caused by viruses and peaks between 4 and 7 years of age. It is rare in children < 1 year of age. Whether caused by a viral or bacterial illness, symptoms of pharyngitis may include pharyngeal erythema, petechiae, and/or exudates. Clinical features that suggest a viral etiology include concurrent coryza, cough, conjunctivitis, hoarseness, oral ulcers, rash, and/or diarrhea.

S. pyogenes (group A *Streptococcus* [GAS]) is the most frequent bacterial cause, but it makes up only 15–30% of cases of acute pharyngitis in children! Other, less common bacterial causes include:

- *Mycoplasma*
- *Arcanobacterium haemolyticum*
- *Neisseria gonorrhea*—consider in the case of sexually active adolescents
- *Corynebacterium diphtheriae*

For more information, see the Infectious Disease section.

Streptococcal pharyngitis frequently begins with nonspecific complaints of headache, abdominal pain, and/or vomiting. Fever is usually quite high. After these initial symptoms, patients develop a sore throat; they can also have exudates, pharyngeal redness, enlarged tonsils, and petechiae of the soft palate. Tender, enlarged anterior cervical lymph nodes are common.

In children > 2–3 years of age, the most helpful clues to *S. pyogenes* infection are physical examination findings of diffuse erythema of the tonsils and tonsillar pillars, petechiae of the soft palate, and absence of URI symptoms (sore throat, conjunctivitis, runny nose, and hoarseness). In patients < 2 years of age, symptoms of streptococcal infections are usually atypical and manifest as a persistent illness called **streptococcosis**. This infection is characterized by coryza with postnasal discharge; fever, which can last up to 8 weeks; pharyngitis; poor appetite; and tender cervical lymphadenitis.

Diagnose with a rapid detection method (e.g., optical immunoassay, chemiluminescent DNA probes). The AAP recommends following up with a throat culture if the rapid test is negative.

Be most concerned with the 2 complications of *S. pyogenes* infection:

1) Rheumatic fever, which can be prevented if antibiotic treatment is given within 9 days after onset

of symptoms (Remember: Rheumatic fever occurs only after pharyngitis—not skin infections. See the Cardiology section for more information.)

2) Poststreptococcal glomerulonephritis, which can occur regardless of therapy and regardless of source of primary infection (i.e., pharynx or skin)

Treat with penicillin V. Children defervesce within 24 hours of antibiotic initiation, and penicillin shortens the disease course by an average of 1.5 days. Amoxicillin 1×/day (50 mg/kg, max 1200 mg × 10 days) also has been shown to be effective. Use erythromycin, clindamycin, or azithromycin for those allergic to penicillin.

A common question: How soon can children go back to school? In other words, when are they no longer infectious? The answer: The child should not return to school until after the fever is gone and at least 12 hours after antibiotics have been started.

Recurrence is possible and can be retreated with the same antimicrobial agent, an alternative oral drug, or an IM dose of penicillin G (especially if nonadherence to oral therapy is likely). GAS pharyngeal carriers may require nontraditional regimens and combination antibiotic therapy.

RETROPHARYNGEAL ABSCESS

Retropharyngeal abscess can occur as a complication in children with bacterial pharyngitis or as an extension from a wound infection following a penetrating injury (e.g., pencil injury to the posterior pharynx or soft palate). The most typical causes are GAS, oral anaerobes (most commonly *Fusobacterium* or *Prevotella*), and *S. aureus.*

Toddlers and children—most typically affected are those 2–4 years of age—present with an abrupt onset of high fever and difficulty swallowing. This occurs during the acute pharyngitis phase. They develop the following symptoms in the midst of the infection: refusal to eat; severe throat pain; neck stiffness, often held in a neutral or slightly extended position; torticollis; resistance to neck movement, especially further extension; and gurgling respirations. Drooling soon develops. Stridor can also occur and simulate croup. Patients might not want to open their mouths because of pain (trismus); however, if they do, an erythematous "bulge" is sometimes visible in the posterior pharyngeal wall.

In cases with no respiratory distress and where suspicion is low, a lateral x-ray of the neck is the initial study and can show a widened retropharyngeal space with anterior displacement of the airway. In addition, the retropharyngeal soft tissue is > 50% of the width of the adjacent vertebral body. However, false positives are common. In high-suspicion cases, a CT with contrast is the preferred method. If the patient is in moderate-to-severe respiratory distress, forego the CT and evaluate the patient in the operating room with a physician present who is experienced in airway management.

A retropharyngeal abscess is a medical emergency. Without prompt treatment, pus can extend into fascial planes or rupture into the pharynx, which can lead to aspiration. If the abscess is fluctuant, drainage is necessary.

Empiric therapy should include coverage for GAS, oropharyngeal anaerobic bacteria, and *S. aureus.* Initial antibiotic therapy often includes either ampicillin–sulbactam or clindamycin. If the patient does not respond to initial treatment or appears septic, consider adding vancomycin or linezolid. If infection with MRSA is of concern, many community-associated MRSA are susceptible to clindamycin. Parenteral treatment should be continued until the patient is afebrile and improving clinically. Continue oral therapy (amoxicillin/clavulanate or clindamycin) to complete a 14-day course. In cases where vancomycin was included in the parenteral regimen, linezolid may be used for oral therapy.

PERITONSILLAR ABSCESS (PTA)

PTAs are often polymicrobial. The predominant bacterial species are GAS, *S. aureus* (including MRSA), and respiratory anaerobes (including *Fusobacterium, Prevotella,* and *Veillonella* species). The abscess occurs either with, or following, an acute pharyngotonsillitis. Fever (as high as 105.0°F [40.5°C]) can abate for several days and then recur or be continuous. The patient, often an adolescent, presents with severe pain and trismus and refuses to speak or swallow. Many describe the patient with PTA as having a "hot potato" voice. The uvula is often displaced to the side opposite the swelling (typically unilateral). The differential diagnosis includes retropharyngeal abscess, which occurs in younger children and lacks peritonsillar and unilateral findings.

Use CT scan with IV contrast to distinguish peritonsillar abscess from peritonsillar cellulitis and to evaluate for the spread of infection to contiguous deep neck spaces. Monitor carefully during transportation and scanning; sedation and positioning can exacerbate mild airway distress. Do not order CT scanning in children with moderate-to-severe respiratory distress, particularly when sedation is necessary. Evaluate these children in the operating room, where an artificial airway can be established if needed.

Management often requires consultation with an ENT specialist. Aspiration with a wide-bore needle may be used for diagnosis and treatment. The aspirate can be sent for culture sensitivity. In some cases, further incision and drainage may not be required. For older cooperative children, intraoral incision and drainage is carried out in a sitting position to prevent aspiration of pus. Most children, however, require sedation and incision and drainage in a controlled operating room setting. Empiric antibiotics should provide coverage for GAS, oropharyngeal anaerobic bacteria, and *S. aureus.* The approach to antibiotic selection is similar to Retropharyngeal Abscess.

OPHTHALMOLOGY / ENT

TONSILLECTOMY

Indications for tonsillectomy:

- Recurrent pharyngitis—7 episodes in the past year, 5 in each of the past 2 years, or 3 in each of the past 3 years
- Marked/severe adenotonsillar hypertrophy—exclude tumor
- Severe sleep apnea—adenotonsillectomy is the 1st line treatment in children with obstructive sleep apnea

Tonsillectomy does not help prevent or treat acute or chronic sinusitis or chronic otitis media. Tonsillectomy does not help prevent URIs!

ADENOIDECTOMY

Indications for adenoidectomy:

- Persistent mouth breathing
- Repeated or chronic otitis media with effusion
- Hyponasal speech
- Adenoid facies
- Persistent or recurrent nasopharyngitis when it seems to be related temporally to hypertrophied adenoid tissue

Do not perform a tonsillectomy for these problems.

NECK

PREVIEW | REVIEW
- What is the most common cause of acute bilateral lymphadenopathy?
- What are some causes of hoarseness in children?
- Which findings indicate possible malignancy when working up a neck mass?

CERVICAL LYMPHADENOPATHY (LA)

Cervical LA is very common in children. LA is defined as enlarged lymph node(s) of the neck (cervical node > 1 cm), with the most common lymph nodes involved being the submandibular and deep cervical nodes. LA includes both inflamed and noninflamed nodes. If the swelling is due to inflammation, the condition is called lymphadenitis. While usually representing a self-limited viral or bacterial infection, it is sometimes a sign of a more serious disease process.

Viral lymphadenitis, which does not require treatment, typically causes acute bilateral LA. Viral causes of cervical LA include URI, cytomegalovirus (CMV), Epstein-Barr virus (EBV), rubeola, varicella-zoster virus, coxsackievirus, herpes simplex virus, HIV, and Kawasaki disease.

Bacterial causes include pharyngitis with GAS (*Streptococcus pyogenes*), *Streptococcus aureus, Mycoplasma pneumoniae, Arcanobacterium haemolyticum*, diphtheria, tuberculosis,

and *Bartonella henselae* (catscratch fever). In very young infants, also consider *Streptococcus agalactiae* (group B *Streptococcus* [GBS]). Remember: GBS is a common cause of postpartum infections and the most common cause of neonatal sepsis.

Acute unilateral disease most commonly results from *S. pyogenes* or *S. aureus* infection and generally responds to oral antibiotics, including amoxicillin/clavulanate or clindamycin. Unilateral subacute/chronic LA is most typically caused by nontuberculous mycobacteria or *B. henselae*, whereas bilateral subacute/chronic disease is usually the result of EBV or CMV.

> 25% of malignant tumors in children occur in the head and neck with the cervical lymph nodes being the most common site. The most common **malignant** causes of cervical LA are:

- Neuroblastoma
- Leukemia
- Rhabdomyosarcoma
- Non-Hodgkin lymphoma

Other causes are:

- Juvenile idiopathic arthritis
- Collagen vascular diseases
- Drugs
- Serum sickness
- Postvaccination

For children with bilateral LA who are toxic-appearing or who have persistent symptoms (> 6–8 weeks without improvement), initial workup includes complete blood count with differential, tuberculin skin testing, and serologic testing for *B. henselae*, CMV, EBV, and HIV. If the above tests do not identify the etiology, arrange excisional biopsy to rule out malignancy or to evaluate for nontuberculous mycobacteria.

LARYNGITIS / HOARSENESS

Hoarseness in children is typically benign and can be caused by nodules, polyps, infection, papillomas, hypothyroidism, foreign body, congenital anomalies, and vocal fold granulomas from gastroesophageal reflux disease, intubation, and vocal cord misuse. Radiologic evaluation is usually not necessary unless a foreign body or mass is suspected. Refer to an ENT specialist if hoarseness lasts > 2 weeks.

NECK MASS

A neck mass can be congenital, inflammatory, or malignant. Examples include:

- Mumps (parotid glands cross angle of jaw)
- Thyroglossal cyst (midline between hyoid bone and suprasternal notch; moves with swallowing)
- Branchial cleft cyst (fluctuant mass at lower anterior sternocleidomastoid muscle)

- Sternocleidomastoid tumor
- Cervical ribs (extra rib arising from C7; occurrence of 1:200 births)
- Cystic hygroma (multilobular cyst filled with lymph; transilluminates well)
- Hemangioma (red or bluish vascular malformation)
- Laryngocele (abnormally large laryngeal saccule, expanding either internally with possible respiratory obstruction or externally forming an air sac on anterior of larynx)
- Dermoid cyst (solid and cystic midline cyst; transilluminates poorly)
- Thyroid mass

A **thyroglossal duct cyst** is a remnant of the thyroglossal tract left during development and presents as a midline mass, which moves with swallowing, often during childhood, especially when the cyst becomes infected. Diagnose with ultrasound or CT scan. Manage by treating the infection followed by surgical removal of the cyst.

A **branchial cleft cyst** is also an embryonic epithelial remnant. It is a remnant of branchial clefts 1–4, which fail to involute completely during embryogenesis. It usually presents in childhood or young adulthood when the cyst becomes infected during an upper respiratory illness. It presents as a solitary rubbery mass anterior to the sternocleidomastoid muscle. Diagnosis and treatment are the same as with thyroglossal duct cysts.

Clues on physical exam suggestive of a **malignant** neck mass include hard, irregular, firm, immobile lymph nodes; nodes > 2 cm; and supraclavicular location. Investigate these findings further with lab work, ultrasound, CT scan, and fine needle biopsy. Treatment is dependent on the results.

Evaluate a **thyroid mass** with thyroid stimulating hormone (TSH) and ultrasound testing. If the TSH is low, order thyroid scintigraphy. If the TSH is normal or elevated, arrange needle biopsy. If biopsy confirms cancer, treatment is thyroidectomy followed by radioactive iodine to destroy any remaining thyroid or cancer cells. Thyroid hormone replacement therapy is required. Sometimes external radiation is also used.

OBSTRUCTIVE SLEEP APNEA (OSA)

PREVIEW | REVIEW

- What are possible long-term complications of untreated obstructive sleep apnea (OSA)?
- What are some risk factors for OSA?
- How is OSA diagnosed?

Sleep-disordered breathing, the disruption of normal respiratory patterns and ventilation during sleep, includes a spectrum of disorders such as central sleep apnea, primary snoring, obstructive hypoventilation, and obstructive sleep apnea (OSA). Obstructive sleep-disordered breathing is characterized clinically by repeated episodes of prolonged upper airway obstruction during sleep despite continued or increased respiratory effort, resulting in partial (obstructive hypoventilation) or complete (OSA) cessation of airflow and disrupted sleep.

The prevalence of OSA, documented by overnight sleep studies, is 1–3% with peak occurrence at 2–6 years of age. Increased weight, anatomic abnormalities, and poor pharyngeal or laryngeal tone increase the risk of OSA. The most common reason for OSA in children remains adenotonsillar hypertrophy, despite the rise in childhood obesity. If left untreated, long-term sequelae of OSA, with frequent episodes of intermittent hypoxia and sleep arousals, include hypertension, pulmonary hypertension, arrhythmias, and heart failure.

Anatomic, physiologic, and metabolic abnormalities that can predispose a child to OSA include:

- Nasal (e.g., choanal stenosis/atresia, deviated septum, rhinitis, polyps)
- Oropharyngeal (e.g., adenotonsillar enlargement, macroglossia, cleft palate repair, masses)
- Craniofacial (e.g., micrognathia, trisomy 21, Pierre Robin sequence, achondroplasia)
- Neuromuscular conditions (e.g., muscular dystrophies, hypotonic cerebral palsy, other hypotonics)
- Metabolic (e.g., obesity, hypothyroidism)

Nocturnal symptoms of OSA:

- Loud, frequent, and disruptive snoring
- Pauses in breathing
- Choking or gasping arousals
- Restless sleep
- Nocturnal diaphoresis
- Partial arousal parasomnias (e.g., sleepwalking, night terrors)

Daytime symptoms of OSA:

- Daytime sleepiness and drowsiness—much less common in children than adults
- Mouth breathing and/or dry mouth
- Chronic nasal congestion or rhinorrhea
- Hyponasal speech
- Morning headaches
- Poor appetite
- Difficulty with morning awakening
- Poor academic performance
- Mood changes such as irritability, mood instability, frustration, depression, and anxiety

Signs and symptoms often overlap with diagnostic criteria for attention-deficit/hyperactivity disorder. See the Behavioral Medicine & Substance Use Disorders section for more information. Diagnosis is often delayed due to absence of symptoms, failure to obtain sleep history, and dismissal of snoring and restless sleep.

OPHTHALMOLOGY / ENT

The gold standard for diagnosis of OSA is an overnight polysomnogram. In children, there is no standard treatment. In those with adenotonsillar hypertrophy, adenotonsillectomy is generally the 1st line therapy. Obesity, hypotonia, and craniofacial anomalies increase perioperative and postoperative risks. Encourage weight loss in obese individuals. Other interventions include continuous or bilevel positive airway pressure (CPAP or BiPAP), topical nasal steroids, short-term use of topical decongestants, antihistamines, and, when indicated, repair of craniofacial anomalies.

THE MEDSTUDY HUB: YOUR GUIDELINES AND REVIEW ARTICLES RESOURCE

For both review articles and current pediatrics practice guidelines, visit the MedStudy Hub at

medstudy.com/hub

The Hub contains the only online consolidated list of all current guidelines focused on pediatrics. Guidelines on the Hub are easy to find, continually updated, and linked to the published source. MedStudy maintains the Hub as a service to the medical community and makes it available to anyone and everyone at no cost to users.

FIGURE SOURCES

Figure 21-1: MedStudy illustration
Figure 21-2: James Heilman, MD, CC BY-SA 3.0
Figure 21-3: Poupig, CC BY-SA 3.0; jd
Figure 21-4: James Heilman, MD, CC BY-SA 3.0
Figure 21-5: (top) Alfonso L. Sabater et al., CC BY 2.0
          (bottom) Tmhlee, Wikipedia, CC BY-SA 3.0
Figure 21-6: Thomas Krzmarzick, MD
Figure 21-8: MedStudy illustration
Figure 21-9: MedStudy illustration
Figure 21-10: MedStudy illustration
Figure 21-11: MedStudy illustration
Figure 21-12: MedStudy illustration
Figure 21-13: MedStudy illustration
Figure 21-15: James Heilman, MD, CC BY-SA 3.0
Figure 21-17: Klaus D. Peter, CC BY 3.0 DE
The remaining figures are from the MedStudy archives.

OPHTHALMOLOGY / ENT

Genetics

SECTION EDITOR

Reem Saadeh-Haddad, MD
Associate Professor; Clinical Geneticist
Department of Pediatrics
MedStar Georgetown University Hospital
Washington, DC

MEDICAL EDITOR

Lynn Bullock, MD
Colorado Springs, CO

Table of Contents

KEY DEFINITIONS IN GENETIC DISORDERS

PREVIEW | REVIEW

- Define the following terms: congenital, hereditary, familial, genotype, phenotype, variable expressivity, mosaicism, heterozygous, homozygous, autosome, and syndrome.

At 1st glance, you might think that congenital, hereditary, and familial all mean the same thing, but they do not. For example, trisomy 21 (a.k.a. Down syndrome), infection with rubella, and amniotic bands are all congenital conditions. **Congenital** refers to a condition or anomaly present at birth. Of the 3, though, only trisomy 21 is a genetic condition. **Hereditary** refers to conditions that are genetically transmitted from parent to offspring. All hereditary conditions are genetic, but some individuals with genetic disorders are a result of a new mutation in the family and are unable to reproduce; thus, not all genetic conditions are hereditary. **Familial** refers to conditions that "cluster" in families and can include genetic as well as nongenetic (e.g., attention deficit hyperactivity disorder, high blood pressure) conditions.

All hereditary conditions are familial, but not all genetic conditions are familial, as shown in the following examples. Achondroplasia is congenital, hereditary, and familial. Breast cancer is not congenital, can be familial, and a small portion is hereditary due to mutations in *BRCA1* or *BRCA2*. Trisomy 21 is congenital and, in the majority of cases, not hereditary and not familial because the individual is usually the 1st case in the family and does not reproduce. (Keep in mind that ~ 5% of trisomy 21 cases are due to unbalanced translocations, which can be hereditary and familial if passed down to > 1 individual.) A balanced translocation occurs with an even exchange of material, resulting in no extra or missing genetic information (and ideally full functionality). An unbalanced translocation occurs when there is unequal exchange of chromosome material, resulting in extra or missing genes.

Genotype refers to the genetic constitution or different forms of a gene (alleles) at a given locus on a chromosome. Although each individual has only 2 alleles, there may be more gene variants in the population. **Phenotype** refers to observed expression—physical, biochemical, or physiological findings—of the genotype or gene mutation. Genotype may or may not be apparent in an individual's phenotype.

Penetrance is the ability of a known disease-causing genotype to exhibit the disease phenotype. Reduced or incomplete penetrance means that some people with the disease-causing genotype do not have evidence of the disease. A common example is retinoblastoma. ~ 10% of people who have an autosomal dominant (AD) retinoblastoma-causing mutation do not develop retinoblastoma. Thus, the penetrance for this condition is 90%.

Variable expressivity is when individuals have the same genetic condition—even the exact same genotype—but have varying degrees of the phenotype. For example, Treacher-Collins syndrome is an AD, craniofacial malformation syndrome. Within the same family, some individuals with the Treacher-Collins gene have cleft palate; others with the same mutation do not.

In genomic imprinting, expression of the gene depends on whether the gene was inherited from the mother or father. Imprinting turns off genes. Thus, if a gene is paternally imprinted, the allele derived from the father is inactive and only the maternally derived allele is expressed. If a gene is maternally imprinted, only the paternal allele is expressed. Examples are Prader-Willi syndrome (paternally derived 15q11–13 deletion) and Angelman syndrome (maternally derived 15q11–13 deletion).

Pleiotropic refers to genes that produce many effects. One example is Marfan syndrome, which can affect the eyes, cardiovascular system, and skeletal system.

Mosaicism is the presence of ≥ 2 genetically different sets of cells in the same person caused by an error in mitosis. Examples are the majority of 45,X (a.k.a. Turner syndrome) cases, other sex chromosome anomalies, and neurofibromatosis Type 1.

Heterozygous refers to 2 different alleles at a gene locus on a pair of homologous chromosomes, whereas **homozygous** refers to identical alleles at a particular gene locus. A mutation is the term used to describe a change in the DNA code.

Autosome refers to all chromosomes except the X and Y chromosomes. There are 22 autosomes, chromosome numbers 1–22, and 2 sex chromosomes, X and Y. The majority of the population has a total of 46 chromosomes: 2 copies of each autosome and either XX (female) or XY (male) to determine the sex of the person.

Nondisjunction occurs when the homologous chromosomes or chromatids fail to separate, resulting in aneuploidy—an abnormal number of chromosomes in the daughter cells.

In clinical genetics terminology, an anomaly is a structural birth defect or congenital malformation. Multiple anomalies can form recognized patterns of malformation known as complex, syndrome, association, or sequence:

- **Complex:** anomalies of several different structures that are near each other during embryonic development (developmental field); e.g., limb-body wall complex
- **Syndrome:** a recognizable pattern of structural defects, due to a known single genetic etiology, with a predictable natural history that remains relatively consistent across unrelated patients; e.g., Cornelia de Lange syndrome, 7q11.23 deletion (a.k.a. Williams syndrome)
- **Association:** anomalies seen together that do not have a known single genetic or developmental etiology; e.g., VACTERL association (vertebral defects, anal atresia, cardiac defects, tracheoesophageal fistula, renal anomalies, limb abnormalities)
- **Sequence:** a pattern of multiple anomalies caused by a single identifiable event in development; e.g., Pierre Robin sequence

GENETICS

RISKS OF GENETIC DISEASE AND DIAGNOSTIC TESTING

PREVIEW | REVIEW

- What are some indications that a genetic disorder is likely?

- A positive prenatal quad screen indicates an increased risk of which 4 disorders?

- What diagnostic testing method is used to detect single gene defects?

GENETIC DISEASE RISK FACTORS

Many parents are concerned about genetic diseases and specific risks for their child. Once a child is born with an abnormality, many parents want to know if this is "genetic" and if the abnormality could happen again.

Clues that a genetic disorder is likely are:

- Previous family history of genetic disorder
- Positive neonatal screen
- Congenital anomalies
- Developmental abnormalities
- Neurologic disorders
- Death in utero or soon after birth
- Growth abnormalities
- Multiorgan dysfunction

Indications for chromosomal analysis are:

- Multiple birth defects
- Developmental delay, intellectual disability, autism
- Growth abnormalities (e.g., short stature, tall stature, abnormalities of one growth parameter [i.e., height, weight, or head circumference])
- Abnormal sexual development
- Recurrent miscarriages

PRENATAL TESTING

Prenatal screening tests tell if a fetus has the possibility of having a genetic disorder. Maternal blood screening (a.k.a. quad screen) is performed between 15 and 18 weeks of gestation. It measures α-fetoprotein, human chorionic gonadotropin, estriol, and inhibin A. The results, measured as a risk ratio, indicate the likelihood of trisomy 18, trisomy 21, neural tube defects, and abdominal wall defects. If this risk ratio is increased, then further diagnostic testing is needed.

Screening for chromosomal disorders also includes cell-free fetal DNA. Remember: This is a screening test with low false-negative and false-positive results.

Prenatal diagnostic testing, on the other hand, tells if a fetus actually has the disorder. Some of the modalities used for diagnostic testing are ultrasound, amniocentesis, chorionic villus sampling (placenta), and umbilical blood sampling. Cells collected from these invasive procedures can be sent for karyotype, gene testing (single genes or short DNA segments), or biochemical testing (protein amounts or activity). However, this information is limited in that the test does not reveal how severe the symptoms will be in the patient. Once diagnosed, many genetic disorders have limited treatment options. Some of the heritable disorders that can be diagnosed prenatally are cystic fibrosis, fragile X syndrome, hemoglobinopathies, and trisomy 21.

POSTNATAL DIAGNOSTIC TESTING

Postnatal diagnostic testing is performed on the baby's blood, cord blood, products of conception, or solid tissue. Large defects in the chromosome (e.g., aneuploidies, large deletions, translocations) can be detected by karyotyping, fluorescent in situ hybridization (FISH), and comparative genomic hybridization (a.k.a. chromosomal microarray, SNP array). FISH uses fluorescent-labeled single-stranded DNA probes that hybridize or fail to hybridize with a target DNA sequence, revealing the defect.

Comparative genomic hybridization compares the DNA of a patient with that of a normal control to detect any abnormalities. It is a 1st line test for patients with intellectual disability, autism, and multiple congenital anomalies. Be aware that this test looks for missing or extra material; however, it does not detect chromosomal rearrangements or indicate where extra material is located.

Single gene sequencing is typically performed with the Sanger method. Multiple gene panels and whole exome sequencing use next-generation sequencing methods. Older methods, such as Southern blots, are still used to detect trinucleotide repeat disorders and methylation disorders.

CHROMOSOMAL DEFECTS

PREVIEW | REVIEW

- What is the genetic abnormality in trisomy 21 (a.k.a. Down syndrome)?

- What is considered to be the etiology of trisomy 21?

- What is the only factor shown to increase the risk of trisomy 21?

- Which screening tests indicate an increased risk of trisomy 21?

- What are some of the classic physical findings in children with trisomy 21?

- What are the common congenital heart defects found in a child with trisomy 21?

- Which gastrointestinal defects are associated with trisomy 21?

- Which glandular disorder should you annually screen for in children/adults with trisomy 21?

- A 30-year-old mother has a child with trisomy 21 with 3 complete copies of chromosome 21. What is her risk of having another child with trisomy 21?

- Is trisomy 18 (a.k.a. Edwards syndrome) more common in boys or girls?

- What are the classic features of a child with trisomy 18?

- What are the classic features of a child with trisomy 13 (a.k.a. Patau syndrome)?

- Describe a girl with 45,X (a.k.a. Turner syndrome).

- Describe a boy with 47,XXY (a.k.a. Klinefelter syndrome).

- Describe a child with 7q11.23 deletion (a.k.a. Williams syndrome).

- What characterizes 11p13 deletion (a.k.a. WAGR syndrome)?

- Describe the classic findings in 20p12 deletion (a.k.a. Alagille syndrome).

- What are the most common cardiac abnormalities in 20p12 deletion?

- List the classic findings in 22q11.2 deletion (a.k.a. DiGeorge syndrome).

OVERVIEW

Large chromosomal abnormalities due to abnormal chromosome number associated with physical and developmental delay are known as aneuploidy. Aneuploidy can be either:

- Monosomy—the loss of 1 chromosome; only 1 is compatible with life in humans:
  - 45,X (a.k.a. Turner syndrome)
- Trisomy—the gain of 1 chromosome; the most common include:
  - 47,+21 (a.k.a. Down syndrome)
  - 47,+18 (a.k.a. Edwards syndrome)
  - 47,+13 (a.k.a. Patau syndrome)
  - 47,XXX
  - 47,XXY (a.k.a. Klinefelter syndrome)
  - 47,XYY

The main risk factor for aneuploidy (except Turner syndrome) is increasing maternal age.

AUTOSOMAL TRISOMY SYNDROMES

Trisomy 21 (Down Syndrome)

Incidence / Screening

Trisomy 21 is the most common autosomal trisomy in humans, occurring in 1/800 live births. The incidence at conception is more than 2× the incidence at birth because

> 50% of those with trisomy 21 at conception spontaneously abort during early pregnancy. ~ 95% of those with trisomy 21 have 3 copies of the whole chromosome 21 (Figure 22-1); ~ 3–4% have only part of the long arm due to translocations with chromosomes 13, 14, or 15; and the remaining 1–2% have mosaicism.

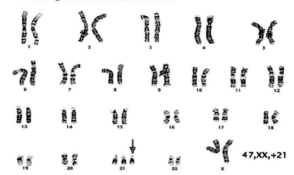

Figure 22-1: Trisomy 21 karyotype

Trisomy 21 is caused by the "extra" copy of chromosome 21, which is thought to be due to nondisjunction during meiosis. The only factor shown to increase the risk of having a child with trisomy 21 from nondisjunction is increasing maternal age—especially mothers ≥ 35 years of age. No environmental factors have been implicated.

Prenatal screening (e.g., **quad screen** [quadruple marker test]) is commonly performed in pregnant women during the 2nd trimester to assess for trisomy 21 risk. A concerning maternal serum screen shows low maternal serum α-fetoprotein, low unconjugated estriol, elevated hCG, and elevated inhibin levels.

Many providers add early ultrasound with measurement of the baby's nuchal translucency (neck thickness) and serum markers to the prenatal screening to improve sensitivity and specificity.

DNA-based maternal blood screening using free fetal DNA found in the mother's blood is available as well. It has much higher sensitivity and specificity than the above screening methods; however, it is not perfect. Use of this technology is rapidly increasing and will likely replace serum marker screening in the future.

Presentation

Trisomy 21 presents with a classic phenotypic pattern; however, if taken singly, many of the findings are minor anomalies or nonspecific. For example, if you have a single transverse palmar crease, as 10% of you do, that does not mean you have Down syndrome. You need the "whole picture" to make an accurate diagnosis.

Typical features are:

- Hypotonia
- Poor Moro reflex
- Intellectual disability

GENETICS

- Brachydactyly—short, broad fingers and toes; especially note the broad space between the 1st and 2nd toes! (See Figure 22-2.)
- Upslanted palpebral fissures
- Flat midface
- Full cheeks
- Protruding tongue
- Epicanthal folds
- Single transverse palmar crease (Figure 22-3)
- Brushfield spots—whitish spots in a ringlike configuration at the surface of the iris
- High-arched palate
- Hypoplasia of the middle phalanx of the 5th finger/clinodactyly

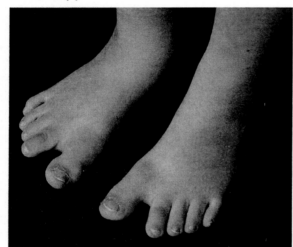

Figure 22-2: Trisomy 21, brachydactyly and broad space between 1st and 2nd toes

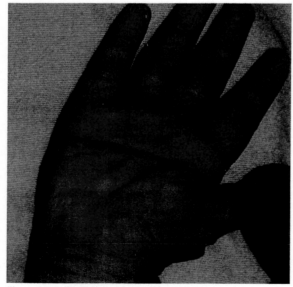

Figure 22-3: Single transverse palmar crease

Heart Defects

Heart defects are common in trisomy 21, occurring in ~ 50% of patients with up to 25% of these having > 1 anomaly. The most common defects are **atrioventricular (AV) canal defects**, ventricular septal defects (**VSDs**), and atrial septal defects (**ASDs**). Less common lesions include tetralogy of Fallot and patent ductus arteriosus. Remember: AV canal defects frequently do not have an associated murmur. Because ~ 50% of children with trisomy 21 have congenital heart defects, echocardiography is mandatory for all children with suspected trisomy 21.

Gastrointestinal Defects

Duodenal atresia and **Hirschsprung disease** occur in 5–10% of infants with trisomy 21. Look for the classic double-bubble sign (Figure 22-4), indicating duodenal atresia on abdominal x-rays. Additional findings include a predisposition to celiac disease as well as findings of gastroesophageal reflux and, in some individuals, imperforate anus. For more information, see the Gastroenterology section.

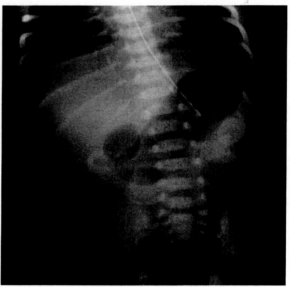

Figure 22-4: Double-bubble sign in duodenal atresia

Ocular Problems

Congenital **cataracts** occur in ~ 5% of newborns with trisomy 21; however, the risk of other problems, such as strabismus, refractive errors, and cataracts, increases with age. Therefore, ensure that careful, routine ophthalmologic evaluations take place.

Developmental Disorders

Children with trisomy 21 have **developmental delay** with mean IQ scores ranging between 50 and 70; however, many develop good social skills. Almost all children learn to walk and communicate. Most progress at a steady but slower pace than usual. Encourage early intervention programs to accelerate milestones in the younger years.

Other Problems of Trisomy 21 in Childhood

Other problems in childhood can include:

- **Hypothyroidism**
- **Atlantoaxial (C1–C2) instability**
- **Leukemia**—particularly acute lymphoblastic leukemia
- **Celiac disease**

Check thyroid function studies at birth (included on newborn screen), at 6 and 12 months of age, and then annually.

Evaluate these patients for signs and symptoms associated with atlantoaxial instability. These include neck pain, radicular signs, weakness, change in tone, gait difficulties, hyperreflexia, change in bowel or bladder function, or other signs/symptoms of myelopathy. If the patient is having symptoms or the exam is abnormal, order cervical imaging and consult a neurosurgeon or orthopedist. Spinal cord injury may result when atlantoaxial instability results in subluxation or dislocation of the 1st and 2nd cervical vertebrae. It is a manifestation of the generalized poor muscle tone and joint laxity common in trisomy 21.

Transient Myeloproliferative Disorder

A unique condition that can occur in patients with trisomy 21 is **transient myeloproliferative disorder** (a.k.a. transient leukemia). This type of leukemia occurs in up to 10% of all infants with trisomy 21 and occurs within the first 3 months of life. A mutation in the *GATA 1* gene is the cause. Transient myeloproliferative disorder is characterized by the presence of blast cells (most commonly megakaryoblasts) in the peripheral blood, which can number as high as 200,000/μL. In contrast to acute megakaryoblastic leukemia, the percentage of blasts in patients with transient myeloproliferative disorder is lower in bone marrow than in peripheral blood. Bone marrow cytogenetic analysis is negative for all clonal abnormalities other than trisomy 21.

Most patients are asymptomatic apart from vesiculopustular skin lesions, which contain cells similar to blast cells. Patients usually undergo spontaneous resolution within the first 3 months of life as the numbers of blast cells gradually decrease. A small number of patients, especially those born prematurely, can experience severe complications, including hepatic fibrosis, generalized edema, multiple effusions, and cardiopulmonary failure. In these patients, treatment with chemotherapy is warranted. Closely monitor patients with a history of transient myeloproliferative disorder as they grow older because there is a 10- to 20-fold increased risk of developing acute myeloid leukemia.

Problems of Older Patients with Trisomy 21

Patients with trisomy 21 can develop problems later in life—in their 30s, 40s, or 50s. Because many pediatricians remain the primary care physician for some patients with trisomy 21 after they advance to adulthood, remember to vigilantly monitor for these long-term complications:

- Type 2 diabetes mellitus
- Thyroid disorders—both hypothyroidism and hyperthyroidism
- Atlantoaxial subluxation—perform screening x-rays in symptomatic patients.
- Cataracts
- Leukemia
- Seizures
- Cognitive dysfunction—during the patient's 40s
- Dementia or early-onset Alzheimer disease

Health Supervision Guidelines

The American Academy of Pediatrics publishes health supervision guidelines with anticipatory guidance for children with trisomy 21. As of 2020, these include but are not limited to:

- All routine immunizations
- Cardiac evaluation with echocardiography in the newborn period
- Ophthalmologic evaluation before 6 months of age
- Hearing evaluation during newborn screening and again by 6 months of age
- Thyroid studies—screening for hypothyroidism in newborns, at 6 and 12 months of age, then annually
- Vision screening at 4 years of age

Cervical spine x-ray for atlantoaxial subluxation is recommended only in the symptomatic child who exhibits signs of myelopathy. Current evidence does not support screening the asymptomatic child; however, a discussion about cervical spine positioning and the risks of contact sports is recommended.

Future Risk of Sibling with Trisomy 21

If the child has 3 complete copies of chromosome 21 and the mother is < 35 years of age, her risk of having another child with trisomy 21 is 1%. If the mother is ≥ 35 years of age, the risk is similar to the age-specific risk. (Remember: Risk for having a child with trisomy 21 increases with increasing age of the mother.)

If the child with trisomy 21 has Down syndrome due to an unbalanced translocation, the future risk depends on whether 1 of the parents has an abnormal chromosome. For example, if a parent has a 21:21 translocation, the risk of having an offspring with Down syndrome is 100%. Besides the 21:21 translocation, if the father has a balanced translocation between 21 and another chromosome, the recurrence risk is 1–2%; if the mother has a balanced translocation, the recurrence risk is 10–15%.

Although trisomy 21 is most commonly a sporadic condition (95%), it is hereditary when due to an unbalanced translocation inherited from the parent. Obtain a karyotype to determine the recurrence risk.

Trisomy 18 (Edwards Syndrome)

Trisomy 18 is the 2nd most common autosomal trisomy and occurs in ~ 1/6,000 live births, with a much higher incidence of stillbirths. The ratio of girls to boys born with trisomy 18 is 4:1.

The characteristics are:

- Intrauterine growth restriction
- Intellectual disability
- High forehead
- Microcephaly
- Small face and mouth
- Rocker bottom feet (Figure 22-5)
- Overlapping fingers (i.e., fingers 2 and 5 over fingers 3 and 4) and clenched fist (Figure 22-5)
- Short sternum
- Hypoplastic nails
- Structural heart defects (90%)—most often a ventricular septal defect with multiple dysplastic valves

Figure 22-5: Trisomy 18, rocker bottom feet and overlapping fingers (fingers 2 and 5 over 3 and 4) with clenched fist

The risk of having an offspring with trisomy 18 increases as maternal age increases, especially mothers ≥ 35 years of age. However, statistics vary. ~ 80% of cases are due to 3 copies of chromosome 18. The other 20% are due to mosaicism or partial trisomy of the long arm of 18. The risk of recurrence for future pregnancies is < 1%, which is less than for full trisomy 21 cases, for mothers < 35 years of age. It is age specific for older mothers.

About 50% of affected children die in the 1st week of life. Another 40% die by 1 year of age. Most die because of central apnea. Children with trisomy 18 do not learn to walk or develop language skills. Those who survive > 1 year of age typically function at the level of a 6- to 12-month-old child, although some develop skills up to the level of a 2-year-old child.

Trisomy 13 (Patau Syndrome)

Trisomy 13 is the 3rd most common autosomal trisomy in humans and occurs in ~ 1/20,000 to 1/25,000 live births. 80% of children with trisomy 13 have 3 complete copies (i.e., meiotic nondisjunction) and the remaining have 3 copies of the long arm of 13 due to an unbalanced translocation. Very few trisomy 13 children are mosaic. Recurrence risk for trisomy 13 is presumed to be very low and similar to trisomy 18: < 1% for a mother < 35 years of age and age specific for older mothers.

Common clinical findings include (think midline defects!):

- Orofacial cleft—often midline cleft lip (Figure 22-6)
- Microphthalmia
- Low-set, dysplastic ears
- Spinal cord abnormalities
- Postaxial (a.k.a. ulnar) polydactyly of the limbs (i.e., duplication of little finger; Figure 22-7)
- Holoprosencephaly—cyclopia to premaxillary agenesis
- Heart malformations—80%
- Hypoplastic or absent ribs
- Genital anomalies
- Abdominal wall defects—omphalocele and visceral defects
- Aplasia cutis congenita
- Rocker bottom feet
- Clenched hands

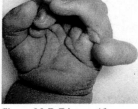
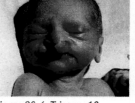
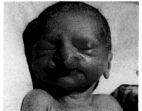

Figure 22-6: Trisomy 13, cleft lip

Figure 22-7: Trisomy 13, postaxial polydactyly

Trisomy 13 shares many characteristics with trisomy 18. When trying to differentiate, there are some traits unique to trisomy 13:

- Holoprosencephaly
- Microphthalmia
- Polydactyly
- Aplasia cutis congenita

Survival is poor. The median survival time is 7–10 days. ~ 70% die in the first 3 months of life; 90% die in the first year of life. Survivors have severe intellectual disability, seizures, and failure to thrive. They rarely live > 10 years of age.

SEX CHROMOSOME SYNDROMES

Incidence

~ 1/500 neonates have an abnormality of either the X or the Y chromosome. 80% of this group is made up of 47,XXY (a.k.a. Klinefelter syndrome); 47,XYY; and 47,XXX. In comparison, 45,X (a.k.a. Turner syndrome) is much less common, occurring in only ~ 1/2,500 to 1/5,000 female neonates.

45,X (Turner Syndrome)

Most girls with Turner syndrome have a 45,X chromosomal abnormality. Other chromosomal variations can also cause Turner syndrome, including mosaics such as 45,X/46,XX. Turner syndrome is discussed in the Endocrinology section. See Figure 22-8 and Figure 22-9. This is the 1 aneuploidy that does not correlate with maternal age.

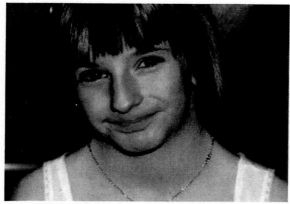

Figure 22-8: 45,X (a.k.a. Turner syndrome)

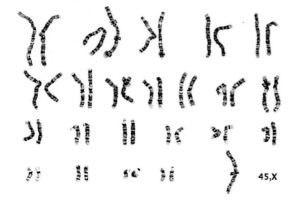

Figure 22-9: 45,X karyotype

These girls are phenotypically female, have short stature and have ovarian failure/gonadal dysgenesis, with subsequent lack of secondary sexual development. Although most patients with Turner syndrome have primary amenorrhea, some with mosaicism can have menses followed by secondary amenorrhea. A small percentage can have normal menses.

Remember: ~ 50% of these girls have cardiovascular anomalies, including bicuspid aortic valves, and 15–20% have coarctation of the aorta. Other findings are:

- At birth—broad, webbed neck (from fetal cystic hygroma), shieldlike chest, posteriorly rotated ears, lymphedema of the hands and feet, short 4th metacarpals, and cubitus valgus
- In childhood or adulthood—chronic autoimmune thyroiditis (a.k.a. Hashimoto disease), alopecia, carbohydrate intolerance, vitiligo, and gastrointestinal disorders, including celiac disease

- Renal anomalies—including horseshoe kidney, duplicate collecting system, or abnormal vasculature
- Hearing loss—including progressive sensorineural, which can occur in up to 25% of adults with Turner syndrome

~ 5–10% have some Y chromosome material in all or some cells, which puts them at risk for gonadoblastoma. These patients require removal of internal streak gonads.

Diagnosis is made by karyotype analysis. 99% of fetuses with Turner syndrome spontaneously abort.

47,XXY (Klinefelter Syndrome)

47,XXY (a.k.a. Klinefelter syndrome) presents with a male phenotype and an extra X chromosome (Figure 22-10).

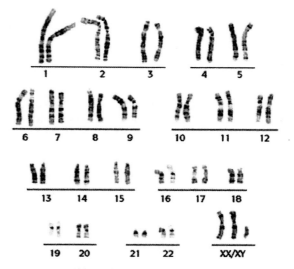

Figure 22-10: 47,XXY karyotype

Meiotic nondisjunction is a common cause, with the extra X chromosome mostly of maternal origin. Typically, these patients are quite tall with gynecomastia. Secondary sex development is delayed. They almost always have azoospermia and small testes. They are infertile. Klinefelter syndrome is discussed in more detail in the Endocrinology section.

Other Extra X Chromosome Syndromes

There are many other syndromes in which ≥ 1 extra X chromosome occurs: 47,XXX; 48,XXXX; 49,XXXXX; 48,XXXY; and 49,XXXXY. Frequently, they are mosaic with a "normal" 46,XX and an abnormal cell line (e.g., 46,XX/47,XXX). As the number of X chromosomes increases, the degree of phenotypic abnormality increases; specifically, the neurologic problems are worse.

47,XYY Male

47,XYY occurs in ~ 1/1,000 live births. This is no longer considered a true syndrome. XYY males are generally taller than average; otherwise, these males are not different from the general population.

GENETICS

Some early studies suggested XYY males were usually impulsive, antisocial, and more likely to commit crimes—with a much higher incidence of being in prison, mental institutions, or juvenile detention than typical 46,XY males. Studies from 2012 suggest these earlier studies were biased.

Boys with a 47,XYY karyotype tend to be tall (due to multiple copies of the *SHOX* gene) and have severe nodular-cystic acne. Developmental delay and behavioral problems are common. These males tend to have a prolonged PR interval and, rarely, radioulnar synostosis (fusion).

MICRODELETION SYNDROMES

Microdeletions are small deletions of contiguous genes on particular parts of chromosomes that are too small to detect, even with the highest quality standard karyotype. They require additional technology such as fluorescence in situ hybridization (FISH), which looks specifically at a predefined region (you need to know what you are FISHing for), or chromosomal microarray (CMA), which is also referred to as comparative genomic hybridization (CGH). CMA provides whole genome coverage but does not detect rearrangements or location of extra chromosomal material.

Oligonucleotide microarray (usually ~ 60 base pairs long) technology and the single nucleotide polymorphism (SNP) array can identify extremely small deletions or duplications anywhere in the genome. These usually provide at least 10× better resolution than a high-quality standard karyotype. However, unlike a standard karyotype, they cannot detect balanced rearrangements—where there is no actual gain or loss of material.

These microdeletions often involve several genes (contiguous gene deletion syndromes) and cause a fairly classic syndrome. They can also cause a more complex version of a typical "single gene" disorder, such as deletions involving the gene that causes neurofibromatosis Type 1, which have a more severe phenotype than those caused by gene mutations. Microdeletions can also "uncover" a recessive gene if the gene on the nondeleted matching chromosome is mutated.

15q11–13 Deletion (Angelman and Prader-Willi Syndromes)

See Atypical Patterns of Inheritance on page 22-12 for more on these disorders.

7q11.23 Deletion (Williams Syndrome)

Children, due to microdeletion on the long arm of chromosome 7, have the following characteristic features and facies (Figure 22-11):

• Broad forehead; medial eyebrow flare; shortened, upturned nose associated with a flattened nasal bridge; elongated philtrum with prominent, downturned lower lip (i.e., "elfin-like" facial features)

• Friendly, "cocktail party" personality; loquacious
• Stellate pattern of the iris
• Strabismus
• Supravalvular aortic stenosis
• Intellectual disability
• Hypercalcemia
• Hypersensitivity to loud sounds
• Connective tissue anomalies—joint laxity, soft skin
• Growth delay and short stature
• Wide mouth with full lips
• Periorbital fullness

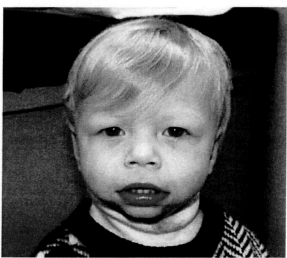

Figure 22-11: 7q11.23 deletion (a.k.a. Williams syndrome)

In ≥ 95% of the cases studied, individuals having Williams syndrome are missing the elastin gene from 1 of their 2 copies of chromosome 7. Supravalvular aortic stenosis and connective tissue anomalies arise from this deletion.

The absent elastin gene is detected using FISH. A blood sample from the child is treated with 2 specifically colored markers that fluoresce when exposed to ultraviolet light. 1 of the markers attaches to each of the 2 copies of chromosome 7 in a cell. The other colored marker attaches to the elastin gene. In the normal state, each chromosome 7 shows 2 fluorescence markers: 1 identifying it as chromosome 7 and the other indicating the elastin gene is present. In the case of Williams syndrome, 1 of the chromosome 7s is completely missing the fluorescence at the elastin location.

Williams syndrome is also readily detected by CMA. For more on CMA, see Microdeletion Syndromes.

11p13 Deletion (WAGR Syndrome)

11p13 deletion results in WAGR syndrome: **W**ilms tumor, **a**niridia, **g**enitourinary malformations, and **r**educed intellectual abilities. It occurs due to the absence of 2 genes, *PAX6* and Wilms tumor 1 (*WT1*).

The characteristics are:

- Wilms tumor—occurs in up to 50% of cases, most often by 3 years of age
- Aniridia—absence of the iris
- Male genital hypoplasia—hypospadias, cryptorchidism, small penis, and/or hypoplastic scrotum
- Intellectual disability—varies widely from IQ < 35 to normal functioning
- Gonadoblastoma
- Long face
- Upward-slanting palpebral fissures
- Ptosis
- Beaked nose
- Poorly formed ears

20p12 Deletion (Alagille Syndrome)

20p12 deletion symdrome has autosomal dominant inheritance and is caused by absence of or mutation in the Jagged-1 (*JAG1*) gene.

The characteristics include:

- Triangular facies with pointed chin
- Long nose with broad midnose
- Bile duct paucity with cholestasis
- Pulmonary valve stenosis and peripheral pulmonic stenosis
- Ocular defects: posterior embryotoxon—a developmental abnormality marked by a prominent white ring of Schwalbe and iris strands that partially obscure the chamber angle
- Skeletal defects: butterfly vertebrae

Hepatic involvement usually presents in the first 6 months of life as cholestasis, jaundice, and pruritus. Some patients develop liver failure. Biopsy shows a paucity of bile ducts.

Cardiac manifestations include peripheral and branch pulmonic stenoses (67% of patients) and tetralogy of Fallot (7–16% of patients).

The ocular defects and butterfly vertebrae do not generally cause symptoms.

22q11.2 Deletion (DiGeorge Syndrome)

The 22q11.2 deletion syndrome includes phenotypes referred to as DiGeorge syndrome. (This is also covered in the Allergy & Immunology section.) It is the most prevalent microdeletion syndrome. ~ 1/6,000 live births are affected.

A good mnemonic is **CATCH 22** (cardiac defects, abnormal facies, thymic hypoplasia, cleft defects hypocalcemia, chromosome **22**)—but this is another old term and should not be used with patients. This is a developmental defect of derivatives of the 3rd and 4th pharyngeal pouches,

resulting in agenesis or hypoplasia of the thymus and parathyroid gland, conotruncal heart defects, and branchial arch defects (i.e., small chin, cleft lip/palate and other palatal abnormalities, abnormal ears). A majority of patients with 22q11.2 deletion have hypotonia in infancy and learning disabilities, with nonverbal learning disability in ~ 66% of patients and intellectual disability in ~ 20–30%. Presentation varies widely even within families, ranging from isolated psychiatric disorders or learning problems to severe congenital heart defects.

The characteristics include:

- Cleft lip/palate, velopharyngeal incompetence
- Tubular-shaped nose
- Hooding of the eyelids
- Hypoplastic alae nasae
- Thymus agenesis or hypoplasia—immunodeficiencies (See the Allergy & Immunology section.)
- Parathyroid gland agenesis or hypoplasia—hypocalcemia with possible tetany and seizures
- Hypoplasia of the auricle and external auditory canal
- Cardiac abnormalities—in decreasing order of frequency—tetralogy of Fallot > interrupted aortic arch > ventricular septal defect > truncus arteriosus
- Short stature
- Behavioral problems

Given that this is a microdeletion condition, diagnostic confirmation relies on abnormal CMA. FISH can be used. However, it may miss up to 1/3 of cases of 22q11.2 deletion because it does not detect nested or distal deletions.

DUPLICATION

Duplication syndromes, as the name indicates, are disorders caused by duplication of a small chromosomal segment that requires special testing to detect. Phenotypic characteristics in patients with a duplication are typically less severe than the corresponding microdeletion syndrome.

22q11.2 Duplication

22q11.2 duplication syndrome is a condition caused by an extra copy of a small portion of chromosome 22 and is inherited in an autosomal dominant pattern. There is a wide variability in features, even within the same family. While many people with this duplication have no apparent physical or intellectual disabilities, patients can present with hypotonia, heart defects, developmental delay, intellectual disability, and short stature. Heart defects are similar to those of deletion of this same region—ventricular outflow tract defects and other conotruncal abnormalities. Diagnose by chromosomal microarray. Individualize treatment depends on the patient's symptoms.

GENETICS

SINGLE GENE DEFECTS

PREVIEW | REVIEW

- Know how to differentiate a pedigree: autosomal dominant, autosomal recessive, and X-linked disorders.
- What is germline mosaicism?
- Which form of classic Mendelian inheritance does not have male-to-male transmission?
- Which form of classic Mendelian inheritance has a father passing the disease allele to all of his daughters and none of his sons?
- What is genomic imprinting?
- Explain the genetic mechanisms that cause Prader-Willi and Angelman syndromes.
- Describe a child with Prader-Willi syndrome.
- Describe a child with Angelman syndrome.
- How is mitochondrial inheritance unique?

PATTERNS OF INHERITANCE

Classic Mendelian Inheritance

Mendelian inheritance refers to the strong link between genotype and phenotype in single gene traits. A botanist, Gregor Mendel, made observations of plants during cross-breeding experiments that revealed predictable, reproducible results and described the Mendelian inheritance patterns of phenotype. These patterns include autosomal dominant (AD), autosomal recessive (AR), X-linked dominant, and X-linked recessive.

Autosomal Dominant (AD) Disorders

AD disorders are caused by a mutation in 1 of the 2 alleles (Figure 22-12). Although AD disorders are common as a group, each individual disorder is still rare; therefore, it would be uncommon—but not impossible—for 2 people with the same AD disorder to mate. A heterozygous parent has a 50% chance of passing the disorder to each child. Classic examples of AD disorders include:

- Alagille syndrome
- Achondroplasia
- Osteogenesis imperfecta
- CHARGE syndrome (See the Allergy & Immunology section.)
- Neurofibromatosis Type 1 (NF1)
- Marfan syndrome
- Most familial cancer syndromes

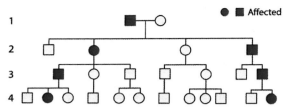

Figure 22-12: Autosomal dominant inheritance

Spotting AD inheritance on **this** pedigree:

- Both sexes are equally affected.
- Both sexes transmit to offspring.
- Present in all generations. Know: An individual may have been undiagnosed due to mild phenotype, incomplete penetrance, or age-related penetrance (e.g., *BRCA* mutations present in adulthood at incomplete penetrance).
- Every affected child has a parent with the disorder. Any affected individual has a 50% risk of passing on the gene mutation to offspring.
- Fathers can transmit to sons. This excludes X-linked and mitochondrial inheritance.

AD disorders have a high "spontaneous" mutation rate. 50% of NF1 cases are due to new dominant mutations. These individuals do not have an affected parent. Some factors, such as older paternal age, increase the risk of new dominant mutations. For example, the older the father is, the more likely he is to have a child with achondroplasia, neurofibromatosis, or Marfan syndrome.

A de novo mutation needs to be considered when an apparently new AD trait develops—one affected child, unaffected parents, and no other affected family members. This is most likely a "spontaneous" mutation, but there is another possibility. Individuals with germline mosaicism do not show signs of the disease because the parent carries the gene mutation in gonadal tissue and germline cells but not in the somatic cells. However, future offspring are at an increased risk (up to 50%) to inherit this condition. Suspect germline mosaicism when an apparently normal parent has more than 1 child affected with the same AD condition. Note: Germline mosaicism can occur with any pattern of inheritance; however, it appears to be less common in recessive disorders.

Autosomal Recessive (AR) Disorders

AR disorders produce a disease phenotype only when both alleles carry mutations (Figure 22-13). AR disorders are more common than AD disorders in most populations. Furthermore, heterozygote carriers of AR conditions (having only 1 mutated allele and clinically normal) are much more common in the general population. Common examples of AR disorders include:

- Cystic fibrosis
- Hemoglobinopathies
- Most inborn errors of metabolism

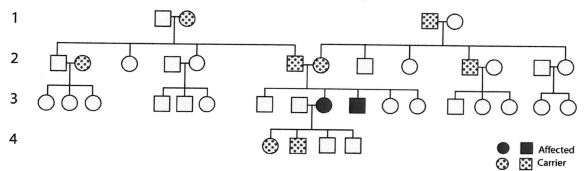

Figure 22-13: Autosomal recessive inheritance

Spotting AR inheritance on a pedigree:

- History of disease may skip generations.
- Males and females are equally affected.
- Males and females can each transmit the altered allele.
- The risk for 2 heterozygotes to have an affected offspring is 1/4. (However, 2 heterozygotes also can have offspring who are all affected or all unaffected!)
- Consanguinity increases the risk of having an offspring with an AR disorder (Figure 22-14).

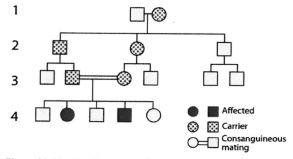

Figure 22-14: AR with consanguinity

Know how to calculate probabilities for various diseases. Here's how to do some of these calculations.

What is the probability of 2 carriers (heterozygotes) producing a child with white hair, a child who is heterozygous, and a child who is homozygous for black hair? Refer to the Punnett square (Figure 22-15) as you answer these questions.

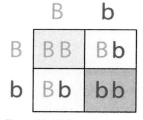

Figure 22-15: Punnett square

Here, we know that mom is *Bb* and dad is *Bb*. Thus, mom's egg is either a *B* egg or a *b* egg, and dad's sperm is either a *B* sperm or a *b* sperm.

So, the chance that junior will be white-haired (*bb*) is (the chance that dad's sperm is *b*) × (the chance that mom's egg is *b*), which is $1/2 \times 1/2 = 1/4$; in other words, a 25% chance.

If mom and dad already have 2 children with white hair (*bb*), what is the chance that the next baby will have white hair (*bb*)? Exactly the same: 1/4, or 25%—the mom's egg and the dad's sperm for making this new baby are not affected by what happened to the earlier kids.

Again, this risk calculation (for the 3rd child) is different from the risk calculation for all 3 as a group; i.e., asking before they have any children: "What is the chance that if they have 3 kids, all 3 will have white hair?" Answer: $1/4 \times 1/4 \times 1/4 = 1/64$.

Here, we have been talking about white or black hair, but in genetics the Punnett square can be used to determine if someone is affected with a genetic condition or is a carrier or neither. In those instances, we use the 2 small letters to represent someone affected with an AR condition. For example, *bb* would be an affected child, *Bb* would represent the heterozygous carriers, and *BB* would indicate that the child is neither affected nor a carrier.

A trick question on an exam might ask the probability of an unaffected child being a carrier. In the Punnett square, there are only 3 squares that are unaffected. Out of those 3, 2 are carriers. So, the probability is 2 of 3 or 2/3.

X-Linked Disorders

X-linked traits can have either a dominant or recessive pattern of inheritance. X-linked recessive is more common and predominantly affects **males**. X-linked dominant traits are seen in both sexes but are typically more severe in the male population due to the absence of a normal X chromosome.

The X chromosome is double the size of the Y chromosome. The X chromosome has thousands of genes compared to the Y chromosome, which has ~ 25 identified genes localized to it, including 1 especially important gene—the sex-determining region Y *(SRY)* gene. Many well-known pediatric diseases are caused by mutations in genes on the X chromosome, including:

- Hemophilia A
- Duchenne and Becker muscular dystrophy
- Red-green color blindness

GENETICS

Over 100 different phenotypes associated with intellectual disability have been mapped to the X chromosome (e.g., fragile X syndrome).

So, you are wondering: "Females have 2 copies of X and males have only 1 copy of X, so do females have a lot more X-linked gene products?" The answer is "no" because of **dosage compensation**, which is due to the inactivation of 1 of the X chromosomes in each cell early in female embryonic life. It usually begins ~ 2 weeks after fertilization. This is a random process, so the inactivated X chromosome could come from either the mother or the father. Somatic cells in the female embryo each have a 50% chance that the active X came from the mother and 50% chance that it came from the father. Somatic mosaicism is the result, with females having 2 different populations of cells (with only 1 population of cells harboring the mutation). In some cases, the mosaicism is visible in the patient. For example, women who are "carriers" for X-linked ocular albinism have patches of pigmented and nonpigmented cells, depending on whether it is the disease-bearing X chromosome (nonpigmented) or the normal X chromosome (pigmented) that is active in that cell.

In some cases, the "extra" X chromosome is not completely inactivated, and the genes in several regions continue to be transcribed. So, at a given locus, females can be homozygous for a disease, heterozygous (1 disease allele and 1 normal allele), or homozygous normal.

Hemizygous refers to having only 1 copy of a gene instead of 2. Males are hemizygous for every allele at each locus on the X chromosome since they have only 1 X chromosome. Thus, if a male inherits an X-linked recessive allele for a disease, he will be affected—but a female inheriting such an allele would not be affected unless she also received a 2nd copy from her father. On the other hand, an X-linked dominant pattern can cause disease in either males or females since only 1 copy of an altered allele is needed to cause disease. Rett syndrome is an example of an X-linked dominant disease. It is typically seen in females because it is most often lethal in males. See the Behavioral Medicine & Substance Use Disorders section for more on Rett syndrome.

Duchenne muscular dystrophy is an example of a disorder with X-linked recessive inheritance. Important features are:

- Progressive muscle weakness, starting with the gluteal, pelvic, and pectoral muscles, with delayed motor milestones
- Calf hypertrophy
- Gowers sign at ~ 2 years of age
- Wheelchair dependency generally by 12 years of age

Other findings are cardiomyopathy, progression to respiratory failure, and risk for cognitive delays.

Spotting X-linked recessive inheritance on a pedigree (Figure 22-16):

- There is never male-to-male transmission.
- If a generation has only females, it will appear that the disease has "skipped" that generation.

- An affected father transmits the disease allele to all his daughters but to none of his sons. (The daughters are obligate carriers but typically are unaffected.)
- Carrier females have a 50% chance of transmitting the disease to each son.

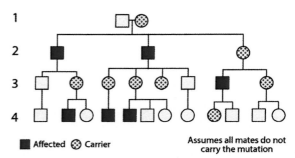

Figure 22-16: X-linked recessive inheritance

Why do some female "carriers" have some or all manifestations of an X-linked recessive disorder? There are 3 possibilities:

1) Remember: Because inactivation of the X chromosome occurs randomly within each cell, differing proportions of normal alleles versus disease alleles are affected. If a much greater proportion of X chromosomes with normal alleles are inactivated, females will manifest a given disease (called manifesting heterozygotes) but usually have a milder form compared to males with the condition. A common example is seen in hemophilia A, where 5% of women who carry 1 of the alleles for hemophilia A have Factor 8 levels low enough to exhibit mild forms of the disease.

2) Some females have only a single X chromosome (Turner syndrome).

3) Deletions or rearrangements in an X chromosome and another non-X chromosome (autosome) can result in affected females, which is rare.

Atypical Patterns of Inheritance

Some single gene disorders do not follow the AD, AR, or X-linked patterns of inheritance (classic Mendelian inheritance). In classic Mendelian inheritance for autosomal chromosomes, the expression of the disease is independent of which parent contributed the disease-causing allele. The following situations, described in Genomic Imprinting, are examples of when it does matter which parent gave the child the autosomal allele.

Genomic Imprinting

Genomic (genetic) imprinting refers to differences in gene expression that depend on whether the disease allele is inherited from the mother or the father.

For example, when deletion of a 2–4 Mb portion of chromosome 15 is inherited from the father, the child is born with **Prader-Willi syndrome** (Figure 22-17), and when deletion of genes from that same locality is inherited from the mother, the child is born with **Angelman syndrome**. Genomic imprinting explains only 70% of the cases of Prader-Willi syndrome and Angelman syndrome. These can also be caused by either true uniparental disomy (see Uniparental Disomy), which results in only maternal alleles at that locus, or functional uniparental disomy (either by a deletion at 15q11–13 or a methylation abnormality), which results in the presence of only an active maternal allele.

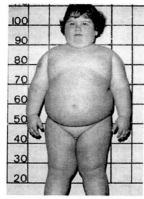
Figure 22-17: Prader-Willi syndrome

Children with Prader-Willi syndrome present with:

- In infancy:
  - Severe hypotonia at birth
  - Feeding difficulties
  - Narrow forehead
  - Almond-shaped eyes
- In childhood:
  - Hyperphagia with development of severe obesity
  - Short stature
  - Small hands and feet
  - Hypogonadism
  - Usually, mild intellectual disability
  - Behavior disorders

Children with Angelman syndrome appear normal at birth; however, as time passes, they develop:

- Seizures
- Severe intellectual disability
- Microcephaly
- Ataxia
- Hand-flapping behaviors
- Outbursts of laughter
- "Puppet-like" gait

The old phrase "the happy puppet" can be offensive and it should not be used to describe children with Angelman syndrome.

Uniparental Disomy

Uniparental disomy occurs if both copies of a chromosome—or a piece of a chromosome—are inherited from only 1 parent. Considering the case in the discussion about genomic imprinting (see Genomic Imprinting), if a child inherits 2 copies of the maternal chromosome 15 (without any deletions), the child lacks the paternally active genes and develops Prader-Willi syndrome. On the other hand, if the child gets both copies from the father, the child lacks maternally active genes and develops Angelman syndrome. Uniparental disomy arises because of nondisjunction of chromosomes during meiosis in the gametes, which results in trisomy (with subsequent loss of 1 chromosome) or monosomy (with subsequent duplication of the chromosome). In both cases, the resulting disomic cell line then has 2 chromosomes originating from only 1 parent. Another condition, which can be caused by uniparental disomy or imprinting defects, is Beckwith-Wiedemann syndrome. Refer to Table 22-8 on page 22-27; also see the Endocrinology section.

Mitochondrial Disorders

Mitochondria have the only genetic material outside of the nucleus. However, the mitochondrial genome contains only 1 copy of each gene (haploid), not 2 (diploid) like in the nucleus. Mitochondrial inheritance is unique because the zygote receives all the mitochondria from the ovum, not the sperm; therefore, a mother carrying a mitochondrial DNA (mtDNA) mutation passes it on to all her offspring, whereas the father carrying the mutation passes it to none of his offspring (Figure 22-18).

Each mitochondrion contains 2–10 copies of the mtDNA genome, and each cell has hundreds to thousands of mitochondria. At cell division, mtDNA replicates and randomly separates into the daughter cells. If there is an mtDNA mutation, then this results in different mitochondria carrying different amounts of normal and mutated (disease-causing) mtDNA. Also, each cell contains different amounts of normal and mutated mtDNA. This leads to an extremely complex type of mosaicism (**heteroplasmy**) in which the mutation load can vary from mitochondrion to mitochondrion, from cell to cell, and from tissue to tissue. **Homoplasmy** occurs when all the mtDNA in an individual is the same.

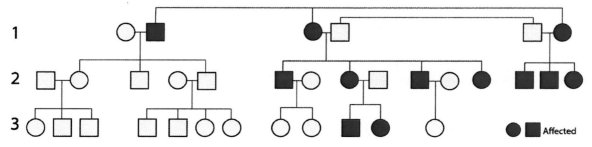
Figure 22-18: Mitochondrial inheritance

You can see why mitochondrial disorders are so confusing and so highly variable! Common presentations for mitochondrial disorders include metabolic encephalopathy, cardiac failure, liver failure, and/or lactic acidosis. Although mtDNA disorders are not common, they account for many cases of cerebrovascular accidents, deafness, and diabetes in children.

A few disorders caused by mutations in the mitochondrial genome are:

- Myoclonic epilepsy and ragged-red fibers (**MERRF**) is associated with progressive myoclonic epilepsy, myopathy, dementia, and hearing loss.
- Mitochondrial encephalopathy, lactic acidosis, and stroke-like episodes (**MELAS**) present anytime from toddlerhood to adulthood.
- **Leigh syndrome** presents with basal ganglia defects, hypotonia, and optic atrophy in infancy or early childhood.
- **Kearns-Sayre syndrome** presents with ophthalmoplegia, retinitis pigmentosa, myopathy, and cardiac conduction defects.
- **Pearson syndrome** presents with anemia, neutropenia, pancreatic dysfunction, and myopathy in infants. Most die in infancy. Patients who survive beyond infancy develop Kearns-Sayre syndrome.

See also the Metabolic Disorders section.

Trinucleotide Repeat Diseases

A DNA triplet is defined as a series of 3 bases in DNA or RNA coding for a specific amino acid. They frequently occur in repeated sequences, 10–20 at a time. Although normally these repeated sequences ("repeats") are steadily transmitted, sometimes they "expand," copying themselves over and over during DNA replication—occasionally causing 100–1,000+ sequential repeats. Size of the repeat is influenced by the sex of parent transmitting. The size of the repeat correlates with the severity and age onset of disease. This "triplet-repeat expansion" leads to several diseases, including **Friedreich ataxia** and **Huntington disease**.

Fragile X Syndrome

Fragile X syndrome is the most common inherited intellectual disability syndrome. The estimated occurrence of the full mutation is 1 in 4,000 males and 1 in 6,000–8,000 females. A "fragile site" on chromosome Xq27.3 was originally identified by cytogenetic analysis in a folate-deficient medium. Although X-linked, its inheritance pattern displays unusual features not seen in other X-linked conditions because it has a trinucleotide repeat that can expand unpredictably, leading to different versions of the disorder in different generations and increasing severity with transmission (**anticipation**).

Fragile X is caused by an unstable cytosine-guanine-guanine (CGG) repeat in the 5′ untranslated region of the fragile X intellectual disability (*FMR1*) gene on the X chromosome:

- Normal: ~ 5–40 repeats
- Premutation: ~ 55–200 repeats
- Full mutation: > 200 repeats

Diagnosis is made by DNA testing for defects in the *FMR1* gene with either Southern blot analysis or polymerase chain reaction (PCR) analysis.

Full mutation blocks transcription and results in methylation of the CpG (cytosine and guanine separated by a phosphate) island.

Full mutation—common clinical findings in males:

- Intellectual disability
- Large head
- Long face with prominent jaw and large ears
- Large hands and feet
- Macroorchidism after puberty
- Hyperextensible joints

Note: ~ 30% of female heterozygote "carriers" of the full mutation can have this phenotype—except macroorchidism.

Premutation—3 distinct clinical disorders:

1) Mild cognitive and/or behavioral deficits on the fragile X spectrum—male and female
2) Premature ovarian failure—female
3) Fragile X–associated tremor/ataxia syndrome:
    - Neurodegenerative disorder of older adult permutation carriers
    - Mostly in male carriers—usually > 50 years of age for onset
    - > 30% of male carriers develop symptoms
    - Significant variability in progression of symptoms
    - Clinical criteria—intention tremor and gait ataxia, parkinsonism
    - Less common in females

Findings that are unique to females with premutation:

- Increased risk of emotional problems—mild form of anxiety and perseverative thinking, depression, interpersonal sensitivity
- Premature ovarian failure in ~ 20% of cases
- Ovarian dysfunction in 20% of cases
- Mild decrease in FMR1 protein
- Risk of expansion when passed down to offspring

The prevalence of an individual having a premutation is much higher than the rate of having fragile X syndrome.

Myotonic Dystrophy

Myotonic dystrophy is another triplet-repeat disease with mutations affecting the CTG repeat in the 3′ untranslated region of the myotonin kinase gene on chromosome 19. A normal individual has 5–35 repeats. Affected individuals with mutations have ≥ 50 to several thousand repeats. Myotonic dystrophy has these clinical features:

- Autosomal dominant, with variable age of onset and variable severity
- Myotonia with progressive weakness and wasting; involvement of facial and jaw muscles (e.g., ptosis, atrophy of sternocleidomastoid muscles); distal muscle groups affected more than proximal muscle groups; myotonia on grip testing. (These are the individuals who grip your hand to shake it; however, they have difficulty letting go because their muscles cannot easily relax of the grip.)
- Other involved organ systems:
  ◦ Eye—cataract
  ◦ Endocrine—testicular atrophy, diabetes mellitus
  ◦ Brain—intellectual disability
  ◦ Skin—premature balding
  ◦ Cardiac—conduction abnormalities
- Congenital myotonic dystrophy results in marked hypotonia, intellectual disability (60–70% of cases), neonatal respiratory distress, feeding difficulties, and talipes—and can cause neonatal death.

Severity varies with the number of repeats. Anticipation—worsening of genetic disease in subsequent generations—is seen due to expansion with transmission. Parent of origin effect: The repeat is more likely to severely expand when passed from the mother. Therefore, the most severely affected babies typically inherited the expansion from their mothers.

MULTIFACTORIAL INHERITANCE

PREVIEW | REVIEW

- What factors suggest multifactorial inheritance has occurred?

Most genetic disorders are due to multiple genetic and environmental factors, not to a "single gene" mutation. Multifactorial inheritance is the most common cause of isolated major anomalies observed in the newborn. Examples include neural tube defects, heart defects, schizophrenia, cleft palate, and clubfoot. Many of these are present at birth. Some, such as diabetes and autism, often do not manifest for years. As a general rule, empiric risks of recurrence for most isolated major anomalies are typically in the range of 2–6%.

In general, a multifactorial disease occurs when enough "bad" factors overcome the "good" factors. Some refer to these bad factors as "liability" factors. Enough liability factors must be present to exceed a threshold to result in the disease. For some diseases, this threshold varies depending on the gender.

An example is pyloric stenosis, which occurs in ~ 1/1,200 females and ~ 1/300 males. This indicates that the "threshold" for this disease is much higher in females than in males. In other words, for a female to get pyloric stenosis, she would need to have an unusually high number of liability factors present, especially compared to the case for a male. When a female does get pyloric stenosis, it means she has more of these "bad" factors. The consequence is that her offspring are much more likely to have this disorder—even more likely than the offspring of an affected male, who presumably would have pyloric stenosis with fewer liability factors present.

Knowing this, consider a woman with a history of pyloric stenosis as a child. Are her boys or her girls more likely to be affected? Boys! Why? Because it takes fewer liability factors—"fewer hoops to jump through"—for males to develop the disease. When the mother is transmitting enough of these factors (remember, we said this is a mother with a history of pyloric stenosis), her son is more likely than her daughter to reach the threshold.

Key features of multifactorial inheritance:

- No discernable pattern
- Recurrence risk increases as more individuals are affected in the family; e.g., the recurrence risk of a disorder is estimated at 2% if 1 sibling has the disorder; it increases to 12% if 2 siblings have the disorder. (Remember: In contrast to multifactorial inheritance, the subsequent risk does not change with single gene disorders; the genetic roulette wheel does not remember what has previously occurred.)
- Recurrence risk is higher if the affected individual belongs to the less commonly affected sex. This also holds true for infantile autism, in which males are 4× more likely than females to be affected. If a girl in the family has autism, the recurrence rate is double in a sibling versus when a boy is the one with the autism.
- Recurrence risk is higher if the affected individual has a more severe form/case.
- Recurrence risk drops dramatically as the degree of relationship decreases from the affected individual. For example, if a woman has clubfoot, her 1st degree relative has ~ 2.5% risk of clubfoot. This drops to 0.5% for a 2nd degree relative and to 0.2% for a 3rd degree relative. The general population has a risk of 0.1%.
- Recurrence risk correlates with the prevalence in the general population. However, in single gene disorders, the recurrence risk is independent of the general population: If 1 parent is heterozygous for a very rare autosomal dominant disorder and the other parent is unaffected, the risk is 50% that their child will get the disorder. The risk of siblings having inherited multifactorial disease is lower than the risk for having single gene mutations. However, the risk for siblings inheriting multifactorial disease is greater than that for the general population.

- Environmental factors can play a role. For example, folic acid supplementation both prior to and through early pregnancy has been proven to prevent neural tube defects and possibly reduce the risk of other birth defects.

TWINS FACTS

PREVIEW | REVIEW

- Are dizygotic twins more likely, less likely, or equally likely to have genetic traits similar to those of a nontwin sibling?
- Name 4 diseases or abnormalities that are more likely to be concordant in monozygotic than dizygotic twins.

Remember: There are monozygotic (identical) and dizygotic (fraternal) twins. Monozygotic twins share 100% of their genes. Dizygotic twins are caused by the fertilization of 2 different egg cells by 2 different sperm cells. Therefore, they share 50% of their genes. From a genetic perspective, dizygotic twins are no more similar than nontwin siblings.

Traits that are strongly influenced by genes show higher levels of concordance in monozygotic twins than in dizygotic twins. Examples are:

- Autism (60% concordance in monozygotic twins vs. 0% in dizygotic twins)
- Cleft lip/palate (38% vs. 8%)
- Clubfoot (32% vs. 3%)
- Spina bifida (72% vs. 33%)

GENETIC CONDITIONS ORGANIZED BY PRESENTING SYMPTOMS

PREVIEW | REVIEW

- Noonan syndrome has what kind of inheritance pattern?
- What is the most common heart defect seen in Noonan syndrome?
- Know Pierre Robin sequence.
- What anomalies are seen in children with craniofacial microsomia?
- What type of head growth is seen with early fusion of the sagittal sutures? Coronal and sphenofrontal sutures? Metopic sutures?
- What is positional plagiocephaly?
- Describe the findings in achondroplasia.

- What skull structural abnormality can occur in infants with achondroplasia?
- What is the most commonly affected bone in infantile cortical hyperostosis (a.k.a. Caffey disease)?
- Describe a child with osteogenesis imperfecta (OI) Type 1.
- Which type of OI is the most severe and usually results in death in infancy?
- Which type of OI has the highest risk of neurologic complications?
- What are the classic scleral findings in OI Type 4?
- What causes most deaths in Marfan syndrome?
- Describe the classic findings in a patient with Marfan syndrome.
- Describe the typical findings in classic Ehlers-Danlos syndrome.
- What are the classic skin findings in neurofibromatosis Type 1 (NF1)?
- How frequently is NF1 due to a new mutation?
- Describe how neurofibromatosis Type 2 (NF2) differs from NF1.
- What abnormalities do vestibular schwannomas cause in NF2?
- Describe the skin findings in tuberous sclerosis.
- What cardiac tumors are common in infants with tuberous sclerosis?
- What tumors are commonly seen in patients with von Hippel-Lindau syndrome?

CHROMOSOMAL INSTABILITY SYNDROMES

At the end of this section are tables listing common congenital anomaly syndromes. See Table 22-5 on page 22-26.

Poor Growth / Short Stature

Cornelia de Lange syndrome is inherited as autosomal dominant (AD) and typically is a new mutation. Patients present with intrauterine growth restriction, poor growth, microcephaly, hirsutism, downturned mouth, heart defects, microbrachycephaly, micrognathia, low hairline, synophrys, long eyelashes, thin upper lip, low-set ears, micromelia (hands/feet) or phocomelia, and 2/3 syndactyly of toes (Figure 22-19). Reflux is a major issue and needs to be treated aggressively. These children also have significant intellectual disabilities, autism, and behavioral concerns such as self-destructive behaviors. They are at risk for hearing loss, myopia, renal anomalies, genital abnormalities, and cardiac defects. Multispecialty management is necessary for the many associated issues.

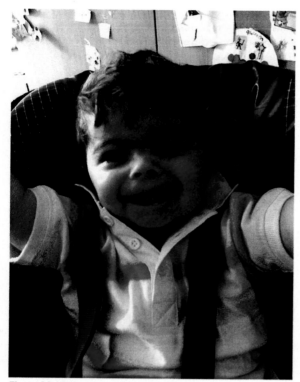

Figure 22-19: Cornelia de Lange syndrome

Russell-Silver syndrome typically occurs sporadically and is most often due to paternal imprinting or uniparental disomy. This disorder is characterized by pre- and postnatal low weight and height with normal head circumference, triangular face, café au lait spots, delayed bone age, and reflux. As compared to the overgrowth syndromes where one may see hemihypertrophy, in Russell-Silver one would expect to see hemihypotrophy with diminished growth on the affected side. Manage these patients with a multidisciplinary approach.

Turner syndrome is due to a loss of chromosome 45,X. See 45,X (Turner Syndrome) on page 22-7 and the Endocrinology section for more information.

Noonan syndrome is inherited as AD. Patients present with short stature, congenital heart defects (most commonly, pulmonary valve stenosis), pectus excavatum, webbed neck, low-set ears, hypertelorism, lymphedema, and bleeding diathesis. Treatment aims at improving final height through the use of growth hormone. Cardiac manifestations are handled on an individual basis.

Williams syndrome is a microdeletion syndrome and is discussed under 7q11.23 Deletion (Williams Syndrome) on page 22-8.

Bone Marrow Dysfunction

Most of these disorders have a predisposition to cancers. They are covered in the Hematology section and the Allergy & Immunology section and include:

- Ataxia-telangiectasia
- Bloom syndrome
- Fanconi anemia
- Diamond-Blackfan anemia
- Thrombocytopenia-absent radius syndrome
- Bruton X-linked agammaglobulinemia
- Chronic granulomatous disease
- X-linked severe combined immunodeficiency

CRANIOFACIAL MALFORMATIONS

Cleft Lip / Palate Disorders

Cleft lip and cleft palate are among the most common craniofacial malformations you will see in your practice. Incidence varies from 1/250 to 1/3,000, depending on the culture and race being reviewed. Native Americans have the highest rates; African Americans have the lowest rates.

Most cases of cleft lip/palate are sporadic. However, there can be recurrence in families, and hereditary factors have been documented. If the first-born child has a cleft lip/palate, the risk of the next sibling having cleft lip/palate is 3–4%. If either parent had cleft lip/palate as a child, the risk increases further. There are nearly 300 syndromes associated with cleft lip/palate—make sure you know all 300 very well. (Just kidding!)

There is evidence suggesting that maternal folate deficiency contributes to this disorder. More studies are underway.

Airway management and feeding difficulties are the usual problems at birth. These children are at risk for recurrent otitis media and persistent middle-ear effusions.

In general, cleft lip repair is done between 2 and 6 months of age. Repair of cleft palate is generally done between 9 and 18 months of age.

"Sequence" refers to a pattern of anomalies that result from a single identifiable event in development. There is no known gene involved in either of the 2 sequences discussed in Pierre Robin Sequence.

Pierre Robin sequence and amniotic band syndrome are important to know!

Pierre Robin Sequence

Pierre Robin sequence presents with a primary embryologic defect of mandibular hypoplasia. This leads to a displacement of the tongue, which in turn interrupts the closure of the lateral palatine ridges and results in a U-shaped cleft palate. Patients have micrognathia and retrognathia, glossoptosis (displacement of the tongue into the airway), respiratory distress, and feeding problems. Respiratory compromise can lead to pulmonary hypertension. Macroglossia is not part of the syndrome.

GENETICS

Amniotic Band Sequence

Amniotic band sequence can present with disruptive clefts of the face and palate resulting from amniotic bands adhering to this area. Bands can also form in other parts of the fetal body. Other defects can include constriction rings of the limbs and/or digits and amputations (Figure 22-20).

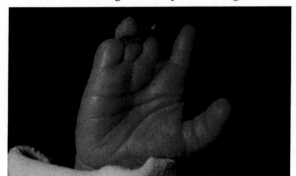

Figure 22-20: Amniotic band sequence defects

Craniofacial Microsomia

Findings

The 2nd most common craniofacial malformation is the association of:

- External ear anomalies
  - Microtia—smallness of the auricle of the ear with a blind or absent external auditory meatus
  - Anotia—congenital absence of 1 or both auricles of the ears
  - Canal atresia
  - Preauricular tags
  - Hearing loss
- Facial asymmetry even in those with bilateral features
- Maxillary and/or mandibular hypoplasia

The malformations can occur as isolated events or be part of a malformation syndrome. Cervical vertebral anomalies occur in nearly 33% with craniofacial microsomia, and cardiac anomalies occur frequently as well.

Be aware that renal anomalies occur in ~ 15% of individuals with these ear malformations, so consider a renal ultrasound for further evaluation. (The ears and kidneys are developed at approximately the same time in embryology. For this reason, it is common practice to evaluate the kidneys in any newborn with ear anomalies.)

Goldenhar syndrome (see Goldenhar Syndrome) and craniofacial microsomia are considered to be the same disorder; however, use the term "Goldenhar syndrome" only if epibulbar dermoids are present.

Goldenhar Syndrome

A child with Goldenhar syndrome (a.k.a. oculoauriculovertebral spectrum) has all the findings of craniofacial microsomia mentioned in Findings. The patient presents with craniofacial microsomia, epibulbar lipodermoids

(lateral-inferior, fibrous-fatty masses on the globe), vertebral defects, cardiac anomalies (ventricular septal defect or outflow tract malformations), and renal anomalies. Preauricular and facial tags and conductive hearing loss are common. This syndrome typically occurs as a "sporadic" finding, but some researchers propose AD inheritance in certain families. The cause is unknown. Some cases are reported to be due to vascular interruption during embryonic development.

Other Facial Anomaly Syndromes

Branchio-Oto-Renal (BOR) Syndrome

BOR syndrome presents with branchial cleft fistulas or cysts, preauricular pits, cochlear and stapes malformation, mixed sensory and conductive hearing loss, and renal dysplasia/aplasia. Occasionally, patients have pulmonary hypoplasia. It is inherited as an AD disorder.

Treacher-Collins Syndrome

Treacher-Collins syndrome (a.k.a. mandibulofacial dysostosis) is an AD disorder and presents with micrognathia (mandibular and maxillary hypoplasia), zygomatic arch clefts, and various forms of ear malformations (e.g., microtia, anotia, atresia). Other characteristic findings include downward-slanting palpebral fissures, scalp hair that extends into the preauricular region like sideburns, and colobomata (defects) of the lower eyelids with absent eyelashes. Conductive hearing loss is a frequent occurrence.

Craniosynostosis

Craniosynostosis is the early, pathologic fusion of calvarial sutures. Craniosynostosis occurs sporadically in 1/2,000 live births; 1/25,000 cases are hereditary. The most common, single-suture fusion is sagittal synostosis. The others, in descending order, are coronal > metopic > lambdoid. Isolated lambdoid is very rare, occurring in only 2–3% of cases. Sagittal synostosis is more common in males than in females by a ratio of 5:1.

What head shapes form from the different early fusions? Refer to Figure 22-21 as you review the results of early suture fusion:

- Sagittal sutures—cause excessive anterior/posterior growth resulting in a long and narrow head, known as **scaphocephaly** or **dolichocephaly**
- Coronal and sphenofrontal sutures—result in flattening of the forehead on the affected side, with elevation of the ipsilateral orbit and eyebrow, and a prominent forehead bulge on the opposite side, known as **frontal plagiocephaly**; more common in girls than in boys
- Metopic sutures—result in a prominent ridge running down the triangular-shaped forehead with widening of the back of the head, known as **trigonocephaly**
- Coronal, sphenofrontal, and frontoethmoidal sutures—cause a cone-shaped head, known as **turricephaly**

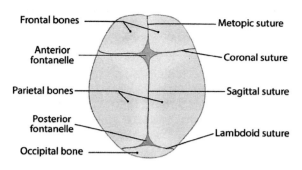

Figure 22-21: Normal newborn skull

Syndromic hereditary forms exist, including Apert syndrome and Crouzon syndrome, which are briefly discussed in Table 22-9 on page 22-28. Many of these forms can be distinguished from each other by specific hand malformations. Surgical intervention is required to correct the risk of intracranial hypertension, as well as to repair facial asymmetry and make the shape of the head more normal.

There is more on craniosynostosis in the Neonatology section.

Plagiocephaly

See the Growth & Development section for more information on plagiocephaly.

Positional plagiocephaly is the postnatal flattening of the skull that is caused by the infant's preference of sleeping/resting position. Infants with torticollis frequently have flattening of the occipitoparietal area. It is sometimes severe enough to cause ipsilateral frontal prominence or anterior displacement of the ipsilateral ear.

Plagiocephaly can look like lambdoid synostosis; however, you can differentiate one from another by physical examination and, if necessary, skull CT. Lambdoid synostosis shows sclerosis of the lambdoid suture. Know that positional plagiocephaly is common; lambdoid synostosis is rare.

Things to look for in positional plagiocephaly:

- Anterior displacement of the ipsilateral ear (posterior/inferior for lambdoid synostosis)
- Ipsilateral frontal prominence (absent in lambdoid synostosis); most easily noted when looking down at the child from above the head
- Absent contralateral occipitoparietal prominence (present in lambdoid synostosis)
- No lambdoid ridge or submastoid prominence (present in lambdoid synostosis)

Positional plagiocephaly stops progressing after 7 months of age because children generally can roll over and move their head more. Lambdoid synostosis continues to progress after 7 months of age.

Positional plagiocephaly has become more common since the implementation of the Safe to Sleep recommendations to help prevent sudden infant death syndrome. Positional plagiocephaly improves with tummy time. Special helmets for sleeping are available in severe cases.

SKELETAL DYSPLASIAS

Achondroplasia

Achondroplasia, the most common skeletal dysplasia, occurs in 1/20,000 live births and consists of:

- Disproportionately short stature with rhizomelic shortening (short lengths of the most proximal, or "root," segment of the upper arms and legs compared to the distal segments)
- Lumbar lordosis
- Trident hands
- Macrocephaly
- Characteristic craniofacial findings, including a flat nasal bridge, prominent forehead (frontal bossing), and midfacial hypoplasia (Figure 22-22)

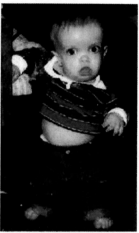

Figure 22-22: Achondroplasia

Achondroplasia is an AD disorder in which most individuals have a de novo mutation of *FGFR3* (fibroblast growth factor receptor 3) on chromosome 4p16.3; the mutation rate increases with advancing paternal age. This gain-of-function mutation results in decreased endochondral ossification, chondrocyte proliferation, and cartilage matrix production.

The hands have a "trident" appearance—hands are short and fingers are quite broad, with digits 3 and 4 splayed more distally than proximally. These children are on the growth curve at birth, but by 2–3 months of age, their length has fallen to < 5th percentile. Children with achondroplasia typically do not have malformations apart from those mentioned above, and they are of normal intellect.

Foramen magnum stenosis and/or craniocervical junction abnormalities can occur in infancy and cause compression of the upper cord—resulting in apnea, quadriparesis, growth delay, hydrocephalus, and even death. It is necessary to measure the size and shape of the fontanelle and monitor the occipitofrontal circumference (with growth curves standardized for achondroplasia) at every pediatric visit. A detailed neurological examination is also very important. Currently, baseline neuroimaging and polysomnography are recommended and repeated if necessary based on recurrent assessments.

Children with achondroplasia are at increased risk for serous otitis media, motor milestone delay, bowing of the legs, and orthodontic problems. Adults are at risk for obesity and, more seriously, spinal stenosis. Most males have final heights of 46–57 inches and females have final heights of 44–54 inches.

GENETICS

The diagnosis can be confirmed clinically or molecularly if needed. Characteristic x-ray findings include squared-off iliac wings, flat and irregular acetabulum roofs, thick femoral necks, and "ice-cream-scoop shaped" femoral heads, as well as the rhizomelic shortening mentioned at the start of this concept. Since all the mutations that result in achondroplasia occur in the same place in the *FGFR3* gene, genetic testing is straightforward and conclusive.

Cleidocranial Dysostosis

Cleidocranial dysostosis is an AD disorder with 60–70% of cases involving *RUNX2* mutation. These patients present with brachycephaly, frontal bossing, wormian bones (abnormal intrasutural bones), delayed eruption of deciduous and permanent teeth, supernumerary and fused teeth, hypoplastic/absent clavicles, and joint laxity. Diagnose by genetic testing of the gene *RUNX2*. Management is based on the patient's symptoms.

Infantile Cortical Hyperostosis (Caffey Disease)

Infantile cortical hyperostosis is transmitted as an AD trait with incomplete penetrance. It is characterized by extreme irritability, fever, anorexia, and soft tissue swelling caused by subperiosteal cortical thickening of underlying bone. Soft tissue swelling is painful and indurated but without suppuration and only minimally warm and red. Typically, changes in the bones begin before 6 months of age and resolve by 24 months of age. The mandible is involved in > 95% of cases and is the most commonly affected bone. Other frequently involved bones include the clavicles, ribs, long bones, and scapulae.

Mandibular involvement is most helpful in differentiating infantile cortical hyperostosis from nonaccidental trauma. Always consider nonaccidental trauma during any encounter with a pediatric patient where you see subperiosteal elevation on imaging studies. Typical radiographic abnormalities in infantile cortical hyperostosis include layers of cortical diaphyseal subperiosteal new bone formation and cortical thickening. Laboratory findings include leukocytosis, elevated erythrocyte sedimentation rate, and increased levels of alkaline phosphatase.

BONE FRAGILITY DISORDERS — OSTEOGENESIS IMPERFECTA (OI)

All Types

OI refers to a disorder characterized by osseous fragility, short stature, and skeletal findings that vary based on the type. The 4 most commonly recognized forms of OI are caused by the abnormal structure of Type 1 collagen, due mainly to mutations in the *COL1A1* and *COL1A2* genes. None of these forms causes retinal hemorrhage or subdural hematomas, which distinguishes osteogenesis imperfecta from nonaccidental trauma.

Note: The nomenclature continues to evolve for the 4 OI types. It is difficult to predict how quickly the terms will make it into standard exam questions. OI types are currently referred to as follows:

- Type 1—classic nondeforming OI with blue sclerae
- Type 2—perinatally lethal OI
- Type 3—progressively deforming OI
- Type 4—common variable OI with normal sclerae

Type 1

OI Type 1 (a.k.a. brittle bone disease) is an AD disease. It is the mildest and most common type of OI, caused by a decrease in collagen synthesis that results in a reduced amount of normal Type 1 collagen. Common characteristics include:

- Multiple fractures—most fractures occur before puberty and mimic child abuse
- Blue sclerae
- Delayed fontanelle closure
- Hyperextensible joints
- Hearing loss
- Decreased stature—usually low normal or near normal
- Dentinogenesis imperfecta—a disorder of tooth development with discolored, weak teeth

Fractures rarely occur at birth; however, they are frequent in childhood, even with minor trauma. By adolescence, fracture frequency diminishes. X-rays show mild osteopenia of the long bones and wormian bones (multiple small bones found in the cranial sutures). Other associated manifestations of scoliosis and hearing loss appear in the patient's 20s and 30s.

Type 2

OI Type 2, the most severe form, results in death during the newborn period due to respiratory insufficiency. These children have numerous fractures and severe bone deformity. The skull is very soft, and the limbs are short and bowed. X-ray shows long bones with a crumpled appearance, and the ribs are beaded due to callus formation. Almost all cases are due to de novo AD mutation of the *COL1A1* gene. The types of mutations that result in OI Type 2 and other severe cases of OI alter the entire structure of OI Type 1 collagen, which weakens bone significantly.

Type 3

OI Type 3 presents in the newborn with numerous fractures. This is also called the progressively deforming type. Short stature is severe. Many cannot ambulate because they are unable to bear their own weight. Blue sclerae occur at birth but lighten with age—unlike those in OI Type 1, which stay dark blue. Most cases are due to a point mutation of the *COL1A1* gene that is similar to the OI Type 2 mutation. Neurologic complications are most common with OI Type 3, including hydrocephalus and basilar skull invagination.

Type 4

OI Type 4 is a milder form, like OI Type 1. The sclerae are typically white or near-white. Fontanelle closure is delayed, and fractures are often present at birth. These individuals have shorter-than-average stature. Tibial bowing is the hallmark of OI Type 4. This type is due to AD collagen 1 mutations or due to autosomal recessive mutations in genes that assist in collagen processing.

CONNECTIVE TISSUE DISORDERS

Marfan Syndrome

Marfan syndrome is an AD disorder that affects 1/5,000 to 1/10,000 individuals. Boys and girls are affected equally. The affected organ systems include the eyes, circulatory system, skeleton, skin, lungs, and dura. Most deaths occur due to cardiovascular complications, namely **aortic root dilatation** and rupture.

The major criteria in Table 22-1 and the scoring system in Table 22-2 are the main clinical clues in a patient with Marfan syndrome. Look for the child with tall stature, high-arched palate, upward lens dislocation, joint hypermobility (Figure 22-23), pectus carinatum or pectus excavatum (Figure 22-24 on page 22-22), spontaneous pneumothorax, and mitral valve prolapse.

Table 22-1: Revised Ghent Criteria for Marfan Syndrome

Negative Family History Plus 1 of the Following Combinations	Positive Family History in 1 of the Following Combinations
Ao (Z ≥ 2) + EL	FH MFS + EL
Ao (Z ≥ 2) + *FBN1*	FH MFS + Syst ≥ 7
Ao (Z ≥ 2) + Syst ≥ 7	FH MFS + Ao (Z ≥ 2 over 20 years old) or FH MFS + Ao (Z ≥ 3 under 20 years old)
EL + *FBN1* + Ao	FH MFS + *FBN1*

Major criteria:
- Ao, aortic dilation or dissection
- EL, ectopia lentis
- *FBN1* mutation
- Systemic features (See Table 22-2.)
- FH MFS, family history of Marfan syndrome

Z = z score, which indicates how many standard deviations a data point is from the mean

Table 22-2: Scoring System for Systemic Features in Marfan Syndrome

Points	Features		Points	Features
3	Wrist and thumb signs	or	1	Wrist or thumb signs
2	Pectus carinatum	or	1	Pectus excavatum or chest asymmetry
2	Hindfoot deformity	or	1	Plain pes planus
2	Pneumothorax			
2	Dural ectasia			
2	Protrusio acetabuli			
1	Skin striae			
1	Myopia > 3 diopters			
1	Mitral valve prolapse			
1	Scoliosis or thoracolumbar kyphosis			
1	Reduced elbow extension			
1	All 3 of the following features: • Reduced upper-to-lower segment ratio • Increased arm span to height ratio (≥ 1.05) • No severe scoliosis			
1	Facial features (≥ 3): • Dolichocephaly • Enophthalmos • Down-slanting palpebral fissures • Malar hypoplasia • Retrognathia			

Total Score ≥ 7 indicates systemic involvement.

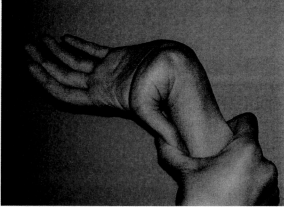

Figure 22-23: Marfan syndrome, joint hypermobility

GENETICS

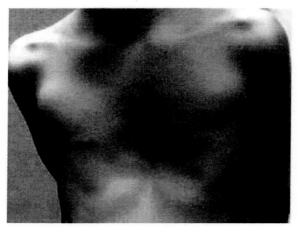

Figure 22-24: Marfan syndrome, pectus excavatum

Diagnosis is made by clinical findings known as the Ghent criteria. Diagnosis is made if there are 2 of the following major criteria:

- Ectopia lentis
- Aortic dilation or dissection
- Family history

If there is only 1 major finding, then either a mutation in the *FBN1* gene (encodes the protein fibrillin-1) or ≥ 7 (out of 20) systemic points are required to make the diagnosis. The systemic points include the wrist and thumb signs, chest wall deformity, scoliosis, myopia, pneumothorax, and striae.

Always rule out homocystinuria, which has many features similar to Marfan syndrome but carries a significant risk of stroke and other embolic events. Homocystinuria has a much different treatment strategy. For more information on homocystinuria, see the Metabolic Disorders section. Homocystinuria features intellectual disability and a downwardly dislocated lens. In Marfan syndrome, the lens dislocates upward.

Because cardiovascular complications are the most serious, annual or semiannual echocardiography to monitor aortic root diameter is the norm. Antihypertensives are used to treat and prevent aortic root dilatation. Evidence for the best medical management (β-blocker and/or angiotensin receptor blocker) is ongoing, with prospective trials demonstrating that combination therapy offers better protection against aortic root enlargement than single drugs alone. Individuals should avoid weightlifting and strenuous exercise, but regular aerobic exercise is important for heart health—as it is for everyone.

Pregnancy greatly increases the risk of accelerated aortic dilatation in women with Marfan syndrome. Pregnant women require extremely close monitoring.

Ehlers-Danlos Syndrome

Ehlers-Danlos syndrome is a group of AD connective tissue disorders that generally include hyperextensible skin, hypermobile joints, easy bruising, and dystrophic scarring. There are 6 major variants. The classic type is the type typically found on exams.

The skin findings are classic. Know! Some describe the skin's texture as "wet chamois," a "fine sponge," or "doughy." "Extra" skin is common over the hands, feet, and stomach. The skin is very stretchy and returns to its normal configuration on release, much like a rubber band. The skin is unusually fragile and can split with the slightest trauma, especially at the shins, knees, elbows, and chin. Skin tears generally do not bleed a lot and have a gaping "fish-mouth" appearance. Scarring is abnormal, and scars that appear are typically thin and shiny. Increased bruising occurs, especially in children, as does bleeding from the gums after toothbrushing. All coagulation tests (including PT, PTT, and bleeding time) are normal, except for capillary fragility testing. Wrinkled palms and soles are common, as are pseudotumors at the heels, elbows, and knees from abnormal scarring.

Joint hypermobility is common but does not occur in certain types of Ehlers-Danlos syndrome. Both large and small joints can be involved. Dislocations or subluxations can occur and can be present at birth. Knees and elbows can be extended past 180°, and the fingers can be extended past 90°. Joint mobility decreases with increasing age, and adults can develop arthritis or chronic joint pain.

Mitral valve prolapse and proximal aortic dilatation occur; screen for these with echocardiography, CT, or MRI.

Aim treatment at prevention with the use of shin guards, high-topped boots, and kneepads. Avoid physical contact sports.

NEUROCUTANEOUS SYNDROMES

Neurofibromatosis Type 1 (NF1)

NF1 (formerly von Recklinghausen disease) is the most common neurocutaneous disease and affects ~ 1/3,000 individuals worldwide. The most common features are **café au lait spots** and benign cutaneous **neurofibromas**. Specific diagnosis requires 2 of 7 criteria. See Table 22-3 for a list of the clinical criteria. Most children meet formal clinical criteria by 10 years of age.

Table 22-3: Clinical Criteria for Neurofibromatosis Type 1
≥ 6 café au lait spots of ≥ 5 mm in greatest diameter in prepubertal children and ≥ 15 mm in postpubertal children
≥ 2 neurofibromas of any type or ≥ 1 plexiform neurofibroma
Freckling in the axillary or inguinal areas
Optic glioma
≥ 2 Lisch nodules (iris hamartomas)
Sphenoid dysplasia or thinning of the long bone cortex, with or without pseudoarthrosis
1st degree relative (parent, sibling, child) with neurofibromatosis Type 1

Café au lait spots (Figure 22-25) ordinarily appear in the first 2 years of life; however, do not forget that these can also appear with other syndromes such as McCune-Albright syndrome and Russell-Silver syndrome. Axillary freckles appear by adolescence in 75% of cases (Figure 22-26). Lisch nodules (benign iris hamartomas) are identified by slitlamp exam in ~ 75% of prepubescent children; however, they usually are not present in early childhood. Optic pathway gliomas occur in 15% of children < 6 years old and sometimes cause visual loss or precocious puberty. Always refer to an ophthalmologist if you suspect NF1.

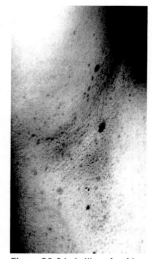

Figure 22-25: Neurofibromatosis Type 1, café au lait spots

Neurofibromas are benign, peripheral nerve sheath tumors that are a collection of Schwann-like cells, fibroblasts, and extracellular matrix. The cutaneous neurofibromas appear at puberty, whereas the plexiform neurofibromas are congenital. Cutaneous neurofibromas can cause discomfort and are cosmetically bothersome. Plexiform neurofibromas have a 10% risk of malignant transformation.

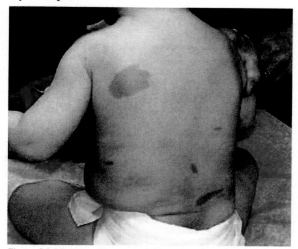

Figure 22-26: Axillary freckles

Focal areas of T2-weighted signal intensity (FASI) on brain MRI were previously described as unidentified bright objects (UBOs). FASI are believed to represent areas of abnormal myelination. They are most often located in the basal ganglia, along the optic tracts, and in the brainstem, thalamus, and/or cerebellum. They are not associated with a mass effect, malignant potential, or contrast enhancement. Commencing in late adolescence, FASI begin to disappear. FASI are generally absent by 30 years of age.

Bony changes can occur in early childhood years and include sphenoid wing dysplasia, long bone bowing—most commonly of the tibia—and dysplastic scoliosis.

~ 50% of affected children have learning disorders, ADHD, and speech disorders. Other features to look for include short stature, macrocephaly, hypertension, constipation, and headaches. Individuals with NF1 are also at risk for seizures, optic gliomas, and intracranial tumors.

50% of cases are sporadic or de novo autosomal dominant mutations. The phenotypic expression is quite variable from one affected individual to another, even among family members. The *NF1* gene encodes the protein neurofibromin and maps to chromosome 17.

Neurofibromatosis Type 2 (NF2)

NF2 is an AD disorder. It is characterized by the presence of **bilateral vestibular schwannomas** (acoustic neuromas). NF1 and NF2 are very distinct and different disorders, with no commonality regarding genetic factors and essentially no clinical overlap. NF2 is less common than NF1. NF2 has an incidence of ~ 1/30,000.

The mean age for clinical presentation is 30 years, but children are frequently diagnosed with the disorder. The vestibular schwannomas cause **sensorineural hearing loss**, tinnitus, imbalance, and facial weakness. The mean age of onset of these schwannomas is 18–24 years. By 30 years of age, all affected individuals have developed bilateral vestibular schwannomas. Other CNS tumors occur in ~ 50% of cases and include intracranial meningiomas, spinal schwannomas, cranial nerve schwannomas (most commonly involving CN 5), and ependymomas. Lens opacities or cataracts occur as one of the 1st signs and can be used for screening in children.

Diagnostic criteria are:

- bilateral vestibular schwannomas or
- unilateral vestibular schwannoma accompanied by 2 of the following: meningioma, schwannoma, neurofibroma, glioma, cataract in the form of subcapsular lenticular opacities, or cortical wedge cataract.

For relatives at risk, do MRI screening to detect vestibular schwannomas small enough to be surgically removed, thereby preserving hearing.

Tuberous Sclerosis

Tuberous sclerosis is an AD disorder that affects 1/6,000 people. There are many features of tuberous sclerosis. The classic findings are:

- Hypopigmented macules (a.k.a. **ashleaf spots**)—the most common presentation in ~ 90% of cases (Figure 22-27)

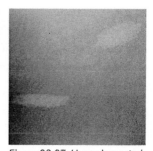

Figure 22-27: Hypopigmented macules (a.k.a. ash-leaf spots)

GENETICS

- **Shagreen patches**—oval-shaped nevoid plaques, skin-colored or occasionally pigmented, smooth or crinkled, appearing on the trunk or lower back
- Facial angiofibromas
- Forehead plaques
- Ungual (nail) and gingival fibromas
- Cortical tubers and subependymal nodules
- Renal angiomyolipomas or renal cysts
- Rhabdomyomas
- Polycystic kidney disease associated with *TSC2* (on chromosome 16)

Tuberous sclerosis has wide variability, both between and within families, much like the variability seen with NF1. Some of the features found in early childhood disappear by adulthood, making diagnosis more difficult. For example, nearly 50% of infants have multiple cardiac rhabdomyomas; however, these regress over time. Another associated complication is infantile spasms. If they occur, they indicate a 50% chance that tuberous sclerosis is present. The hypopigmented macules usually enhance with a Wood lamp, and this can be helpful in diagnosis.

Tuberous sclerosis is caused by mutations in *TSC1* (found on chromosome 9) or *TSC2* (found on chromosome 16).

The focus of clinical management is controlling seizures and cardiac arrhythmias associated with the cardiac rhabdomyomas. Treat infantile spasms with vigabatrin. Good seizure control improves intellectual outcome.

FAMILIAL CANCER SYNDROMES

Key features of cancer genetics are:

- Genes involved in familial cancer syndromes are also commonly involved in sporadic tumors.
- Gene types involved in oncogenesis include protoon-cogenes, tumor suppressor genes, and genes involved in DNA repair, apoptosis, and genomic integrity.

Features of cancer syndromes are:

- Family history—multiple members in family
- Early age of onset
- Bilateral/Multifocal
- Clustering of specific types
  - Breast and ovarian
  - Retinoblastoma and osteosarcoma
- Multiple tumor types in same person
- Unusual type

Breast and Ovarian Cancer

BRCA1, the first identified breast cancer gene, is localized to chromosome 17q21. The *BRCA2* gene is localized to 13q12. Mutations in these genes:

- Increase a woman's risk of breast cancer in her lifetime to 50–85%, with a 50% risk of occurrence before 50 years of age; the general population risk of sporadic breast cancer is 12%.
- Increase a woman's risk of ovarian cancer to 27–40%; the general population risk of ovarian cancer is 1.5%.
- Increase a man's risk of male breast cancer and prostate cancer; however, the incidence is not as high as for female cancers.
- Increase an individual's risk for pancreatic cancer, and with *BRCA2* mutation, of melanoma
- Are found in all populations, but the incidence is higher in those of Ashkenazi Jewish ethnicity.

Keep in mind that the majority of breast and ovarian cancers are sporadic rather than hereditary. Only ~ 5–10% of breast cancers and ~ 10–25% of ovarian cancers are hereditary. Mutations in the *BRCA1* and *BRCA2* genes are responsible for > 50% of hereditary cases. Mutations in other genes are responsible for the remaining hereditary cases.

Recommendations include frequent surveillance to identify cancer in its early stages. A bilateral mastectomy reduces the risk of breast cancer by > 90%. To address the risk of ovarian cancer, it is recommended that women have a bilateral salpingo-oophorectomy once they are over 40 years of age.

Familial Adenomatous Polyposis

Familial adenomatous polyposis is an AD disorder with a 100% risk of colon cancer. See the Gastroenterology section for more information.

Multiple Endocrine Neoplasia (MEN) Syndromes

MEN syndromes are a group of rare genetic disorders in which 2 or more endocrine glands develop tumors or grow excessively. Symptoms vary depending on the glands involved. See the Endocrinology section for more information.

von Hippel-Lindau (VHL) Syndrome

VHL syndrome is a highly penetrant, AD, multisystem cancer disorder that presents with various benign and malignant tumors of the eyes, CNS, kidneys, pancreas, adrenal glands, and reproductive glands. It occurs in ~ 1/36,000 live births.

It is caused by a mutation in the *VHL* tumor suppressor gene on chromosome 3. Molecular genetic testing of the *VHL* gene detects mutations in nearly 100% of patients.

Diagnosis depends on:

- Finding ≥ 2 hemangioblastomas in the CNS (particularly the cerebellum) or retina or
- Finding 1 single hemangioblastoma plus 1 of the following:
  - Pheochromocytoma
  - Endolymphatic sac tumors
  - Cysts in the kidney/pancreas

- Renal cell carcinoma
- Cystadenomas and neuroendocrine tumors of the pancreas or
- Having a 1st degree relative with VHL and 1 manifestation listed above

The most classic presentation is a cerebellar hemangioblastoma in adolescence or a retinal angioma by 10 years of age. Renal cysts are common. Renal cell carcinoma presents in the patient's 40s and is the leading cause of mortality in VHL, occurring in nearly 40% of patients.

PTEN Hamartoma Tumor Syndrome (PHTS)

PHTS includes Cowden syndrome and Bannayan-Riley-Ruvalcaba syndrome. See the Gastroenterology section for more information.

CONGENITAL ANOMALY SYNDROMES

Table 22-4 on page 22-26 through Table 22-12 on page 22-29 describe some congenital anomaly syndromes. Syndromes shown with a pink background are frequently staples for exams—review these well.

Remember clues that might indicate a genetic syndrome—especially if more than 1 occurs:

- Micro- or macrocephaly
- Congenital heart defects
- Short or very tall stature
- Abnormal skin findings
- Developmental delay or intellectual disability
- Failure to thrive
- Limb or back/spine anomalies

GENETICS

APPENDIX — CONGENITAL ANOMALY SYNDROMES

Especially if you are testing for initial certification, know the disorders listed with a pink background in Table 22-4 through Table 22-12 on page 22-29.

Table 22-4: Trisomy Disorders

Syndrome	Signs and Symptoms	Inheritance Pattern/Gene Mutation
Trisomy 21 (Down syndrome)	Brachydactyly, upslanted palpebral fissures, flat midface, epicanthal folds, single transverse palmar crease, heart defects, duodenal atresia, developmental delays/intellectual disabilities Associations: hypothyroidism, atlantoaxial instability, leukemia	Trisomy 21
Trisomy 18 (Edwards syndrome)	IUGR, microcephaly, rocker bottom feet, overlapping fingers & clenched fist, hypoplastic nails, heart defects, intellectual disability	Trisomy 18
Trisomy 13 (Patau syndrome)	Holoprosencephaly, microphthalmia, polydactyly, aplasia cutis congenita, orofacial cleft, heart defects, rocker bottom feet, clenched hands	Trisomy 13

Table 22-5: Chromosomal Instability Syndromes

Syndrome	Signs and Symptoms	Inheritance Pattern/Gene Mutation
Ataxia-telangiectasia	Ataxia, telangiectasia, especially of sclera, frequent infections, malignancies, growth failure, worsening CNS function, carriers are at an increased risk of breast cancer	AR > 95% *ATM* mutation
Bloom syndrome	IUGR, microcephaly, malar hypoplasia, facial telangiectasia, malignancies	AR > 90% *RECQL3* mutation
Fanconi anemia	Pancytopenia, hypoplastic thumb and radius, hyperpigmentation, abnormal facial features, malignancies	AR (multiple genes)
Xeroderma pigmentosa	Photosensitivity, skin atrophy, pigmentary changes, malignancies	AR (multiple genes)

Table 22-6: Syndromes with Severe Neurologic Manifestations

Syndrome	Signs and Symptoms	Inheritance Pattern/Gene Mutation
Sturge-Weber syndrome	Capillary hemangioma in trigeminal nerve distribution, glaucoma, seizures, meningeal hemangiomata	Sporadic
Rett syndrome	Most affected are females; apparently normal psychomotor development for ~ 6–18 months, followed by rapid regression in language and motor skills; repetitive, stereotypic hand movements replace purposeful hand use (hand wringing); autistic features; episodic apnea and/or hyperpnea; gait ataxia; tremors; seizures; acquired microcephaly.	X-linked dominant Majority are female; rare in males (but more severe phenotype); almost all (99%) are new mutations. 80% *MeCP2* mutation and 8% deletion/duplication
Prader-Willi and Angelman syndromes	(See Table 22-8.)	

Table 22-7: Syndromes with Short Stature

Syndrome	Signs and Symptoms	Inheritance Pattern/Gene Mutation
Turner syndrome	Short stature, webbed neck, coarctation of the aorta, bicuspid aortic valves, lymphedema of hands and feet, short 4th metacarpals, shield-like chest	Monosomy: 45,X
Noonan syndrome	Short stature, congenital heart defects (commonly pulmonary valve stenosis), pectus excavatum, webbed neck, low-set ears, hypertelorism, lymphedema, bleeding diathesis	AD ~ 50% PTPN11 mutation
Williams syndrome	Growth delay, intellectual disability, stellate iris, hypoplastic nails, periorbital fullness, anteverted nares, supravalvular aortic stenosis, friendly with "cocktail party personality" (i.e., very social)	7q11.23 microdeletion
Cornelia de Lange syndrome	IUGR, microcephaly, hirsutism, downturned mouth, heart defects, microbrachycephaly, micrognathia, low hairline, synophrys, long eyelashes, thin upper lip, low-set ears, micromelia (hands/feet) or phocomelia; 2,3 syndactyly of toes	AD > 50% have a gene mutation (NIPBL). Multiple other genes in the cohesion complex make up the rest.
Russell-Silver syndrome	Low weight and height with normal head circumference, triangular face, hemihypotrophy, café au lait spots, delayed bone age, and reflux	Typically occurs sporadically and is most often due to paternal imprinting or uniparental disomy

Table 22-8: Syndromes with Growth Abnormalities

Syndrome	Signs and Symptoms	Inheritance Pattern/Gene Mutation
Prader-Willi syndrome (paternal)	Severe hypotonia at birth, obesity (usually after 2 years of age), short stature, hypogonadism, mild intellectual disability, small hands and feet	15q11–13 deletion (paternal) in 70% of cases Maternal uniparental disomy in 25% of cases
Angelman syndrome (maternal)	Jerky ataxic movements, microcephaly, characteristic gait, hypotonia, midface hypoplasia, prognathism, seizures, uncontrollable bouts of laughter, severe intellectual disability	15q11–13 deletion (maternal) in 70% of cases UBE3A mutation (maternal) in 11% of cases Paternal uniparental disomy in ~ 5% of cases
Beckwith-Wiedemann syndrome	Large for gestational age (LGA), generalized overgrowth, macroglossia, ear lobe creases, posterior auricular pits, omphalocele, Wilms tumor, cryptorchidism, hemihypertrophy	AD 11p15.5 deletion Multiple gene mutations (KCNQIOTI, H19, CKNIC) Paternal uniparental disomy in ~ 20% of cases
Sotos syndrome	LGA, macrocephaly, prominent forehead, hypertelorism, intellectual disability, large hands/feet	AD 80–90% NSD1 mutation or 5q35 deletion
Proteus syndrome	Macrodactyly, soft/connective tissue hypertrophy, hemihypertrophy, nevi, lipomas, lymphangiomata, hemangiomata, accelerated growth	Sporadic; due to somatic mosaicism for activating AKT1 mutations

GENETICS

Table 22-9: Craniofacial Syndromes		
Syndrome	**Signs and Symptoms**	**Inheritance Pattern/Gene Mutation**
Treacher-Collins syndrome	Cleft palate, malar hypoplasia, micrognathia, lower eyelid missing medial lower lid lashes, hearing loss, ear anomalies	AD 100% *TCOF1* mutation
Waardenburg syndrome I	Partial albinism, white forelock, premature graying, telecanthus (lateral displacement of inner canthi of eyes), heterochromia of iris, cleft lip/palate, cochlear deafness, occasional absent vagina, occasional Hirschsprung disease	AD > 90% *PAX3* mutation
Stickler syndrome	Pierre Robin sequence (micrognathia, cleft palate, glossoptosis [dorsal displacement of the tongue], airway obstruction, feeding difficulty), high myopia, retinal detachment, midface hypoplasia, hearing loss	AD 70–80% *COL2A1* mutation 10–20% *COL1A1* mutation Some forms are AR and due to other genes.
Crouzon syndrome	Craniosynostosis with turricephaly, proptosis, hypertelorism, strabismus, maxillary hypoplasia	AD 100% *FGFR2* mutation
Apert syndrome	Craniosynostosis, brachycephaly, acrocephaly, hypertelorism, proptosis, strabismus, maxillary hypoplasia, narrow palate ("cathedral ceiling"), syndactyly, broad thumbs (most commonly with mitten-hand deformity: complete fusion of 2, 3, or 4 fingers with common nail bed ["single nail"])	AD 100% *FGFR2* mutation
Cleidocranial dysostosis	Brachycephaly, frontal bossing, wormian bones (abnormal intrasutural bones), delayed eruption of deciduous and permanent teeth, supernumerary and fused teeth, hypoplastic/absent clavicles, joint laxity	AD 60–70% *RUNX2* mutation

Table 22-10: Syndromes with Limb Abnormalities with/without Hematologic Abnormalities		
Syndrome	**Signs and Symptoms**	**Inheritance Pattern/Gene Mutation**
Rubinstein-Taybi syndrome	Short stature and limbs, microcephaly, beaked nose, broad thumbs and great toes, congenital heart disease, intellectual disability	AD *CREBBP* mutation 30–50% Microdeletion (detected by FISH) ~ 10% *EP300* mutation 3–8%
Fanconi anemia	See Table 22-5 on page 22-26.	AR multiple genes
Diamond-Blackfan anemia	Triphalangeal thumb, radial hypoplasia, hypoplastic anemia, congenital heart defects	AD multiple genes
Thrombocytopenia-absent radius (TAR) syndrome	Thrombocytopenia, absent radii, normal thumbs, petechiae, congenital heart defects	AR > 95% *RBMA8* deletions/duplications ~ 3% *RBMA8* mutation
Holt-Oram syndrome	Upper extremity anomaly of the radius or carpal bones with absent thumbs, congenital heart defects, cardiac conduction defects	AD, 70% will have mutation in *TBX5*

Table 22-11: Metabolic Syndromes with Congenital Anomalies

Syndrome	Signs and Symptoms	Inheritance Pattern/Gene Mutation
Menkes disease	Progressive neurologic deterioration, sparse/broken hair (pili torti), skeletal changes, decreased serum copper and ceruloplasmin	X-linked
Wilson disease	Kayser-Fleischer rings, abnormal copper metabolism with accumulation of copper in tissues; neurological, liver, or psychological manifestations; low ceruloplasmin but elevated urine copper	AR
Zellweger spectrum disorder	Hypotonia, flat occiput, epicanthal folds, hepatomegaly, camptodactyly (flexion of 1 or both interphalangeal joints of 1 or more fingers, usually the little finger), cerebral defects, retinal lesions, renal cysts, peroxisomal defects	AR
Glutaric acidemia Type II	Hepatomegaly, facial dysmorphism, renal cysts, GU anomalies	AR
Smith-Lemli-Opitz syndrome	Short stature; microcephaly; ptosis, anteverted nares; syndactyly of toes 2,3; cryptorchidism; hypospadias; intellectual disability; cholesterol metabolism defect	AR
Kallmann syndrome	Short stature, variable degrees of intellectual disability, hypogonadotropic hypogonadism, anosmia	X-linked

See the Metabolic Disorders and Endocrinology sections for more information.

Table 22-12: Common Associations and Other Miscellaneous Syndromes

Syndrome	Signs and Symptoms	Inheritance Pattern/Gene Mutation
VATER/VACTERL	Vertebral, anal atresia, cardiac, tracheal, esophageal, renal, limb defects	Sporadic
CHARGE	Coloboma, heart defects, atresia of the choanae, restricted growth and development, genital anomalies (hypogonadism), ear anomalies and/or deafness	AD CHD7 mutation
McCune-Albright syndrome	Multiple bony fibrous dysplasia, café au lait spots, precocious puberty	Sporadic, somatic mutations in GNAS
Neurofibromatosis Type 1	Café au lait spots, axillary freckling, neurofibroma, plexiform neurofibroma, sphenoid bone dysplasia, malignancies (< 5%), optic glioma, Lisch nodules, learning disability, macrocephaly	AD NF1 mutation
Opitz syndrome (G/BBB syndrome)	Hypertelorism, telecanthus, high nasal bridge, cleft lip/palate, hypospadias, laryngotracheoesophageal cleft	X-linked dominant/AD
Alagille syndrome	Bile duct paucity with cholestasis, peripheral pulmonic stenosis, posterior embryotoxon, butterfly vertebrae, characteristic triangular-shaped facies with long nose, broad midnose, and pointed chin	AD 89% JAG1 mutation 7% JAG1 deletion (detected by FISH) 1–2% NOTCH2 mutation

GENETICS

FIGURE SOURCES

Figure 22-2: Loranchet, CC BY 3.0
Figure 22-4: JasonRobertYoungMD, CC BY-SA 4.0
Figure 22-7: Chen et al., CC BY 2.0
Figure 22-12: MedStudy illustration
Figure 22-13: MedStudy illustration
Figure 22-14: MedStudy illustration
Figure 22-15: MedStudy illustration
Figure 22-16: MedStudy illustration
Figure 22-19: Joris, CC BY-SA 3.0
Figure 22-20: Moscowmom
Figure 22-21: MedStudy illustration
Figure 22-23: Magnolia Dysnomia, CC BY-SA 3.0
The remaining figures are from the MedStudy archives.

Metabolic Disorders

SECTION EDITOR

Pamela Trapane, MD
Clinical Professor
Chief, Division of Pediatric Genetics
Department of Pediatrics
University of Florida College of Medicine-Jacksonville
Jacksonville, FL

MEDICAL EDITOR

Lynn Bullock, MD
Colorado Springs, CO

Table of Contents

INBORN ERRORS OF METABOLISM

PREVIEW | REVIEW

- What are the 3 mechanisms that typically cause metabolic disorders?
- How are most inborn errors of metabolism inherited?
- Mitochondrial disorders are inherited from which parent?

METABOLISM REVIEW

Figure 23-1 presents an overview of the metabolic processes discussed in this section. Metabolism encompasses all the enzyme-catalyzed reactions that occur in our body. These reactions can be considered either catabolic or anabolic reactions. **Catabolism** is the breaking down of proteins, carbohydrates, and fats into simple molecules (amino acids, simple carbs, and fatty acids).

These simple molecules can be used for **anabolic** processes (making required tissue proteins and fats, and for glycogenesis and gluconeogenesis).

These same simple molecules can alternately be further catabolized to make energy needed for anabolic processes.

These interrelated metabolic processes consist of protein, carbohydrate, and fat metabolism.

A genetic defect causing a problem in an enzyme in a metabolic pathway is called an **inborn error of metabolism** (IEM).

CAUSES OF INBORN ERRORS OF METABOLISM (IEMs)

Most IEMs result from a single gene defect causing deficiency in the production or function of a single enzyme or cofactor. Names for the IEMs typically reflect the primary affected metabolite.

IEM signs and symptoms are caused by the resulting upstream or accessory pathway buildup of toxic product or by the insufficient production of a required metabolite. Some disorders combine these effects.

There are many IEMs. Before we jump into them, let's give some structure and priority to what you will be reviewing.

Except for a review of newborn screening at the end, the rest of the section is broken up into 3 main topics based on the general mechanisms of the defect. Intoxications, energy utilization defects, and complex-molecule defects are the 3 mechanisms that typically cause metabolic disorders.

METABOLIC DISORDERS

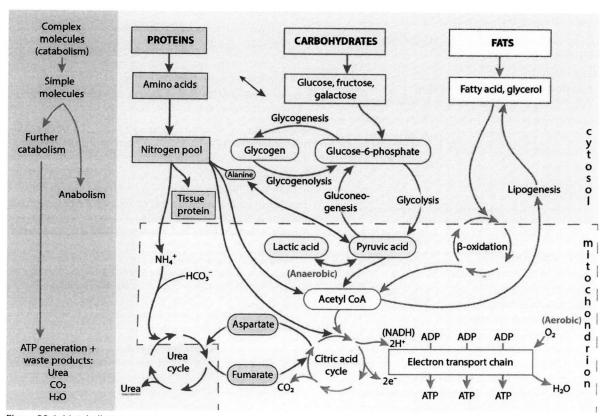

Figure 23-1: Metabolism summary

Intoxications are due to toxic buildup upstream of the affected enzyme. These occur mainly in the protein catabolism pathway, although there are some in the carbohydrate pathway (galactose and fructose disorders). (For more information, see Intoxications.)

Energy utilization defects cause problems with converting food into energy or problems with utilizing normal sources of stored energy (i.e., glycogen, fat; see Energy Utilization Defects on page 23-12 for more information). So, it makes sense that these disorders involve:

- defects in fatty acid oxidation,
- glycogen storage diseases, and
- mitochondrial disorders.

The last one makes sense if you remember that all chemical energy production required by the cell occurs in the mitochondria. In fact, virtually all the processes below the dashed line in Figure 23-1 on page 23-1 occur within the mitochondria (except some urea cycle reactions occur in the cytosol).

Complex-molecule defects occur when the deficiency in a particular enzyme results in abnormal or unregulated synthesis of complex molecules. These complex molecules include mucopolysaccharides, mucolipids, glycoproteins, and sphingolipids. There are also disorders of peroxisomes, mineral absorption and metabolism, porphyrin production (porphyrias), purine metabolism, and lipoproteins and lipids. Symptoms from these disorders are permanent and progressive. (For more information, see Complex-Molecule Defects on page 23-19.)

The following conditions are the must-know topics in this section:

- **Intoxications**
  - Disorders of amino acid metabolism
    – Classic Phenylketonuria (PKU) on page 23-5
    – Maple Syrup Urine Disease (MSUD) on page 23-6
    – Glutaric Acidemia Type 1 on page 23-7
    – Homocystinuria on page 23-7
  - Urea Cycle Disorders on page 23-8
    – Carbamoyl phosphate synthetase 1 (CPS1) deficiency
    – Ornithine transcarbamylase (OTC) deficiency
  - Organic acidemias
    – Isovaleric Acidemia (IVA) on page 23-10
  - Sugar intolerances
    – Galactosemia on page 23-11
    – Hereditary Fructose Intolerance on page 23-12
- **Energy utilization defects**
  - Defects in fat metabolism
    – Medium-Chain Acyl-CoA Dehydrogenase (MCAD) Deficiency on page 23-15
  - Glycogen storage diseases (GSDs; the most prevalent ones are autosomal recessive [AR])
    – Type 1 GSD (von Gierke Disease) on page 23-16
    – Type 2 GSD (Pompe Disease) on page 23-17

- **Complex-molecule defects**
  - Mucopolysaccharidoses (MPSs; all AR, except MPS Type 2, is X-linked recessive)
    – MPS Type 1 (Hurler Syndrome) on page 23-20
    – MPS Type 2 (Hunter Syndrome) on page 23-21
  - Sphingolipidoses
    – Gaucher Disease (GD) on page 23-22
    – Niemann-Pick Disease (NPD) on page 23-23
    – Tay-Sachs Disease on page 23-24
    – Fabry Disease on page 23-24
  - Peroxisomal disorders
    – Zellweger Spectrum Disorder (ZSD) on page 23-25
  - Disorders of minerals
    – Menkes Disease (Kinky Hair Disease) on page 23-26
  - Purine disorders
    – Lesch-Nyhan Syndrome on page 23-26

Notice that the previous disorders are all autosomal recessive (AR) except MPS Type 2, Fabry disease, Menkes disease, and Lesch-Nyhan syndrome.

INHERITANCE PATTERNS

When faced with a critically ill child, it is crucial to identify an IEM vs. infection vs. nutritional disorder vs. exogenous intoxication. However, most of us find this extremely challenging. In the early 1900s, when IEMs were first described by Archibald Garrod, there were only 4 diagnoses. Today, there are > 400!

Here are a few orienting points on inheritance of IEMs:

- Most IEMs have autosomal recessive inheritance.
- Next most common are those that are X-linked.
- Only a few are autosomal dominant (AD) disorders.
- A few of the described diseases are caused by mutations in the mitochondrial genome.

IEMs are rare, with most occurring in < 1/15,000 births, but they account for ~ 20% of diseases in sick, full-term newborns!

Certain populations have a markedly higher prevalence of individual disorders. If an exam question specifically mentions a patient's ethnicity or genetic background, it is probably a clue to consider an IEM! Example: Compared with the general population, persons of Ashkenazi Jewish ancestry are more typically carriers of gene mutations causing Tay-Sachs disease or Type 1 Gaucher disease. The incidence of Type 1 Gaucher disease is nearly 1/900 in the Ashkenazi population (vs. 1/40,000 in the non-Jewish population). The incidence of Tay-Sachs disease is 1/4,000 in the Ashkenazi population vs. 1/100,000 in the non-Ashkenazi population.

For discussion of inheritance types, please refer to the Genetics section. We briefly discuss mitochondrial inheritance, due to its relevance and complexity, under Mitochondrial Inheritance.

MITOCHONDRIAL INHERITANCE

Mitochondria supply the chemical energy for the cell. It might surprise you that each cell contains from hundreds to ~ 2,000 mitochondria!

Mitochondria are coded for by nuclear genes from both parents, but, unlike any other animal organelle, mitochondria contain their own genome, termed mitochondrial DNA (mtDNA). Disorders in mitochondria can arise from mutations of nuclear DNA (usually AR), but they can also arise from a defect in the mtDNA, which comes solely from the mother. This mtDNA is a circular DNA strand with only 37 genes. Most are related to the oxidative phosphorylation (in the electron transport chain). A few genes are involved with forming tissue proteins.

Due to this maternal transmission pattern, women who have a genetic mutation in the mitochondria pass it to all their children, whereas men never pass it on.

Heteroplasmy describes mitochondria having > 1 genome. Each mitochondrion contains 2–10 copies of the mtDNA. But this is only the start! Because of the random nature of distributing these strands during cell division and because the mitochondria themselves are randomly distributed during cell division, we can end up with cells with a wide variation in the number of affected mitochondria. For this same reason, each oocyte (egg) from the mother has varying numbers of affected mitochondria. And, getting to the point of this paragraph, this is why, even though all of the mother's children may inherit the mtDNA defect, the expression can vary widely between siblings. This variability in expression can make family history unreliable.

INTOXICATIONS

PREVIEW | REVIEW

- Disorders of intoxication present in what 3 forms?
- When should you suspect an inborn error of metabolism (IEM) in an infant with acute encephalopathy?
- Why are infants who have an IEM with acute encephalopathy generally normal at birth?
- How does chronic encephalopathy present?
- What are the most useful diagnostic tests for disorders of amino acid metabolism?
- What is phenylketonuria (PKU)?
- How do patients with PKU present?
- Which subset of children with hyperphenylalaninemia presents with severe neurologic disease, even with dietary treatment that maintains normal phenylalanine levels?
- What is the treatment for children with hyperphenylalaninemia who have neurologic symptoms that progress despite dietary treatment that maintains normal phenylalanine levels?

- What is tyrosinemia?
- Which disease is nitisinone used to treat?
- Name the 3 branched-chain amino acids.
- How do you diagnose maple syrup urine disease?
- Differentiate the lens findings in Marfan syndrome vs. homocystinuria.
- What molecule is the problem in all urea cycle disorders?
- How are almost all urea cycle disorders inherited? Which one is not inherited in this manner? How is it inherited?
- You are presented with an infant with elevated ammonia, no liver abnormalities, and no ketoacidosis. Which type of defect should you consider?
- What is the importance of a citrulline level?
- What is the importance of ordering a urinary orotic acid level?
- How does propionic acidemia present in early infancy?
- An infant with encephalopathy presents with a smell of sweaty feet. What is a possible diagnosis?
- What is the triad of symptoms associated with carboxylase deficiency?
- Describe galactosemia.
- What is a common screening test for galactosemia?
- What is the only manifestation of galactokinase deficiency?
- What is the significance of fructokinase deficiency?
- How might hereditary fructose intolerance (aldolase B deficiency) present?

OVERVIEW

Everything in biochemistry must go from compound A to compound B to compound C:

$$A \longrightarrow B \longrightarrow C$$

If the enzyme between B and C does not work properly, we get an accumulation of A and B and a deficiency of C:

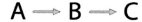

IEM intoxications are caused by upstream or accessory pathway buildup of toxic chemicals (see Table 23-1 on page 23-4):

1) Disorders of **amino acid metabolism**

2) **Urea cycle disorders**—problems with nitrogen excretion

METABOLIC DISORDERS

3) **Organic acidemias**—problems with small molecules generated from the metabolism of selected amino acids, carbohydrates, and fatty acids

4) **Sugar intolerances**

Generally, the enzyme block is in protein degradation and disposal or sugar breakdown and results in buildup of ketoacids or nitrogen (ammonia). These are the metabolites that cause the clinical problems. A state of catabolism or increased protein intake makes the disease worse.

We'll go over the IEM intoxications one by one, but first, let's look at how they present.

INTOXICATION PRESENTATIONS

The hallmark for intoxication disorders is a period of normalcy. These infants are not ill at birth and symptoms present from hours to years later. The illness may be acute, intermittent, or insidious in onset. Diagnose by abnormalities on screening tests:

• Expanded newborn screen
• Urine organic acids
• Plasma amino acids
• Plasma acylcarnitine profile

Keep in mind that abnormalities on the screening tests will be more striking when the patient is symptomatic and some results may normalize when the patient is well.

The goal for treatment is to identify patients before they develop symptoms if possible (on newborn screen) and restrict the diet to remove precursors that build up and poison the cells. It is also important to avoid catabolism to decrease the rate of unrestricted protein breakdown.

There are many causes of IEM intoxications, but their clinical presentations can be characterized as:

• acute encephalopathy,
• chronic encephalopathy, or
• acid-base disturbances.

Acute Encephalopathy

Suspect IEM intoxication if acute encephalopathy occurs without warning in previously normal neonates or young infants—and progresses rapidly.

Symptoms can include:

• Unexplained seizures
• Coma
• Lethargy
• Hypertonia
• Hypotonia

Because of the acute onset, focal neurologic deficits are usually not present.

Most of these infants are normal at birth, following uneventful pregnancies. However, once the infant disengages from the maternal circulation, extra substrates start to build up due to the infant's own metabolic impairment, and large increases in brain-diffusible molecules (small molecules such as glucose, ammonia, and amino and organic acids) cause toxic effects on the brain.

After a symptom-free interval, the infant begins to have feeding problems, lethargy, irritability, and vomiting. The toxic effect is usually much more pronounced when the infant/child is under stress or in an increased catabolic state (such as with viral/bacterial illness or fasting), or, in some types, with an increase in protein ingestion.

Generally, 4 categories of "small-molecule defects" present with acute encephalopathy. Table 23-1 outlines key things to look for in exam questions. We discuss each in more detail later in this section.

Table 23-1: Inborn Errors of Metabolism — Intoxications	
Disorder	**Initial Laboratory Testing**
Amino acid disorders (e.g., MSUD)	Plasma amino and urine organic acids High anion gap metabolic acidosis with ketonuria
Urea cycle defects (e.g., OTC deficiency)	Plasma ammonia markedly increased Minimal metabolic acidosis Respiratory alkalosis
Organic acidemias (e.g., isovaleric acidemia)	High anion gap metabolic acidosis with ketonuria Plasma ammonia mildly to moderately increased Hypoglycemia Increased glycine Abnormal urine organic acid Plasma amino acids
Sugar intolerances (e.g., galactosemia, fructose)	Newborn screening enzymatic testing Urine organic acids Liver enzyme analysis

MSUD = maple syrup urine disease
OTC = ornithine transcarbamylase

Once you identify these infants, work quickly to prevent further damage. The key strategy in the acute phase is to:

1) stop catabolism by providing adequate calories and

2) dilute toxins and promote excretion with generous hydration.

Intravenous fluids (typically 10% dextrose in 0.45% saline, with 20 mEq/L of potassium [if urine output is adequate]) are run at 1.5× maintenance—or sometimes even faster. Sodium bicarbonate is used only if the serum bicarbonate level is < 15 mEq/L—and then only with great care. Perform hemodialysis or hemofiltration in severe cases to remove the toxic small molecules. Once you identify the specific problem, proceed with appropriate therapy (i.e., dietary restriction, disease-specific medications).

Chronic Encephalopathy

Chronic encephalopathy presents in a slowly progressive manner as toxic metabolites build up. The symptoms are not immediately life-threatening; however, this usually changes over time as more and more damage occurs.

The most common examples are **phenylketonuria** and **homocystinuria**. Both cause symptoms after a period of exposure. With phenylketonuria, the buildup of phenylalanine eventually kills brain cells, causing loss of developmental milestones and, eventually, permanent brain damage. Homocystinuria causes problems after exposure to high levels of homocysteine and subsequent damage to the blood vessels, resulting in clots and stroke.

Acid-Base Disturbances

IEM intoxications can present as an acid-base disturbance. Acid-base abnormalities are generally due to either accumulation of fixed anions or loss of bicarbonate (which is almost always due to renal tubular dysfunction).

Accumulation of Fixed Anions

In the case of accumulation of fixed anions, the plasma chloride concentration is normal and the anion gap is increased (> 10 mEq/L). These disorders become more pronounced with increased catabolic states, such as after surgery, during illness, or with dietary changes involving increased protein intake. The child usually presents with feeding difficulties and failure to thrive (FTT). This category of disease includes organic acidurias, ketoacidosis, and lactic acidosis +/– pyruvate elevations.

Loss of Bicarbonate

Kidney injury results in renal loss of bicarbonate. Only a few metabolic disorders involve proximal renal tubular dysfunction with bicarbonate loss.

DISORDERS OF AMINO ACID METABOLISM

The most valuable diagnostic tests for amino acid metabolism disorders are examination of plasma amino acids and urine organic acids. You need to do both. These disorders are typically single-gene deficiencies. Systemic manifestations are typical because of the large amount of small-molecule metabolites in the circulation, frequently resulting in intellectual disability. These disorders fall into the intoxication classification of disorders. Presentation can be either acute or chronic, depending on the disorder.

Phenylalanine-Tyrosine Disorders

Classic Phenylketonuria (PKU)

PKU is an AR disorder in which phenylalanine cannot be converted to tyrosine. The enzyme defect is in phenylalanine hydroxylase (PAH). This results in high levels of phenylalanine (Phe) in the blood and large amounts of phenylpyruvic acid in the urine. PKU occurs in 1/10,000 to 1/20,000 births. See Figure 23-2.

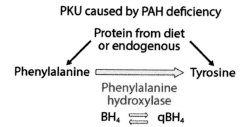

Figure 23-2: PKU caused by PAH deficiency

Clinical findings vary, depending on when treatment is initiated and on the degree of metabolic control. Phe in high amounts is toxic to the CNS. Those who remain untreated have severe intellectual disability with IQs of < 30. The damage becomes irreversible by 8 weeks of age. PKU infants appear normal at birth, but early symptoms occur in > 50% of those affected. The most common presentations in infants include vomiting, irritability, an eczematoid rash, and a peculiar odor—"mousy," "wolflike," or musty in character—that is due to the phenylacetic acid in the urine. Nearly all of those affected are fair haired and fair skinned, compared to their unaffected relatives. EEGs are abnormal.

Diagnosis, made by demonstrating an elevated serum concentration of Phe, must occur in the neonatal period to prevent serious consequences. In the U.S., universal newborn screening for PKU in the 1st few days of life occurs in all 50 states. The next step following a positive screen is a quantitative analysis of the concentrations of Phe and tyrosine. Phe will be elevated, and tyrosine will be low. These patients also have high levels of urinary Phe metabolites and normal plasma concentration of tetrahydrobiopterin cofactor.

Most patients identified by newborn screening are false positives due to delayed maturation of amino acid–metabolizing enzymes. These patients will also have a high tyrosine level (compared to those with PKU who have a low tyrosine level).

Therapy is straightforward: Limit the dietary intake of Phe for life. Start dietary treatment by 14 days of age. All infants should be supervised by a dietician familiar with PKU, and Phe levels need to be frequently monitored to determine how much dietary restriction is necessary. You must give Phe for normal growth and development, even in PKU infants. Even after infancy, CNS damage occurs if the Phe levels get too high. Tyrosine is an essential amino acid in PKU patients due to their inability to convert Phe to tyrosine.

Maternal PKU refers to the teratogenic effects of elevated Phe on the developing fetus in a mother with untreated PKU. Infants do not actually have PKU, but they can have growth deficiency, microcephaly, intellectual disability, and congenital heart defects—very similar to fetal alcohol syndrome. This is managed by strict dietary control of Phe in the mother.

METABOLIC DISORDERS

Hyperphenylalaninemia

Patients with hyperphenylalaninemia are without classic PKU but have elevated levels of Phe in the blood. Most of these infants have a milder deficiency of the PAH enzyme and can tolerate higher amounts of Phe.

A subset of these patients, however, has a defect in the synthesis or recycling of biopterin. These patients have neurologic symptoms that progress despite dietary treatment that maintains normal Phe levels. They have a defect in either the synthesis of tetrahydrobiopterin (BH_4), a cofactor for PAH, or they have a defect in the enzymes that regenerate tetrahydrobiopterin from dihydrobiopterin. Both of these result in diminished conversion of Phe to tyrosine. Tetrahydrobiopterin is also a cofactor for the hydroxylation of tryptophan and tyrosine, so you get interference in the synthesis of important compounds such as serotonin, dopa, and norepinephrine.

Clinically, these infants present with severe neurologic disease with marked hypotonia, spasticity, and posturing. Drooling is common, and psychomotor developmental delay is marked.

Treatment includes Phe restriction and supplementation of biopterin and biogenic amine precursor (i.e., 5-hydroxytryptophan and dopa).

Tyrosinemia

Tyrosinemia refers to a group of disorders in which blood tyrosine levels are elevated. The most common form, particularly in premature infants, is a **transient tyrosinemia** due to delayed maturation of tyrosine-metabolizing enzymes. Tyrosinemia can also occur in scurvy and liver diseases. We discuss the 3 inborn errors of tyrosine metabolism; they all are AR.

Hereditary tyrosinemia Type I (a.k.a. hepatorenal tyrosinemia) is due to a deficiency of fumarylacetoacetate hydroxylase, which is the final step in tyrosine metabolism. It is common in the French-Canadian population. The severe symptoms result from accumulation of succinylacetone; although tyrosine itself has some toxicity, this is mild compared with succinylacetone.

Infants are affected early, and most have a rapid course to death; some, however, progress more slowly. FTT, hepatomegaly with hepatic adenomas that progress to hepatoblastomas, and liver failure are the most common presentations. These infants are not intellectually disabled. They have renal tubular acidosis resembling Fanconi syndrome, as well as x-ray findings of rickets.

You can diagnose this type by finding elevated levels of tyrosine in the plasma, but the definitive pathognomonic diagnostic finding is succinylacetone in the urine.

Nitisinone (NTBC [2-[2-nitro-4-(trifluoromethyl)benzoyl] cyclohexane-1,3-dione]) is the treatment for tyrosinemia Type I. This blocks tyrosine metabolism before the fumarylacetoacetate hydrolase enzyme, which prevents the accumulation of toxic metabolites (i.e., succinylacetone). Because NTBC blocks tyrosine breakdown, tyrosine levels are elevated, causing symptoms like tyrosinemia Type II if not treated. Patients must be on a diet low in tyrosine and Phe.

Tyrosinemia Type II (a.k.a. Richner-Hanhart syndrome; oculocutaneous tyrosinemia) is a deficiency of tyrosine aminotransferase, which is the 1st step of tyrosine metabolism. Patients present with corneal ulcers or dendritic keratitis, along with red papular or keratotic lesions on their palms and soles; 50% have intellectual disability. They do not have the liver toxicity seen in Type I disease since they do not build up succinylacetone. The eye and skin lesions are from deposition of tyrosine itself. Treat with a diet low in tyrosine; however, even this is not always curative.

Tyrosinemia Type III is very rare. It is due to deficiency of 4-hydroxyphenylpyruvate dioxygenase, and patients can have intellectual disability. Patients respond well to a diet low in tyrosine.

Maple Syrup Urine Disease (MSUD)

If you have a newborn with the odor of maple syrup, think of MSUD. It is a defect in the breakdown of the branched-chain amino acids (BCAAs) during the oxidative decarboxylation of ketoacids (the ketoacids are what smell sweet).

Note that this disorder comes after catabolism of BCAAs into ketones (problems with downstream catabolism of BCAAs [propionic and methylmalonic acidemias] are discussed under Organic Acidemias on page 23-9). Hence, MSUD may be discussed as one of the organic acidemias in other sources.

Two different genes (*BCKDHA* and *BCKDHB*) are associated with MSUD, each inherited in an AR fashion. The incidence is ~ 1/150,000. It occurs more frequently in populations with consanguinity, such as the Pennsylvania Mennonites.

Classic MSUD presents with CNS disease early in infancy, and the urine (or hair or skin) smells like maple syrup. Infants are well at birth but start having symptoms by 3–5 days of life, with rapid progression to death in 2–4 weeks without treatment. Babies have feeding difficulties, irregular respirations, or loss of the Moro reflex. Severe seizures, opisthotonos (head, neck, and back held in abnormal position), and rigidity are typical presenting signs. Death follows decerebrate rigidity from cerebral edema.

Milder forms of the disease have intermittent, branched-chain aminoaciduria, characterized by ataxia and repeated episodes of lethargy, progressing to coma but without intellectual disability. Stressors, such as infection, frequently induce this form.

These patients have a high anion gap metabolic acidosis with ketonuria. Diagnose by finding increased amounts of the 3 BCAAs—**leucine**, **isoleucine**, and **valine**—in the plasma and urine. Finding alloisoleucine, an abnormal amino acid, is diagnostic and pathognomonic for MSUD.

Therapy: Aim for dietary control of leucine, isoleucine, and valine. If therapy is started early, before damage has occurred, normal IQ is possible. There is a very rare form of MSUD that responds very well to thiamine.

Glutaric Acidemia Type 1

Glutaric acidemia Type 1 is an AR enzyme defect (glutaryl-CoA dehydrogenase) in the catabolic pathway of lysine, hydroxylysine, and tryptophan; it is the only clinically relevant disorder in the lysine-hydroxylysine-tryptophan group of disorders.

Note that glutaric academia Type 1 is often discussed as one of the organic acidemias due to the abnormal production of glutaric acid.

Affected infants present with macrocephaly at birth but generally have normal development until they have a febrile illness or metabolic stressor, at which time they suddenly develop hypotonia and dystonia. CT/MRI shows frontal and cortical atrophy at birth, with increased extra-axial space, and, after symptoms of dystonia develop, degeneration of the caudate nucleus and putamen occurs. Striatal degeneration occurs in some during the 1st few years of life if they have a metabolic decompensation.

This is one of the few metabolic diseases (Menkes disease is another one) that can cause **subdural hematomas** and **retinal hemorrhages**, which can be mistaken for child abuse. Increased extraaxial space causes stretching of the bridging veins, making them susceptible to hematomas.

Diagnosis: Urine organic acids test shows increased excretion of glutaric and 3-hydroxyglutaric acids. Carnitine levels are usually low.

Treat with L-carnitine, riboflavin, and a special diet—and rapid implementation of IV fluids containing glucose when ill, particularly with febrile illnesses. This regimen helps prevent symptoms and striatal degeneration if given early, before symptoms develop.

~ 10% of patients never have problems, and ~ 10% of patients have problems despite good therapy.

Homocystinuria

Homocystinuria is a heterogeneous group of disorders caused by 6 types of genetic defects that disrupt the inter-related pathways of methionine metabolism. Originally, the term was used specifically to indicate disease due to a defect in the cystathionine β-synthase enzyme. This is an AR disorder. All diseases in this group cause elevated levels of homocysteine.

Clinically, patients with cystathionine β-synthase deficiency have marfanoid habitus, developmental delay, **lens dislocation,** and an increased risk of thromboembolism in both arteries and veins. These symptoms can present within the first 10 years of life, and the risk of embolic events persists throughout adult life. Clotting studies are normal, but elevated homocysteine levels cause damage

to collagen and elastic fibers within connective tissue and increased platelet stickiness, increasing the risk of formation of vascular thrombi. Intellectual disability is fairly common. The joints are limited in mobility (not hyper-mobile as in Marfan syndrome) and are osteoporotic.

Suspect homocystinuria in a child with subluxation/dislocation of the ocular lens. Lenticular subluxation is usually downward and medial. Memory aid: Think of downward (downward = low IQ) for homocystinuria, as opposed to Marfan syndrome, which is upward (upward = normal IQ).

Initial testing for diagnosis includes plasma total homocysteine and amino acids in plasma (primarily for the methionine level). Molecular genetic testing may confirm the diagnosis. Newborn screening specifically tests for methionine levels.

Treatment: Large doses of pyridoxine (vitamin B₆) cause a decrease in the total plasma homocysteine levels (in the vitamin-responsive form). Generally, affected individuals also require a diet low in methionine (which gets broken down into homocysteine). These patients need to be followed by a metabolic specialist over time. Betaine is another therapy that helps to convert homocysteine back into methionine, which can then be used for other purposes in the body (Figure 23-3).

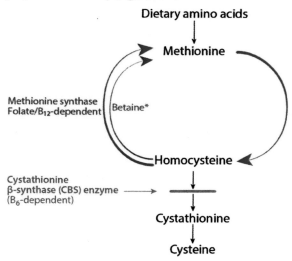

*Alternative pathway with betaine treatment

Figure 23-3: Methionine metabolic pathway

Nonketotic Hyperglycinemia

Nonketotic hyperglycinemia (NKH; a.k.a. glycine encephalopathy) is an AR IEM in which large amounts of glycine build up in body fluids without detectable accumulation of organic acids. The highest levels of glycine are in the CNS. This presents as intractable seizures in the neonatal period or as **hiccups in utero** in the classic form. It can present as seizures and hypotonia in the milder, later-onset form of the disease. Severe intellectual disability is typical in individuals who survive.

METABOLIC DISORDERS

Diagnosis is made by an increased ratio of CSF glycine to serum glycine. Prenatal diagnosis is possible by biochemical analysis of chorionic villus biopsy. Sodium benzoate seems to reduce CSF glycine levels and decrease seizures. Dextromethorphan has also been used with some success.

UREA CYCLE DISORDERS

The urea cycle converts nitrogen waste to urea, which is water soluble and safely excreted by the kidney. Nitrogen waste comes from catabolism of proteins as ammonium (NH_4^+) and from muscle breakdown.

The urea cycle (Figure 23-4) occurs in the liver and the periportal hepatocytes, in a series of reactions distributed between the mitochondria and the cytosol.

Before we get started on the enzymes, know that the bad effects of not breaking down NH_4^+ are increases in ammonia (NH_3) and glycine, both of which easily pass the blood-brain barrier and have a very toxic effect on the brain. Brain edema occurs quickly, and ammonia levels between 100 and 200 µmol/L cause lethargy, vomiting, and confusion. Higher levels result in coma and increased risk of brain herniation.

During normal metabolism, NH_4^+ initially becomes part of glycine, glutamine, and carbamoyl phosphate via different enzymes. A cyclic cascade of reactions follows the formation of carbamoyl phosphate—it is converted to citrulline, which then combines with nitrogen-containing aspartate to become argininosuccinate, then arginine, and, finally, urea. Note that of 2 moles of nitrogen in urea, 1 mole comes from ammonium and another from aspartate—which is supplied by the citric acid cycle (CAC; a.k.a. Krebs cycle).

Any of the enzymes in the urea cycle can be defective due to IEMs. Let's look at these:

1) *N*-acetylglutamate synthetase (NAGS) deficiency

2) Carbamoyl phosphate synthetase 1 (CPS1) deficiency—severe disorder

3) Ornithine transcarbamylase (OTC) deficiency—most common; X-linked; severe disorder

4) Argininosuccinate synthetase (AS) deficiency (a.k.a. citrullinemia)

5) Argininosuccinate lyase (AL) deficiency—accumulation of argininosuccinic acid with argininosuccinic aciduria

6) Arginase deficiency (a.k.a. argininemia)

All of the urea cycle disorders have AR inheritance, except for OTC deficiency, which has X-linked inheritance (and is also the most common!).

Does it matter where the defect is in the cycle? Yes! Usually, the more upstream the defect is, the higher the ammonia levels and the more severe the symptoms.

Review Figure 23-4. The most severe urea cycle defects are **CPS1 deficiency** and **OTC deficiency**. These infants are typically born at term and healthy (because the mom can filter out the excess ammonia easily during pregnancy). But by 5 days of age, in the **classic form** of the disease, the elevated ammonia levels result in clinical symptoms of lethargy, hypotonia, vomiting, and poor feeding. These infants progress rapidly to coma and death if the hyperammonemia is not quickly identified and treated.

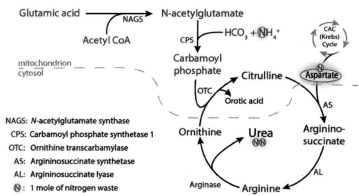

NAGS: *N*-acetylglutamate synthase
CPS: Carbamoyl phosphate synthetase 1
OTC: Ornithine transcarbamylase
AS: Argininosuccinate synthetase
AL: Argininosuccinate lyase
Ⓝ: 1 mole of nitrogen waste

Figure 23-4: The urea cycle

With either CPS1 or OTC deficiency, plasma ammonia levels can be > 1,000 µmol/L (normal < 35 µmol/L). In addition to elevated ammonia levels, a key diagnostic clue is that these infants usually have a respiratory alkalosis, not a metabolic acidosis, as would be expected with sepsis or other metabolic disorders. Liver functions are normal.

Late-onset urea cycle defects do occur and typically are partial enzyme deficiencies (there is some residual enzyme activity), precipitated by infection or some other stressor. Symptoms include loss of appetite, lethargy, vomiting, and behavioral changes. Some females with OTC deficiency experience later onset; their symptoms can be precipitated by pregnancy and childbirth. Also, be aware that valproate and haloperidol can unmask partial urea cycle defects.

Diagnosis: Once you clinically suspect the child has a urea cycle defect, order ammonia level (obtained on free-flowing blood and sent immediately to the lab on ice), quantitative plasma amino acids, and urinary organic acids to establish the specific defect in urea synthesis.

Table 23-2 lists specific laboratory findings seen with the urea cycle disorders. As you read the following, consult both the table and Figure 23-4; it all makes sense!

Table 23-2: Metabolite Levels in Urea Cycle Disorders					
Deficiency	Glutamine, Alanine, Asparagine	Citrulline	Orotic Acid (Urine)	Ammonia	Arginine
NAGS/CPS1	High	Absent or low	Low	Very high	Low
OTC			Very high		
AS		Very high	High	High	
AL					
Arginase		Normal	Normal	Normal	Very high

AL = argininosuccinate lyase
AS = argininosuccinate synthetase
CPS1 = carbamoyl phosphate synthetase

NAGS = N-acetylglutamate synthetase
OTC = ornithine transcarbamylase

Look for these metabolite levels:

- Glutamine, alanine, and asparagine are elevated—because they are storage forms for nitrogen, which cannot be excreted.
- Citrulline is absent or very low in proximal disorders such as OTC and CPS1 defects because citrulline is the direct product of these reactions.
- Orotic acid is a byproduct of the OTC-catalyzed reaction and is a very sensitive indicator of OTC deficiency. It helps differentiate between OTC and CPS1 deficiency. With OTC deficiency, carbamoyl phosphate is shuffled to an alternate pathway for orotic acid synthesis, thus resulting in elevated orotic acid levels. With CPS1 deficiency, the carbamoyl phosphate level is low, and therefore orotic acid levels are low.
- Plasma arginine concentration is low in all urea cycle defects except for argininemia (i.e., arginase deficiency). Without replacement, affected individuals have hair fragility and rash.

Acute treatment consists of volume replacement with D10W, restricting dietary protein, minimizing catabolism and enhancing anabolism, replacing deficient amino acids, and pushing alternate pathways to eliminate nitrogen waste.

Pushing these alternative pathways is done with an IV solution of sodium benzoate–sodium phenylacetate. Note that not all hospitals stock this prepackaged combination medication, and it is more likely available at tertiary care hospitals.

The alternate pathways for nitrogen removal use sodium benzoate, which is conjugated in the liver with glycine to make hippuric acid and sodium phenylacetate, which conjugates with glutamine to form phenylacetylglutamine. The hippuric acid and phenylacetylglutamine are easily excreted in the urine.

But if the plasma ammonia level is > 200 µmol/L and/or the infant is in a coma, hemodialysis is the best method to clear the ammonia.

Chronic management involves a high-caloric, protein-restricted diet with additional amino acids as needed. More and more patients with infantile-onset disease are having liver transplants with improved long-term outcomes.

ORGANIC ACIDEMIAS

Organic acidemias (a.k.a. organic acidurias) are a group of rare inherited disorders caused by a defect in specific enzymes that process proteins, especially BCAAs.

An organic acid is a chemical compound with ≥ 1 carboxyl groups (COOH) in its structure. The kidneys clear most organic acids, so it is easiest to examine the urine for these disorders—which is why these disorders are also called organic acidurias.

Organic acidemias are characterized by a high anion gap metabolic acidosis (HAGMA) with normal chloride and hyperammonemia. They are, for the most part, AR disorders. Symptoms are a result of buildup of ketoacids. Patients present acutely in the neonatal period or intermittently with illness.

Note that maple syrup urine disease (MSUD) is sometimes considered an organic acidemia, but it also belongs in the amino acid metabolism disorders. It causes a ketonuria and elevated BCAAs (leucine, isoleucine, and valine) in the urine. Glutaric academia Type 1 is also considered an organic acidemia due to the abnormal production of glutaric acid.

All organic acidemias have overlap in complications, including bone marrow suppression and pancreatitis. Diagnose with characteristic organic acid profile followed by specific enzyme diagnosis. Treat with a low-protein diet omitting the offending amino acids and give carnitine.

Propionic Acidemia (PA)

PA is an AR disorder due to a deficiency in propionyl-CoA carboxylase, a biotin-containing enzyme that converts propionyl-CoA to D-methylmalonyl-CoA. Propionyl-CoA is an intermediary in the oxidation of valine, methionine, isoleucine, and threonine. This is ketotic hyperglycinemia. A mnemonic to remember these amino acids is VoMIT—which is what kids with PA do when they get sick. The vomiting can be so severe that babies with PA get worked up for pyloric stenosis.

In the early neonatal period, PA can present as severe ketoacidosis with or without hyperammonemia. The infant will have encephalopathy, vomiting, and bone marrow depression. A milder presentation is ketoacidosis precipitated by infection or vomiting. Other major problems include malnutrition with FTT, dermatitis, recurrent infections, cardiomyopathy, and pancreatitis.

The patient has a high anion gap metabolic acidosis. Diagnose by examining urine organic acids. Look for large amounts of 3-hydroxypropionic and methylcitric acids. Plasma amino acids reveal an elevated glycine. Abnormal ketone bodies are common, too.

Treatment is dietary restriction of protein (usually < 1 g/kg/day). To decrease intake of the amino acids that are prone to produce more propionyl-CoA, nontoxic amino acids are supplemented in a special formula. Carnitine is helpful in increasing excretion of propionyl-CoA. During crisis, make sure the patient is getting a lot of glucose.

Methylmalonic Acidemias (MMAs)

There are a group of inherited disorders that cause MMA (a.k.a. methylmalonic aciduria). All ultimately inhibit methylmalonyl-CoA mutase function. These either affect mutase activity or interfere with the formation of **cobalamin** (vitamin B_{12}).

Disorders affecting mutase activity are mut(0)—no activity—and mut(–)—residual but low activity.

Disorders affecting cobalamin formation are termed cblA, cblB, cblC, cblD, cblF, cblH, and cblJ.

Clinically, patients present early with hyperammonemia, ketoacidosis, and thrombocytopenia—or later with chronic ketotic hyperglycinemia, vomiting, and FTT. A late-onset complication is renal failure of uncertain origin, and cardiomyopathy can also occur.

Diagnose with organic acid analysis of urine, which shows increased methylmalonic acid and abnormal ketone bodies, as with PA. Homocystinuria is also present if the patient has the enzyme deficit in the pathway that blocks the synthesis of methyl-B_{12}, resulting in increased methylmalonic acid and increased levels of homocysteine.

Treatment relies on restricting dietary protein. Carnitine is useful. Liver and kidney transplantation can be beneficial. If the patient has both methylmalonic aciduria and homocystinuria, treat with betaine (which provides another methyl donor for the conversion of homocysteine to methionine) and IM vitamin B_{12}.

Isovaleric Acidemia (IVA)

IVA is an AR disorder and a defect in the 3rd step of **leucine metabolism**.

If you have a newborn with the odor of **sweaty feet**, think of IVA, especially if the infant has encephalopathy. The enzyme defect is in isovaleryl-CoA dehydrogenase. Patients cannot convert isovaleryl-CoA to 3-methylcrotonyl-CoA, so they have increased levels of isovaleryl-CoA.

IVA can present in the newborn period with an acute episode of severe HAGMA and moderate ketosis with vomiting, which can lead to coma and death. More typically, it presents later in infancy or childhood and is precipitated by an infection or increased protein intake. A chronic intermittent form with pancytopenia and acidosis occurs in infants who survive the acute episode.

Diagnose IVA with urine organic acids. Prenatal diagnosis is possible.

Treatment in the acute setting is aimed at the acidosis, which usually responds to IV glucose and bicarbonate. Focus long-term treatment on restricting leucine intake and prescribing carnitine and/or glycine to increase conversion of isovaleryl-CoA to isovalerylglycine, which is excreted easily.

3-Methylcrotonyl-CoA Carboxylase Deficiency

3-Methylcrotonyl-CoA carboxylase (a.k.a. 3MCC, or BMCC) deficiency, an AR disorder, is a defect in the 4th step of **leucine metabolism**. The biotin-containing enzyme, 3-methylcrotonyl-CoA carboxylase, is missing and 3-methylcrotonyl-CoA is not converted to 3-methylglutaconyl-CoA.

Patients present between 1 and 3 years of age with acute metabolic acidosis, hypoglycemia, and carnitine deficiency—typically during a stressful event (e.g., an infection). The majority of affected individuals never have any decompensation or symptoms related to the enzyme defect.

Diagnose with urine organic acid analysis, which shows increased excretion of 3-methylcrotonylglycine and 3-hydroxyisovaleric acid.

Acute treatment consists of IV glucose, fluids, and electrolytes. Long-term therapy consists of oral carnitine to correct carnitine deficiency, if present, and biotin to enhance enzymatic function.

Although the majority of patients identified with this disorder by newborn screening most likely will not have problems, this disease can be serious. Because we cannot tell who is likely to get sick, we treat them all.

Multiple Carboxylase Deficiency

Biotin is the cofactor for 4 essential carboxylases that are important in the metabolism of dietary fats, carbohydrates, and proteins. Two disorders are associated with **biotin** deficiency or inability to incorporate biotin:

1) **Biotinidase deficiency**—biotinidase extracts biotin from food and recycles biotin from carboxylase enzymes. It has variable severity, and symptoms can appear from several days to years after birth.

2) **Holocarboxylase synthetase deficiency**—this enzyme incorporates biotin into the carboxylase enzymes. This deficiency has neonatal onset.

In both biotin disorders, the absence of functional carboxylases results in the inability to properly metabolize propionyl-CoA, 3-methylcrotonyl-CoA, acetyl-CoA, and pyruvate. This leads to the classic triad of carboxylase deficiency:

- Encephalopathy
- Alopecia
- Skin rash

Seizures, hearing loss, and blindness can also be complications of untreated disease.

Biotinidase deficiency typically presents later than holocarboxylase deficiency. It has a perioral dermatitis that looks like acrodermatitis enteropathica.

Diagnose by analyzing urine organic acid and finding increased 3-methylcrotonylglycine and 3-hydroxyisovaleric acid with lactic acids. Multiple carboxylase deficiency can also be found on newborn screening for biotinidase deficiency (and is included in most states). Holocarboxylase deficiency should be detected with the expanded newborn panels.

Treatment is quite effective with free biotin in doses of 5–20 mg/day. This usually reverses all disease manifestations.

SUGAR INTOLERANCES

Galactose Metabolism Disorders

Inadequate metabolism of galactose can be caused by 3 different enzymes necessary for converting galactose to glucose:

1) Galactose-1-phosphate uridyltransferase (GALT)

2) Galactokinase

3) Uridine diphosphate (UDP)-galactose-4-epimerase (GALE)

Galactosemia

Lactose in dairy products is hydrolyzed by lactase in the intestine into glucose and galactose. Galactose is quickly converted to more glucose. Galactosemia occurs when a deficiency of the GALT enzyme causes galactose to be metabolized poorly or not at all. Galactose and its derivative molecules then build up in cells and tissues, especially the liver, kidneys, and brain.

Classic galactosemia is usually what we think about when we say "galactosemia." It is an AR disorder occurring in 1/60,000 births where there is a mutation of both copies of the *GALT* gene resulting in no detectable GALT activity. These patients have 2 copies of severely affected genes (shown as G/G). **Clinical galactosemia** results from similar, but not as severe, damage to both copies of the *GALT* gene (G/G); detectable, but insufficient, GALT function remains. Remember, because this is an AR disorder, both genes must be affected to have any enzyme deficiency.

In untreated classic or clinical galactosemia, infants present clinically in the first few days of life after their first lactose meal with some combination of:

- Jaundice
- Vomiting
- Hepatosplenomegaly
- Seizures
- Cataracts
- Lethargy
- Irritability
- Poor weight gain
- Hypoglycemia
- Vitreous hemorrhage
- Cirrhosis
- Ascites
- Intellectual disability

Those affected are at increased risk for *E. coli* sepsis, which usually precedes the diagnosis of galactosemia.

The **Duarte variant** is a damaged gene that codes for a partially functional GALT. It is the most common galactosemic gene mutation, with 12% of those with Caucasian ancestry and 3% of those with Asian ancestry being carriers. Individuals who are Duarte-variant homozygous (D/D) have ~ 50% of normal red cell enzyme activity but do not have symptoms. Individuals who are compound heterozygous (D/G) have only 25% of activity, with elevated galactose-1-phosphate levels. Patients are usually asymptomatic, but most practitioners restrict lactose intake if the RBC galactose-1-phosphate levels are elevated.

Suspect this disorder in patients with galactosemia symptoms or when you discover a reducing substance in urine while the patient is drinking breast milk, cow's milk, or formula containing lactose. Reducing substances in the urine is usually done by labs as a reflex test when the urine shows no glucose, but this is neither sensitive nor specific enough to confirm or rule out the diagnosis. Definitive diagnosis requires deficient activity of GALT in RBCs or other tissues, while also showing an increased concentration of galactose-1-phosphatase.

Newborn screening for galactosemia is widespread in the U.S. Many states use a fluorescent spot test (Beutler test) for GALT activity, whereas other states examine galactose-1-phosphate levels. Note that the Duarte variant is often not picked up by the latter test.

For classic or clinical galactosemia, elimination of lactose and galactose from the diet reverses growth failure and renal/hepatic problems. Even cataracts regress. Give soy-based formula instead. Unfortunately, for reasons that are unclear, long-term complications are typical, even with treatment. Complications include ovarian failure, amenorrhea, developmental delay, and learning disabilities that worsen with age. Speech disorders are also very common.

Galactokinase Deficiency

Cataracts alone typically characterize this disorder. Otherwise, the infant is asymptomatic. Treatment is dietary restriction of galactose.

Uridine Diphosphate (UDP)-Galactose-4-Epimerase (GALE) Deficiency

The accumulated metabolites are extremely analogous to those seen in galactosemia, but there is also an increase in cellular UDP-galactose. This deficiency may not be detected on a newborn screening.

There are 2 forms of this disease:

1) **Benign** form: Individuals are healthy, and no treatment is necessary. The only evidence is seen in RBCs.

2) **Generalized** form: This clinically resembles galactosemia, with the additional symptoms of hypotonia and nerve deafness. Treatment with dietary restriction of galactose is effective. The GALT activity is normal, unlike in classic galactosemia.

Fructose Metabolism Disorders

Benign Fructosuria

Benign fructosuria is a condition caused by the deficiency of fructokinase. It has no clinical manifestations and requires no treatment. It is an incidental finding when you discover fructose during a urine screen for reducing substances.

Hereditary Fructose Intolerance

Hereditary fructose intolerance, caused by aldolase B deficiency, is a severe disease of infancy that appears when the infant ingests fructose-containing food. The enzyme, which is deficient in these patients, normally causes the hydrolysis of fructose 1-phosphate and fructose 1,6-bisphosphate into 3 sugars: dihydroxyacetone phosphate, glyceraldehyde 3-phosphate, and glyceraldehyde. With the enzymatic deficiency, the accumulation of fructose 1-phosphate leads to severe toxic symptoms in patients who ingest fructose.

The incidence is estimated to be ~ 1/23,000.

Affected individuals are completely healthy until they ingest fructose or sucrose (table sugar, which consists of fructose and glucose). Usually, the culprit is juice or sweetened cereal. It can look much like galactosemia, but onset is generally later when exposed to fructose, as opposed to the 1st week or so of life, when patients are exposed to lactose.

Symptoms after introduction of fructose or sucrose into the diet include jaundice, hepatomegaly, vomiting, lethargy, seizures, and irritability. Laboratory results will show prolonged clotting time, low albumin, elevated bilirubin

and transaminases, and proximal tubular dysfunction. If fructose intake continues, severe hypoglycemia occurs, followed by liver and kidney failure and, ultimately, death. Sugar ingestion causes hypoglycemia!

Suspect this deficiency if you find fructose as a urinary reducing substance during a symptomatic episode.

A definitive diagnosis depends on assaying fructose 1,6-bisphosphate aldolase B activity in the liver. Genetic testing is also available and can make biopsy unnecessary in some patients.

Treatment consists of complete dietary elimination of all sources of fructose and of its progenitors, sucrose and sorbitol. Due to unsuspected sources of these sugars, consultation with an expert nutritionist is mandatory. Treatment reverses liver and kidney damage, and it improves growth. With treatment, intellectual disability is very uncommon. Symptoms improve with age, especially as those affected develop an aversion to sweets (and have lovely teeth because of it).

ENERGY UTILIZATION DEFECTS

PREVIEW | REVIEW

- What events exacerbate energy defect disorders?

- What are some of the ways a patient with an energy utilization defect can present?

- Where does fatty acid oxidation occur? Why is this important?

- What is the most common disorder affecting mitochondrial fatty acid oxidation and ketogenesis?

- How do most patients present with disorders of fatty acid oxidation?

- What are the laboratory tests you would order to detect disorders in fatty acid oxidation?

- How is medium-chain acyl-CoA dehydrogenase deficiency (MCAD) diagnosed?

- Which medical problems occur in patients with LCHAD deficiency that do not develop in those with MCAD or VLCAD deficiency?

- Describe glucose-6-phosphatase deficiency. Which organs are most commonly affected?

- How do patients with Type 1 GSD present?

- Which laboratory findings are common in patients with Type 1 GSD?

- How is Type 1 GSD diagnosed?

- What is the metabolic disorder in Type 2 GSD?

- Which laboratory tests are elevated in Type 2 GSD?

- How does a child with Type 5 GSD present?
- Which laboratory test is elevated at rest and increases after exercise in patients with Type 5 GSD?
- Describe fructose 1,6-diphosphatase deficiency.
- True or false? All mitochondrial DNA disorders are inherited from the father.
- What is the triad of symptoms associated with Kearns-Sayre syndrome?
- In MELAS, which symptom typically occurs long before a stroke?

OVERVIEW

These disorders have symptoms related to the inability to use energy due to disruption of normal metabolic pathways (see Figure 23-1 on page 23-1). The pathway looks like this:

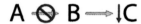

So, when you block the pathway between A and B, C goes down, and that is the problem—the inability to use normal resources of stored energy. Our bodies derive energy in a specific order during fasting:

1) Blood glucose
2) Breakdown of stored glycogen
3) Fatty acid oxidation (a.k.a. β-oxidation) in the fatty acid spiral
4) Breakdown of amino acids for glucose synthesis

Disorders of energy metabolism can occur with a breakdown in any of the above metabolic processes or elsewhere in the adenosine triphosphate (ATP) pathway. Examples of these disorders are:

- Fatty acid oxidation defects
- Glycogen storage diseases (defects in making or breaking down glycogen)
- Mitochondrial disorders (Krebs cycle and mitochondrial respiratory chain disorders)

PRESENTATION

Fasting or illness with increased energy needs can exacerbate an energy defect metabolic disorder and bring on decompensation. There may or may not be hypoglycemia; it is usually the last sign. Patients can present with FTT, hypotonia, cardiac dysfunction, lactic acidosis, or weakness and fatigue.

The presentation is determined by the effect on the cells. If muscle is affected, such as with

mitochondrial defects, then weakness is noted. If the body is unable to utilize the oxidative phosphorylation pathway, lactic acid builds up. See Table 23-3 for a list of findings.

Table 23-3: Presentation of Various Disorders of Energy Metabolism	
Disorder	**Presentation**
Fatty acid (β-) oxidation defects	Hypoketotic hypoglycemia Hypotonia Cardiomyopathy SIDS Reye-like syndrome
Glycogen storage diseases	Hepatomegaly Hypoglycemia Lactic acidosis FTT
Mitochondrial disorders	Lactic acidosis Seizures Cardiomyopathy Hypotonia/myopathy +/– Hypoglycemia

FTT = failure to thrive
SIDS - sudden infant death syndrome

DEFECTS IN FAT METABOLISM

Remember: Fatty acid oxidation (β-oxidation) occurs in the mitochondria, and this process provides the main energy source for the heart and skeletal muscles (Figure 23-5) during fasting from fat breakdown. Fatty acids are initially conjugated to carnitine. Then carnitine is transported across the mitochondrial membrane and released into the mitochondrial matrix as an acyl-CoA before it can be catabolized in the β-oxidation spiral. β-oxidation generates acetyl-CoA, which enters the Krebs cycle and provides energy to other tissues when the supply of glucose is gone. Acetyl-CoA is used to produce ketone bodies.

Diseases that limit β-oxidation do so by:

- Decreasing carnitine uptake by cells
- Inhibiting fatty acids from entering mitochondria
- Blocking β-oxidation

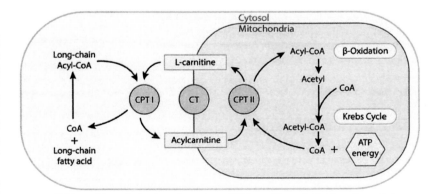

CPT I: carnitine palmitoyltransferase I   CPT II: carnitine palmitoyltransferase II
CT: carnitine-acylcarnitine translocase

Figure 23-5: Fatty acid (β-) oxidation

If β-oxidation is impaired, there is limited energy available for the heart and skeletal muscles at rest; it also limits the ability of the brain to cope with low-glucose settings. Thus, a child with a defect in β-oxidation is the poster child for disorders of energy metabolism. These are nearly all AR disorders.

There are 12 known disorders affecting mitochondrial β-oxidation and ketogenesis, with medium-chain acyl-CoA dehydrogenase (MCAD) deficiency being the most common. Age of onset varies from birth to adulthood. The most common clinical presentations involve the hepatic, skeletal, muscular, and cardiac systems. Neonates can present with arrhythmias, hypoglycemia, or with sudden death. (Makes sense, doesn't it? The heart cannot function correctly because of the lack of energy and hypoglycemia.) Sometimes they have renal cystic dysplasia. Older children can have arrhythmias or cardiomyopathy. Muscle weakness is typical, as is exercise-induced rhabdomyolysis. Patients with these disorders are susceptible to metabolic decompensation in times of stress (e.g., prolonged fasting, infection, surgery).

Evaluation involves these main laboratory studies:

- Routine lab measurements (i.e., CBC, electrolytes, liver function studies, ammonia, lactate, creatine phosphokinase [CPK], urine ketones)
- Free carnitine and acylcarnitine levels in the blood
- Gas chromatography and mass spectrometry analysis of organic acids
- Analysis of plasma acylcarnitine and urine acylglycines by specialized techniques

Lab findings include:

- Hypoketotic hypoglycemia
- Hyperuricemia
- Acidosis
- Hyperammonemia (but mild compared to urea cycle disorders)

Definitive diagnosis of these disorders requires measurement of specific enzyme activity or mutation analysis.

Treat the acute presentation with IV D10½NS or D10NS and possibly L-carnitine. Long-term therapy revolves around keeping the glucose from getting low, which is especially important when the patient is stressed by illness or decreased intake (including the period of fasting while sleeping at night) and catabolism.

We'll now discuss some of the more clinically relevant (and quizzable) disorders.

Primary Carnitine Deficiency

Primary carnitine deficiency (a.k.a. carnitine uptake defect) is an AR defect occurs in the plasma membrane of the cell. This disorder is caused by a deficiency of the carnitine transporter in the kidneys, where free carnitine is recycled for use by the body. When this transporter is not functioning, free carnitine is lost in the urine, resulting in low levels of free carnitine in the serum. Patients present in early infancy or later childhood with cardiomyopathy or recurrent episodes of encephalopathy and hypoketotic hypoglycemia. If the skeletal muscles are involved, weakness is prominent. Conduction defects and arrhythmias are rare with this disorder, in contrast to other disorders.

Diagnose by finding very low levels of carnitine in tissues. In serum, it may be undetectable or < 1 μmol/L. Keep in mind that losses from fatty acid oxygenation defects or organic acidurias can also cause fairly severe carnitine deficiency or secondary deficiency. Treat with L-carnitine, which results in dramatic improvement. Administer orally for chronic maintenance; administer IV for emergencies.

Defects of Fatty Acid Entry into Mitochondria

Short-chain and medium-chain fatty acids can enter mitochondria directly, but CoA esters that are longer than 12 carbons require transport with carnitine palmitoyltransferase I and II (CPT I and CPT II) and by carnitine-acylcarnitine translocase. AR disorders occur and cause defects in these enzymes. Patients present with symptoms similar to long-chain disorders.

All transporter defects can present in infancy with fasting-induced hypoglycemia, liver failure, and cardiomyopathy. However, they can all have later phenotypes as well.

Diagnosis: For CPT I, serum carnitine levels are normal or elevated (key: no other disorder elevates carnitine—elevated carnitine is otherwise seen only in excessive supplementation), and the serum acylcarnitine profile is normal. In CPT II and carnitine-acylcarnitine translocase deficiency, serum carnitine levels are very low with elevated C_{16} esters (an abnormal acylcarnitine profile).

Treat acute cases with IV glucose and aggressive hydration. Avoidance of fasting alleviates symptoms. Give carnitine if serum carnitine levels are low. Medium-chain triglyceride (MCT) oil, which can enter the mitochondria without these enzymes, provides an alternative energy source as well.

Defects in β-Oxidation

Once acyl-CoA is in the mitochondria, it enters the β-oxidation cycle. Here, a series of reactions occur, and defects/deficiencies of the enzymes can cause problems. Different enzymes cleave different lengths of carbon chains. Short-chain disorder is unlikely to cause symptoms and has been removed from many newborn screens.

Three main AR conditions are discussed in this group:

1) Defects in medium-chain acyl-CoA dehydrogenase (MCAD)
2) Defects in long-chain 3-hydroxyacyl-CoA dehydrogenase (LCHAD)
3) Defects in very-long-chain acyl-CoA dehydrogenase (VLCAD)

Medium-Chain Acyl-CoA Dehydrogenase (MCAD) Deficiency

Medium-chain triglycerides (MCTs) are triglycerides whose fatty acids have an aliphatic tail of 6–12 carbon atoms. MCAD deficiency, the most common β-oxidation defect, typically presents in the first 2 years of life. The infant/child will have fasting-induced lethargy and hypoglycemia. Seizures and coma are typical. MCAD deficiency—as well as the majority of other fatty acid oxidation disorders—has been implicated in some cases of Reye syndrome and SIDS. In an acute episode, elevated liver transaminases and CPK with hypoglycemia occur. Liver biopsy shows microvesicular steatosis.

Diagnose MCAD deficiency by finding elevated C6, C8, C10, and C10:1 carnitine esters. Free serum carnitine is low sometimes, but it is not consistently low.

Acute treatment is IV glucose and bicarbonate. Restrict MCTs from the diet because there is no acyl-CoA dehydrogenase to break them down and the resultant buildup of these chains is toxic to the cells.

As preventive maintenance, avoid fasting when healthy. During illness, rapid intervention is most important. A secondary carnitine deficiency may develop as excess acylcarnitines bind to free carnitine and are renally excreted. When carnitine is low, some will prescribe oral replacement; however, evidence of benefit is lacking.

In the U.S., the majority of states mandate screening for MCAD deficiency because it responds so well to treatment. Prior to newborn screening, 25% of infants died with the 1st metabolic crisis.

Long-Chain 3-Hydroxyacyl-CoA Dehydrogenase (LCHAD) Deficiency

LCHAD is the long chain–specific enzyme, and it acts on all acyl groups longer than 8 carbons. LCHAD deficiency affects mainly the liver and heart. Patients usually present in infancy (earlier onset than MCAD) with fasting-induced hypoketotic hypoglycemia, although some will have cardiomyopathy or, later in adulthood, exercise-induced rhabdomyolysis. Sometimes the pregnancy is a clue: Was it complicated with acute fatty liver or **HELLP** (hemolysis, elevated liver function tests, and low platelets) syndrome?

Patients with LCHAD deficiency frequently develop **cholestatic liver disease** and have **retinopathy** with hypopigmentation or focal pigment aggregations later in life. Note: These are not seen in MCAD or VLCAD deficiency!

Therapy for LCHAD deficiency is similar to that for MCAD and VLCAD deficiency. Frequent meals, without prolonged fasting, are recommended, especially for infants. You also can use MCT oil and carnitine. Oral docosahexaenoic acid may reverse retinopathy if it occurs.

Very-Long-Chain Acyl-CoA Dehydrogenase (VLCAD) Deficiency

VLCAD deficiency mainly affects the heart and skeletal muscles with an earlier onset than MCAD. It presents in infancy as arrhythmias with severe cardiomyopathy and sudden death. Occasionally, it is found in older infants and children with hepatic, cardiac, or muscular abnormalities.

Diagnose by finding elevated saturated and unsaturated C_{14-18} esters. Free carnitine is usually low.

Treatment includes frequent meals with a high-carbohydrate diet and avoidance of fasting, especially for infants. If an acute episode occurs, give IV glucose and fluids. You can use MCTs because their oxidation does not involve VLCAD.

Glutaric Acidemia Type 2

Glutaric acidemia Type 2 (a.k.a. multiple acyl-CoA dehydrogenase deficiency) is caused by AR defects in electron-transfer flavoprotein (ETF) and ETF-ubiquinone oxidoreductase. These enzymes transfer electrons from acyl-CoA dehydrogenases involved in fatty acid and amino acid oxidation from flavin adenine dinucleotide coenzymes into the respiratory chain.

The neonate typically presents with severe hypoglycemia, metabolic acidosis, hyperammonemia, and a **sweaty feet odor,** as with IVA (isovaleric acidemia). Frequently, the patient has cardiomyopathy, facial dysmorphism, and severe renal cystic dysplasia.

Diagnose by finding glutarylcarnitine, isovaleryl-carnitine, and straight-chain C_4, C_8, C_{10}, and C_{12} esters. Serum carnitine is low, and ketones are absent. Patients with absolute deficiency die within the first few weeks, usually due to conduction defects. Those with incomplete defects survive into adulthood.

Treatment relies on avoidance of fasting and sometimes requires continuous intragastric feeds. Carnitine is useful. You cannot use MCTs because all of the acyl-CoA dehydrogenases are deficient.

GLYCOGEN STORAGE DISEASES (GSDs)

Mono- and Polysaccharides

GSDs are disorders of carbohydrate metabolism essentially involving 3 monosaccharides (glucose, galactose, and fructose) and 1 polysaccharide (glycogen):

- **Glucose** is the main source of energy. When metabolized, glucose makes ATP via glycolysis (glucose is converted to pyruvate) or mitochondrial oxidative (pyruvate is converted to carbon dioxide and water). Eating, gluconeogenesis, and breakdown of storage glycogen maintain glucose levels.
- **Galactose** is derived from lactose (galactose + glucose), which is in milk and milk products.

- **Fructose** is found in the diet (fruits and vegetables) and is also derived from sucrose (fructose + glucose).
- **Glycogen** is the storage form of glucose. Defects in glycogen metabolism usually lead to buildup of glycogen in tissues, resulting in GSDs.

Important GSD Types to Know

Most of these diseases are inherited as AR traits (except for phosphoglycerate kinase deficiency and one form of phosphorylase kinase deficiency, both of which are X-linked disorders). The frequency of all forms of GSD is ~ 1/20,000.

For an overview of the GSDs, refer to Table 23-4.

We will discuss some important types of GSDs here:

- **Type 1 GSD** (see Type 1 GSD (von Gierke Disease)): This is due to either decreased glucose-6-phosphatase or translocase deficiency and is not to be confused with glucose-6-phosphate dehydrogenase (G6PD) deficiency, a completely different disease.
- **Type 2 GSD** (see Type 2 GSD (Pompe Disease)): This does not present as an energy metabolic defect but is a lysosomal storage disease that has excess glycogen storage.
- **Type 5 GSD** (see Type 5 GSD (McArdle Disease)): Myophosphorylase deficiency—this is the most common adult GSD.

Type 1 GSD (von Gierke Disease)

Type 1 GSD (von Gierke disease) is due to a defect in glucose-6-phosphatase in the liver, kidney, and intestinal mucosa.

There are 2 subtypes (Figure 23-6):

1) **Type 1a**—defect in the glucose-6-phosphatase enzyme
2) **Type 1b**—defect in the translocase that transports glucose-6-phosphate across the cell membrane

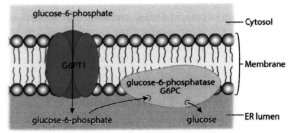

Figure 23-6: The glucose-6-phosphatase system

Both subtypes cause the same deficit, which is failure to convert glucose-6-phosphate to glucose in the liver. The affected individual has excess storage of glycogen in the tissues and suffers from severe and rapid fasting hypoglycemia.

Clinically, these patients present at ~ 3–4 months of age with FTT, protuberant abdomen due to hepatomegaly, doll-like facies, short stature with thin extremities, and/or hypoglycemic seizures. The kidneys are also hypertrophied, but the spleen and heart are normal in size.

Types 1a and 1b are similar, except that Type 1b has associated recurrent bacterial infections due to neutropenia and impaired neutrophil function. Oral and intestinal mucosa ulcers also occur with Type 1b.

In the long term, the liver is the most commonly affected organ, although other organ systems are also affected. Gout usually appears in puberty because of the elevated uric acid. Puberty is usually delayed, but sexual development is otherwise normal. Pancreatitis can occur

Type	Enzyme Deficiency	Tissue	Common Name	Glycogen Structure
0	Glycogen synthase	Liver	Glycogen synthase deficiency	Normal; deficient in quantity
1	Glucose-6-phosphatase	Liver	von Gierke disease	Normal
2	α-1,4-glucosidase	All lysosomes	Pompe disease	Normal
3	Amylo-1,6-glucosidase (debranching enzyme)	All organs	Cori disease	Outer chains missing or very short
4	Amylo-(1,4→1,6)-transglycosylase (branching enzyme)	Liver, probably all organs	Andersen disease	Very long unbranched chains
5	Glycogen phosphorylase	Muscle	McArdle disease	Normal
6	Glycogen phosphorylase	Liver	Hers disease	Normal
7	Phosphofructokinase	Muscle	Tarui disease	Normal
8	Phosphorylase kinase	Liver	X-linked phosphorylase kinase deficiency	Normal
9	Phosphorylase kinase	All organs		Normal

because of the elevated lipids. Note that the triglyceride levels remain elevated even with regular feeding/dietary maintenance.

By 20–30 years of age, most patients develop hepatic adenomas that can bleed and occasionally become malignant. Pulmonary hypertension and osteoporosis can occur. Proteinuria occurs in all patients > 20 years of age. Hypertension, kidney stones, and abnormal creatinine clearance are common. With advanced disease, focal segmental glomerulonephritis develops.

Key lab findings for diagnosis:

- Hypoglycemia—does not make glucose from stored glycogen
- Lactic acidosis—relies on anaerobic metabolism
- Hyperuricemia—breaks down protein for glucose
- Hyperlipidemia (increased VLDL, LDL, and apolipoproteins B, C, and E)—breaks down fat for energy
- Elevated ketones—using fat and protein for energy
- Neutropenia in Type 1b

Note: Even though patients have hepatomegaly, the liver transaminases are usually normal. The plasma can appear milky because of the hypertriglyceridemia. Also, if you give glucagon or epinephrine, blood glucose levels do not rise, but lactate does. Gene-based mutation analysis provides the definitive diagnosis. Liver biopsy is generally not required.

Aim treatment at preventing hypoglycemia with continuous gastric feeds. Initially this is achieved with a nasogastric tube, but most choose placement of a gastrostomy tube for long-term use at home.

Give uncooked cornstarch orally when the patient is old enough for pancreatic enzymes to break it down (> 1 year of age). Fructose and galactose cannot be converted to free glucose, so restrict these in the diet. Use allopurinol to lower uric acid levels. Granulocyte colony-stimulating factor (G-CSF) has been used to correct the neutropenia of Type 1b. Some patients have difficulty with bleeding, especially during surgery, because they have platelet dysfunction. You can correct this with a constant infusion of glucose for 24–48 hours prior to surgery.

Type 2 GSD (Pompe Disease)

Type 2 GSD (Pompe disease) is the main disorder in the skeletal and/or cardiac category. It is an AR condition that is classified as both a GSD and a lysosomal storage disorder. It is due to a deficiency in the lysosomal acid α-1,4-glucosidase (a.k.a. acid maltase), which is responsible for breaking down glycogen in lysosomal vacuoles.

Type 2 GSD does not fall into an energy metabolism defect category. Symptoms are due to the buildup of complex molecules, not primarily from energy problems. It is a lysosomal storage defect with excess storage of glycogen. Type 2 GSD is different from the other GSDs in that the glycogen accumulates in the lysosomes and not in the cytoplasm.

It has a wide variety of phenotypic presentations:

- **Infantile-onset form:** This is the most severe form and presents with cardiomegaly, hypotonia, and death before 1 year of age. The infant is normal at birth but soon develops generalized muscle weakness, hypotonia, macroglossia, hepatomegaly, FTT, and heart failure due to hypertrophic cardiomyopathy. ECG shows a high-voltage QRS and a shortened PR interval.
- **Juvenile/Late-childhood form:** Slowly progressive skeletomuscular manifestations occur without cardiac involvement. Patients present with slowed developmental milestones (e.g., delayed walking). Swallowing difficulties, proximal muscle weakness, and respiratory muscle depression then follow. Death may occur before these individuals reach their 20s.
- **Adult form:** This presents in those 20–70 years of age as a slowly progressive myopathy without cardiac involvement. Clinically, patients have progressive proximal muscle weakness, including in the trunk. Lower extremities are more severely affected than the upper extremities. The pelvic girdle and diaphragm are most seriously affected. Initially, the adult might present with increased sleepiness, morning headache, and exertional dyspnea.

Diagnosis: Look for elevated CPK, aspartate aminotransferase (AST), and lactate dehydrogenase (LDH), especially in the infantile form. Muscle biopsy shows vacuoles full of glycogen on staining. There are reduced or absent levels of acid glucosidase activity in muscle or skin fibroblasts.

Treatment: Enzyme replacement therapy is available. In the juvenile and adult forms, institute a high-protein diet. Nocturnal ventilatory support may be necessary, which improves daytime symptoms.

Note: Type 2 GSD (Pompe disease) is now on the Recommended Uniform Screening Panel (RSUP). See if your state has added Type 2 GSD to its newborn screening: babysfirsttest.org/newborn-screening/rusp-conditions#pompe

Type 5 GSD (McArdle Disease)

Type 5 GSD (McArdle disease) is an AR disorder due to deficiency of muscle phosphorylase. This deficiency reduces ATP (adenosine triphosphate) generation by glycogenolysis and results in glycogen accumulation in the muscle.

Symptoms are usually not present until patients reach their 20s or 30s, although many can remember symptoms from childhood, including exercise-induced muscle cramps and exercise intolerance. The exercise can be either brief and intense (such as sprinting) or sustained and less intense (such as walking up a hill). Many patients report a "second-wind" phenomenon: If they rest, they can resume the exercise. And 50% report burgundy-colored urine after exercise, which is from myoglobinuria due to rhabdomyolysis.

METABOLIC DISORDERS

CPK is elevated at rest and increases after exercise. Exercise also increases ammonia and uric acid in the blood.

What suggests the diagnosis? No increase occurs in blood lactate level, but instead an increased ammonia level is found when the patient exercises. This suggests a defect in the conversion of glycogen or glucose to lactate. Enzymatic assays on muscle tissue or DNA analysis for the myophosphorylase gene provide definitive diagnosis.

Treatment is geared toward avoiding strenuous exercise to prevent rhabdomyolysis. Gradual aerobic training or oral fructose/glucose intake can improve exercise tolerance.

Gluconeogenesis

Fructose 1,6-diphosphatase deficiency is a defect in gluconeogenesis. Patients have severe episodes of metabolic acidosis, hypoglycemia, hyperventilation, seizures, and coma. Decrease in oral intake during an illness or gastroenteritis precipitates events. This contrasts with hereditary fructose intolerance, in which renal and liver functions are normal. Diagnose by finding the enzyme deficiency in liver or intestinal biopsy. Treat with IV glucose. For the long term, patients must avoid fasting and eliminate fructose and sucrose from the diet. Cornstarch is helpful for preventing hypoglycemia.

MITOCHONDRIAL DNA (mtDNA) DISORDERS

Cellular respiration (oxidative phosphorylation) occurs in the mitochondria using a series of enzymes to convert carbohydrates, protein, and fatty acids into ATP. These organelles have their own DNA—mtDNA—and there are multiple mitochondria in each cell. All mtDNA disorders are maternally inherited, but not all mitochondrial disorders are caused by mtDNA mutations. The majority are due to recessive mutations in the nuclear DNA, but they can also be AD or X-linked. By definition, these are energy metabolism (i.e., cellular respiration) defects.

Mitochondria exhibit heteroplasmy, meaning there is a mixture of > 1 type of mtDNA within a cell or individual. Very frequently, mutations affect only some of the copies while the others are unaffected. These disorders have variable presentations with variable age of onset (i.e., they can give rise to any symptoms, in any tissue, at any age). The main phenotype, however, is related to energy deficiency so think about a mitochondrial defect in patients with cardiomyopathy, neuromuscular symptoms, seizures, or poor growth.

Diagnosis can be difficult. Lab findings may include elevated pyruvate and lactic acid (on free-flowing sample) and elevated alanine and proline. The mutation analysis is tricky due to mitochondrial heteroplasmy and to mtDNA vs. nuclear DNA mutations. It is better to have an idea of where the defect is in functioning.

There is no good evidence for treatment although many providers put these patients on a cocktail of vitamins including antioxidants (to reduce free radicals), carnitine, thiamine, pantothenic acid, and riboflavin. Results are subjective.

The diseases that follow are based on phenotype. Note: Different mutations can cause the same phenotype, and similar mutations can cause different phenotypes!

Kearns-Sayre and Chronic Progressive External Ophthalmoplegia (CPEO) Syndromes

The following triad classifies Kearns-Sayre syndrome and CPEO:

- Ptosis
- Ophthalmoplegia
- Ragged-red fiber myopathy

This triad is very specific for the presence of an mtDNA mutation.

Kearns-Sayre syndrome is the most severe and can begin in infancy, childhood, or adolescence. In addition to the triad, multisystem disease is common, particularly cardiomyopathies, diabetes mellitus, cerebellar ataxia, and deafness.

Some present in infancy with a variant called **P**earson syndrome, which has **p**ancytopenia and **p**ancreatitis (think **P**s).

CPEO-plus is a disorder of intermediate severity that begins in adolescence or adulthood and has variable systemic involvement, including the eyelids and eye muscles.

Isolated CPEO is the mildest variant, but clinical signs/symptoms worsen with age. These individuals can progress to CPEO-plus or Kearns-Sayre syndrome.

These 3 variants are usually due to a rearrangement of mtDNA. Most of the mutations are spontaneous events during oogenesis or early embryogenesis and are not inherited. They can also occur as nuclear DNA mutations and be transmitted in an AD or AR fashion.

Myoclonic Epilepsy and Ragged-Red Fiber (MERRF) Disease

MERRF disease usually begins anytime from late childhood to adulthood. The 3 typical traits seen in this disorder are:

- Epilepsy
- Cerebellar ataxia
- Ragged-red fiber myopathy

Myoclonic jerks occur at rest and increase in frequency and amplitude with movement. Most of these are due to an A-to-G mutation of a nucleotide in the transfer RNA (tRNA) used by mtDNA.

Mitochondrial Encephalopathy, Lactic Acidosis, and Stroke-Like Episodes (MELAS)

MELAS can appear at any age, but most cases present before 45 years of age and are known as "stroke of the young." The stroke can be associated with migraines, seizures, or both. It can be difficult to distinguish MELAS from other causes of stroke, especially now that we are seeing more young people with atherosclerotic disease. Look for myopathy, ataxia, cardiomyopathy, deafness, and diabetes mellitus presenting before the stroke. Cerebellar ataxia most commonly occurs long before the stroke. The gene mutation is an A-to-G mutation in tRNA and is maternally inherited.

Note: As many as 1% of patients with adult-onset diabetes mellitus have the mutation, which brings an increased risk of stroke. Think of an oxidative phosphorylation disease in any young person with diabetes mellitus and stroke.

Leigh Syndrome

Consider Leigh syndrome (a.k.a. subacute necrotizing encephalopathy) when you see severe neurological findings (mental and movement), respiratory dysfunction, and ataxia with bilateral hyperintense signals on T2-weighted MRI of the basal ganglia, cerebellum, or brainstem. It typically occurs during infancy/early childhood. mtDNA mutations are usually responsible, although nuclear DNA mutations can also be causative, and it can have AR transmission. Besides the findings listed above, patients can have cardiomyopathy, sensory and motor neuropathies, and muscle weakness.

COMPLEX-MOLECULE DEFECTS

PREVIEW | REVIEW

- True or false? Most infants with mucopolysaccharidosis are normal at birth.
- What are the common features of Hurler syndrome?
- In which 2 ways is Hurler syndrome distinguished from Hunter syndrome?
- Describe Sanfilippo syndrome.
- What is Morquio syndrome?
- What are sphingolipidoses?
- Which type of Gaucher disease (GD) does not have CNS involvement?
- What is GD Type 1?
- How does GD Type 1 present?
- How effective is mutation screening for GD in persons of Ashkenazi Jewish ancestry?
- How does Niemann-Pick disease Type C present?
- Describe a child with Tay-Sachs disease.
- What is the classic eye finding in Tay-Sachs disease?
- How is Fabry disease inherited?
- What happens in children with Fabry disease when they are excessively overheated, as in exercise?
- What is the function of the peroxisome?
- Name the physical features of a patient with Zellweger spectrum disorder.
- Describe Lesch-Nyhan syndrome.
- What do you look for in homozygous children with familial hypercholesterolemia?
- Which disease should you suspect in a child whose father and 3 uncles all have tendon xanthomas?
- If you draw blood from a child with excessive chylomicronemia, spin it down, and leave the plasma in a test tube overnight, what will you see in the morning?
- What complaints would you expect from a child affected by lipoprotein-lipase deficiency?
- What is Smith-Lemli-Opitz syndrome?

OVERVIEW

The complex-molecule defect disorders are broken down into 2 major categories as well as an assortment of other categories:

- **Major categories**
  - Lysosomal storage disorders
    - Mucopolysaccharidoses
    - Sphingolipidoses
    - Pompe disease (classified as glycogen storage disorder)
  - Peroxisomal storage disorders
- **Other categories**
  - Disorders of mineral absorption and metabolism
  - Purine disorders
  - Inborn errors of cholesterol synthesis

Patients with complex-molecule defects exhibit symptoms that are permanent and progressive; symptoms do not wax and wane with general health or nutritional status. Often there is multiorgan involvement with storage of substance going to the soft tissues (e.g., liver, spleen, heart, joints, airway).

Some general screening tests for this group of disorders include urine oligosaccharides and mucopolysaccharides, WBC lysosomal enzyme studies, very-long-chain fatty acids, and serum sialo transferrins. Definitive diagnosis requires enzyme or mutation studies.

There is enzyme replacement for several lysosomal storage disorders; otherwise, treatment is symptomatic. Because these disorders are progressive, new problems evolve with time.

METABOLIC DISORDERS

LYSOSOMAL STORAGE DISORDERS

These are complex-molecule defects because symptoms result from lysosomal storage of large complex molecules. Lysosomes are cytoplasmic organelles where we normally degrade all sorts of compounds. If the body is unable to break down the macromolecules in the lysosomes, they are stored there, and the lysosomes enlarge. All of these disorders are progressive, and most are fatal. Most of these are usually known by their eponym (e.g., MPS 1H = Hurler syndrome).

In most of these disorders, infants are normal at birth, and the phenotypic characteristics of the disease appear over time as storage material accumulates.

Remember: This is where GSD Type 2 (Pompe disease) fits in; it was initially classified as a GSD and has not yet been reclassified.

See Table 23-5.

Table 23-5: Complex-Molecule Defects	
Category	**Examples**
Lysosomal storage disorders	MPS Gaucher disease Niemann-Pick disease Types A, B, and C Tay-Sachs disease Fabry disease
Peroxisomal diseases	Zellweger spectrum disorder X-ALD
Intracellular trafficking and processing defects	Menkes disease (kinky hair disease; copper defect) Wilson disease (copper defect) Hemochromatosis (iron defect) α_1-Antitrypsin deficiency Congenital disorders of glycosylation
Inborn errors of cholesterol synthesis	Smith-Lemli-Opitz syndrome Hypercholesterolemia (AD) Apolipoprotein E deficiency Tangier disease

AD = autosomal dominant
MPS = mucopolysaccharidosis
X-ALD = X-linked adrenoleukodystrophy

Mucopolysaccharidoses (MPSs)

MPSs result from defects in the catabolism of glycosaminoglycans by various lysosomal hydrolase enzymes. Lysosomes are cytoplasmic organelles that have enzymes, which phagocytose (degrade) the micromolecules (mucopolysaccharides, glycoproteins, and various lipids). Depending on the specific MPS disorder, there is accumulation of dermatan sulfate, heparan sulfate, or keratan sulfate in target organs.

Presentation is usually in 1 of 3 forms:

1) Dysmorphic/Coarse features: MPS 1H, MPS 2, MPS 6
2) Learning difficulties, behavior problems, and dementia: MPS 3
3) Severe bone dysplasia: MPS 4

Screen urine first for glycosaminoglycans, but inaccurate/false-negative results are common. WBC and plasma lysosomal enzyme studies can be helpful. Radiographs demonstrating dysostosis multiplex (skeletal abnormalities) are diagnostic. Enzyme replacement therapy is available for some of these disorders.

MPS Type 1 (Hurler Syndrome)

MPS Type 1 is AR and due to a defect in the gene coding for α-L-iduronidase. Disease presentations vary widely. MPS 1 subtypes represent a spectrum and include Hurler, Scheie, and Hurler-Scheie syndromes (not discussed here).

Those severely affected have **Hurler syndrome** (MPS 1H) and are frequently diagnosed within the first 2 years of life. They have coarsened facial features, with midface hypoplasia, large tongues, and **corneal clouding**. Early on, they have frequent URIs and may have inguinal/umbilical hernias. Head circumference is typically larger than the 95th percentile, and communicating hydrocephalus is common. They have severe intellectual disability. Obstructive sleep apnea is also typical, with surgical treatment often needed. Skeletal growth is usually normal during the 1st year, but severe growth restriction soon develops. These kids are at high risk for atlantoaxial subluxation. Evidence of hepatosplenomegaly and cardiac disease is seen systemically. Deafness is common.

Prognosis is generally related to the cardiac involvement, which can be severe and may predict early cardiomyopathy and death. Older children frequently have mitral and atrial valvular involvement. Early coronary artery disease is common.

Less severely affected individuals are often not diagnosed until early adulthood. Usually, they present with bone abnormalities (e.g., spondylolisthesis of L5/S1, degenerative bone loss) or eye problems (e.g., corneal clouding, retinal disease). There is a variant called **Scheie syndrome** (MPS 1S) in which patients have normal intelligence and life span; carpal tunnel syndrome is characteristic in this form.

Treatment of choice is enzyme replacement therapy for those with milder forms and later onset of symptoms. Hematopoietic stem cell transplant (HSCT) is successful in infants/children < 18 months of age to prevent intellectual deterioration—and provides a good chance for long-term survival. However, complex spinal surgery is still required because the HSCT does not correct the skeletal abnormalities. It appears that HSCT is useful only for MPS Types 1H and 6. (Type 6 is very rare and is not discussed here.)

Note: MPS 1 has been added to the Recommended Uniform Screening Panel (RSUP). See if your state has added MPS 1 to its newborn screening: babysfirsttest.org/newborn-screening/rusp-conditions#mucopolysaccharidosis-type-i

MPS Type 2 (Hunter Syndrome)

MPS Type 2 (Hunter syndrome) is X-linked recessive and is due to a defect in the gene that encodes for iduronate-2-sulfatase on the X chromosome. Therefore, only males display the trait (except for the rare affected female patient who has Turner syndrome, a chromosomal translocation, or nonrandom X inactivation).

Clinically, these patients can present with a very wide range of findings. If children are severely affected, it can look like a milder form of MPS 1 because most live into their midteens. In milder forms of MPS 2, normal life span is possible, as is the ability to reproduce and have normal intelligence. When compared, MPS 2 is distinct from MPS 1 in two ways:

1) MPS 2 is inherited as X-linked recessive (the only one that is X-linked).

2) Corneal clouding does not occur with MPS 2. (Remember that you have to be able to see well to hunt: Hunter's = no corneal clouding.)

In those severely affected, diagnosis is usually made by 2 years of age.

Typical findings are:

• Learning difficulties (with challenging behavior, attention deficit hyperactivity disorder [ADHD], or seizures)
• Middle ear disease
• Hernias
• Coarse facial appearance
• Diarrhea
• Joint stiffness
• Hepatosplenomegaly

A nodular rash around the scapulae and the extensor surfaces is pathognomonic (but rare in children). Atlantoaxial instability, as seen in MPS 1, is unusual in MPS 2. However, you can see cervical cord compression leading to cervical myelopathy. Adults with MPS 2 have upper respiratory obstruction and sleep apnea.

Cardiomyopathy is rare in younger patients, but uncomplicated valvular lesions are relatively common. Over time valvular heart leaflets become dysfunctional owing to glycosaminoglycan accumulation. Accumulation also results in thickened myocardium that eventually leads to coronary artery compromise and myocardial disease.

Treat with enzyme replacement therapy, which replaces the protein the body does not make in affected individuals. Enzyme replacement therapy improves most symptoms, including movement, stiff joints, breathing, growth, and facial features. Treatment, however, does not reverse or prevent CNS disease.

Note: MPS 2 has not yet been added to the Recommended Uniform Screening Panel (RSUP). See if your state has added MPS 2 to its newborn screening: babysfirsttest.org/newborn-screening/rusp-conditions#mucopolysaccharidosis-type-ii

MPS Type 3 (Sanfilippo Syndrome)

There are 4 described variants of MPS 3 (Sanfilippo syndrome): A, B, C, and D. MPS Type 3A is the most common. Each variant is AR and due to mutations in different enzymes. All variants are unable to break down heparin sulfate. The disease is usually diagnosed at ~ 4–5 years of age, with severe CNS involvement and mild somatic disease. This disproportionate CNS involvement is unique among the mucopolysaccharidoses. It typically follows a classic triphasic pattern:

• Phase 1—developmental delay with recurrent URIs, diarrhea, and sleep disturbance occurs before 1 year of age.
• Phase 2—severe, challenging behavior presents with hyperactivity and aggression. These children have no concept of danger to themselves and must be watched continuously. Family life is completely uprooted. Major tranquilizers are usually required to sedate the child and modify the aggressive behavior. Precocious puberty is common, as well as progressive loss of motor skills.
• Phase 3—swallowing dysfunction develops with further deterioration to a vegetative state by the midteens. Death occurs by the 20s.

MPS Type 4 (Morquio Syndrome)

MPS 4 (Morquio syndrome) is due to a deficiency of galactose-6-sulfatase, resulting in defective degradation of keratan sulfate. Characteristics include short-trunk dwarfism, fine corneal deposits, and skeletal (spondyloepiphyseal) dysplasia distinct from other types of MPS, along with normal intelligence.

These patients present during the 1st year of life with severe skeletal dysplasia but are not dysmorphic. Vertebral platyspondylisis is typical.

Adults with the severe form are < 3½ feet in height and have:

• Fixed hip flexion
• Genu valgum
• Pes planus
• Sternal protrusion
• Short neck

Odontoid dysplasia is universal and can be life-threatening. Most of the bone deformities cannot be corrected, and most patients eventually require motorized wheelchairs. Dental decay is also common.

METABOLIC DISORDERS

SPHINGOLIPIDOSES

Sphingolipidoses are characterized by defects in the lysosomal breakdown of sphingolipids. Again, these are disorders resulting from lysosomal storage of complex molecules. When the deficient enzymes can't break down the lipids effectively, there is a buildup of ceramide, which is the lipophilic core. There is also a buildup of 1 of 2 hydrophilic compounds: either oligosaccharide (comprising the glycosphingolipids) or phosphorylcholine (which is sphingomyelin).

The glycosphingolipids can be divided into 3 groups:

1) Globosides (RBC membranes and kidney)
2) Gangliosides (gray matter of the brain in synaptic terminals)
3) Galactocerebrosides (cerebral white matter)

Thus, if you know which "-side" is involved, you can figure out where the problem will occur! The glycosphingolipids (globosides, gangliosides, and galactocerebrosides) and sphingomyelin are mainly components of cell membranes. Remember that each of these conditions has a range of ages for onset, from neonatal to adult, depending on the level of enzyme activity. Generally, the more enzyme activity, the later the age of onset.

Gaucher Disease (GD)

Type 1

GD Type 1 is the most common lysosomal storage disease, affecting 1/900 persons of Ashkenazi Jewish ancestry (carrier rate in this group is 1/15). It is due to a deficiency of lysosomal glucocerebrosidase and results in an increased accumulation of glucocerebroside in the reticuloendothelial system. GD Type 1 is a non-CNS disease with only visceral involvement.

Splenomegaly is the most common presentation and is usually found incidentally on a routine physical examination. Abdominal protuberance is common. The hypersplenism predisposes to significant thrombocytopenia, which can result in severe bleeding. Younger children may complain of "growing pains" in the lower extremities, especially at night, and there may be bone infiltration with Gaucher cells (i.e., large macrophages laden with cerebrosides). Growth restriction is typical in those with severe disease.

At examination, look for an anemia-like complexion with increased pigmentation of the skin. Generally, though, these children look well, considering the extent of splenomegaly they have. CBC confirms anemia.

Diagnosis: Bone marrow studies show Gaucher storage cells. Confirm diagnosis by finding a deficiency of β-glucosidase in leukocytes or cultured skin fibroblasts.

Treatment: The best treatment is enzyme replacement therapy. Splenectomy is contraindicated because it causes increased storage in the lysosomes in the bone, resulting in worsened bone disease. Bone crises usually require narcotics. Enzyme replacement therapy is standard, with biweekly infusions of glucocerebrosidase. This reverses the hematologic and early skeletal complications of the disease.

Note: GD has not yet been added to the Recommended Uniform Screening Panel (RSUP). See if your state has added GD to its newborn screening: babysfirsttest.org/newborn-screening/rusp-conditions#gaucher

Type 2

Type 2, the acute neuronopathic form of GD, is also due to a deficiency of lysosomal glucocerebrosidase. This causes increased accumulation of glucocerebroside both in the reticuloendothelial system and the brain. Infants are usually normal initially; however, by 2–4 months of age, they start having feeding difficulties and FTT. They develop strabismus, have difficulty swallowing, and exhibit opisthotonic posturing. They have huge livers and spleens, but their liver function tests are typically only mildly affected. In a few infants, a macular cherry-red spot is visible bilaterally.

A characteristic lab result is an increased plasma tartrate-resistant acid phosphatase. Bone marrow aspiration shows classic Gaucher storage cells—large, mononucleated histiocytes with cytoplasm containing basophilic material that looks like wrinkled tissue paper. Unlike the later-presenting forms of GD, skeletal involvement is minimal.

You can confirm diagnosis by finding a deficiency of β-glucosidase in the leukocytes or cultured fibroblasts. Treatment for Type 2 is supportive. Bone marrow transplant is not helpful. Most of these infants die before 2 years of age due to FTT or pneumonia.

Type 3

Type 3 is the subacute neuronopathic form of GD. It is also due to a deficiency of lysosomal glucocerebrosidase. Previously, it was thought to be uncommon and occurring only in those of Swedish descent. Now we know it crosses all ethnic groups. There are 2 main groups for presentation:

1) **Type 3a** has more prominent neurologic findings with little visceral involvement.
2) **Type 3b** has prominent, severe visceral involvement.

Type 3a presents in early-to-middle childhood with myoclonus, dementia, and ataxia. Look for isolated, supranuclear, horizontal-gaze palsy. You'll see blinking, superimposed upward looping of the eyes, and head thrusting. Myoclonic seizures are typical later, along with spasticity. Hepatosplenomegaly is common but is not as severe as in Type 3b. Patients generally die before 30 years of age.

Type 3b cases appear as though they have severe Type 1 disease at ~ 2–3 years of age (described previously). The degree of hepatosplenomegaly is impressive and rapidly progressive compared to Type 1. Hepatocellular dysfunction is prominent with FTT, ascites, nosebleeds, and easy bruising. Portal hypertension and esophageal varices are common. The progression in the viscera is so rapid that neurologic manifestations are usually masked or never develop. The main finding of neurologic significance can be oculomotor apraxia—eye movements are not well executed.

Bone marrow shows the Gaucher cells. Confirm diagnosis by looking for deficiency of β-glucosidase in leukocytes or cultured skin fibroblasts. Bone marrow transplant is very effective in reversing the visceral and hematologic problems. We do not yet know the impact of bone marrow transplant on neurologic deterioration.

Perinatal Lethal Type

These infants present with severe GD and have thick, shiny, collodion-like skin. They have multiple congenital anomalies, hepatosplenomegaly, hypertonic and hyperreflexic movements, neck retraction, and a poor sucking mechanism. Nonimmune hydrops can be severe. They usually die within days or weeks.

GD Summary

Points to remember about the types of GD:

- Type 1 is the most common and does not have CNS involvement.
- Type 2 has the earliest onset, with neurologic symptoms as well as bleeding tendency.
- Type 3 has neurologic symptoms that are later in onset and more chronic than in Type 2.
- Perinatal lethal type is the most severe type; neonate dies within days to weeks.
- All forms include hepatosplenomegaly, bone lesions, and some lung disease.
- Diagnosis: 97% of mutations in persons of Ashkenazi Jewish ancestry, as compared to ~ 75% in the non-Jewish population, can be detected by screening for the 5 most common mutations.
- Note: Enzyme replacement therapy does not work for the neurologic disease of GD Types 2 and 3!

Niemann-Pick Disease (NPD)

Type A

Type A is a very rare form of NPD, occurring mainly in persons of Ashkenazi Jewish ancestry. Its degenerative and neurovisceral manifestations result from a deficiency of acid sphingomyelinase.

It initially causes vomiting, diarrhea, and FTT. Hepatosplenomegaly is prominent by 3 months of age. Neurologic problems occur at ~ 5–10 months of age with hypotonia, progressive loss of motor skills, and reduction in spontaneous movements. Of those affected, 50% have macular cherry-red spots, but usually these do not appear until after the occurrence of advanced neurologic disease.

Patients develop interstitial lung disease and frequent lung infections. Respiratory failure is a common cause of death, usually by 2–3 years of age.

Diagnose by finding low levels of sphingomyelinase in leukocytes or cultured fibroblasts. Treatment is supportive.

Type B

NPD Type B is due to incomplete deficiency of acid sphingomyelinase, and it is also most common in persons of Ashkenazi Jewish ancestry. It is the same as NPD Type A but has more residual enzyme activity; therefore, it is less severe than Type A—with later onset, longer survival, and little-to-no CNS involvement.

Clinically, it looks and presents just like Type 1 Gaucher disease, with isolated hepatosplenomegaly. Bone marrow studies show the foamy storage histocytes, as seen in NPD Type A; however, in Type B, the marrow also contains sea-blue histiocytes. Treatment is supportive, but severe disease appears to respond to bone marrow transplant.

Type C

Type C is the most common form of NPD and occurs in 250–500 children (1/150,000) each year in the U.S. The defect is not a lysosomal enzyme disorder, but instead is likely due to routing of cholesterol esters within and through the lysosome. Cholesterol accumulates within the lysosomes of the reticuloendothelial system. It is categorized with the lysosomal deficiency disorders because it was classified before we had the molecular genetic know-how to classify it correctly, but it does appear to cause secondary buildup of GM2 (disialotetrahexosylganglioside) gangliosidosis.

Most cases occur between 3 and 5 years of age with signs of ataxia and hepatosplenomegaly. In children 6–12 years of age, presentation usually includes poor school performance and impaired fine motor skills. Organomegaly generally occurs but is not present in up to 10% of cases. Cataplexy (e.g., sudden loss of motor movement after an emotional scare) and narcolepsy (i.e., uncontrolled attacks of sleep during the day) are common. On physical examination, the most common finding is **supranuclear vertical-gaze palsy** (downward, upward, or both). Voluntary, vertical eye movement is lost, but reflex "doll's eye" movements are preserved. Dysphagia is common and, if progressive, results in the need for a feeding tube. Death in the teenage years is common.

Another possible phenotype is isolated organomegaly. This is being further examined and is likely underdiagnosed.

Diagnosis: Demonstrate intralysosomal accumulation of unesterified cholesterol in cultured fibroblasts.

Treatment is supportive, but limited data suggests that substrate reduction therapy may be beneficial for some patients with Type C.

METABOLIC DISORDERS

Note: NPD has not yet been added to the Recommended Uniform Screening Panel (RSUP). See if your state has added NPD to its newborn screening: babysfirsttest.org/newborn-screening/rusp-conditions #niemann-pick-disease

Tay-Sachs Disease

Tay-Sachs disease is an AR disorder that causes mutations in the *HEXA* gene, resulting in disruption of the enzyme β-hexosaminidase A. This enzyme breaks down the glycolipid GM2 ganglioside. As a result of the enzymatic defect, GM2 ganglioside builds to toxic levels in the neurons, especially in the brain and spinal cord, causing progressive destruction of the neurons. Symptoms include blindness, deafness, and paralysis. Increasingly toxic levels can result in death.

Diagnosis is made by demonstrating low hexosaminidase A activity in blood or tissue and is confirmed by DNA analysis.

There are 2 forms of the disease:

1) The **infantile form** usually begins within the 1st few months of life and is due to β-hexosaminidase α-subunit deficiency. It is most prominent in persons of Eastern European Jewish ancestry and in French Canadian and Cajun populations. The 1st symptom, usually at 3–6 months of age, is frequently an enhanced startle reflex to noise or light and quick extension of the arms and legs with clonic movements. Unlike the Moro reflex, this does not diminish with repeated stimuli. Motor skills are progressively lost. Axial hypotonia, extremity hypertonia, and hyperreflexia are common. In > 90% of infants, a **macular cherry-red spot** (Figure 23-7) occurs bilaterally. This is due to storage of lipids that causes white discoloration everywhere in the retina except the fovea, which remains the normal red color of the retina. While the macular cherry-red spot is a feature of other storage disorders that include hepatosplenomegaly, the visceral organs are normal in patients with Tay-Sachs. Macrocephaly is common. Auditory stimuli cause seizures. By 2–3 years of age, the child has decerebrate rigidity, is blind, and is unable to respond to stimuli. Autonomic dysfunction also occurs. Frequently, the child dies by 4–5 years of age.

2) The **juvenile/adult form** occurs in persons of Ashkenazi Jewish ancestry and has an indolent presentation. Early in childhood, the children are labeled "clumsy and awkward." The 1st sign may be an intention tremor (usually by 10 years of age). School problems can occur early on with dysarthria. By adolescence, proximal muscle weakness occurs with fasciculations and atrophy. Psychiatric symptoms are common and include anxiety, depression, and suicide. With appropriate help, patients with this form can continue to ambulate until their 60s.

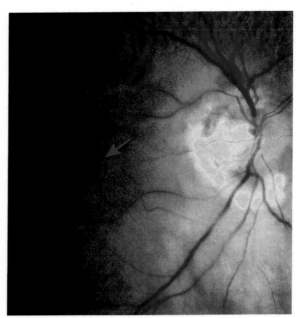

Figure 23-7: Tay-Sachs cherry-red spot

Fabry Disease

Fabry disease is the only sphingolipidosis transmitted as an X-linked recessive disease; thus, it mainly affects boys. However, some heterozygous girls develop similar pain crises. Boys present at puberty with complaints of severe, episodic neuropathic pain in the hands and feet. Fever and increased erythrocyte sedimentation rate (ESR) are common with the pain crises. Heat exposure, especially during physical exertion, initiates the pain crises, and the patient does not sweat or sweats very little (hypohidrosis).

Usually, by the mid-to-late teenage years, affected boys develop angiokeratomata—tiny, red-to-dark blue, papular lesions on the buttocks, scrotum, penis, buccal mucosa, and in the umbilicus. They are individual, ectatic blood vessels covered with a few layers of skin. The lesions are without other symptoms, except they tend to bleed if traumatized.

Corneal opacities are common but do not interfere with vision. Renal disease, coronary artery disease, and stroke occur in early adulthood even in some manifesting heterozygous females. Autonomic nervous system dysfunction occurs and can present as chronic diarrhea, constipation, and the hypohidrosis described above. Cerebrovascular complications include hemiparesis, vertigo, diplopia, nystagmus, headache, ataxia, and memory loss.

Diagnosis: Urine shows casts and Maltese crosses (birefringent lipid globules). Confirm by finding deficiency of lysosomal α-galactosidase in plasma, leukocytes, or cultured skin fibroblasts.

Treatment: Painful peripheral neuropathy appears to respond to carbamazepine or gabapentin. IV infusion of purified α-galactosidase seems to also relieve pain. Enzyme replacement therapy is clinically available and approved by the FDA; however, no consistent recommendations currently exist for its use in females and children. Renal transplant is required for end-stage renal disease.

Note: Fabry disease has not yet been added to the Recommended Uniform Screening Panel (RSUP). See if your state has added Fabry disease to its newborn screening: babysfirsttest.org/newborn-screening/rusp-conditions#fabry

Sphingolipidoses Pearls

Know these key points:

- All disorders are AR, except for Fabry disease (X-linked).
- Enzyme replacement therapy is available for Gaucher's and Fabry's.
- Enzyme replacement therapy is effective in preventing/reversing the hematologic and early skeletal complications of Gaucher's (all types), but it does not affect the neurologic problems of Types 2 and 3.
- Gaucher's and Fabry's are included on some U.S. states' newborn screening.
- See Table 23-6 to help you remember which sphingolipidoses involve the CNS.

Table 23-6: Sphingolipidoses — CNS or Not?	
CNS Diseases	
CNS only	Tay-Sachs
CNS with hepatosplenomegaly	Gaucher Types 2 and 3 NPD Types A and C
CNS with vascular and pulmonary involvement	NPD Type A
Non-CNS Diseases	
Predominantly hepatosplenomegaly	Gaucher Type 1 NPD Type B
Peripheral nervous system +/- skin lesions and cardiac, renal, vascular, or pulmonary involvement	Fabry disease

CNS = central nervous system
NPD = Niemann-Pick disease

PEROXISOMAL DISORDERS

First, what are peroxisomes? These are organelles that have a single membrane and are found in just about all cells except RBCs. Peroxisomes contain > 50 different enzymes, including a group of important enzymes that catalyze β-oxidation of fatty acids. These enzymes differ from the mitochondrial enzymes that break down fatty acids. The peroxisomal enzymes oxidize very-long-chain and long-chain fatty acids, whereas the mitochondrial enzymes oxidize the long-, medium-, and short-chain fatty acids. Another difference is that in peroxisomal oxidation, the 1st step is the production of hydrogen peroxide

(H_2O_2), which is later eliminated by another enzyme in the peroxisomal cascade.

Generally, there are 2 classes of peroxisomal disorders:

1) Peroxisomal biogenesis disorders, which involve a deficiency of multiple peroxisome functions
2) Single-function disorders, in which only 1 peroxisomal function is missing

The peroxisomal biogenesis disorders are all AR, and their combined frequency for the 12+ disorders is ~ 1/50,000. Zellweger spectrum disorder is the classic one usually described. The single-function peroxisome disorders are much less typical and can be AR or X-linked in inheritance. The most commonly described is X-linked adrenoleukodystrophy (X-ALD).

Zellweger Spectrum Disorder (ZSD)

ZSD is at the severe end of the spectrum for disorders of peroxisome function; this includes **infantile Refsum disease** and **neonatal adrenoleukodystrophy**. There is reduced or absent function of all the peroxisome enzymes. Onset of symptoms ranges from birth to 1–2 years of age with loss of skills and a progressive course. These infants have characteristic facies with high forehead, epicanthal folds, broad-based nasal bridge, anteverted nares, and micrognathia. Other prominent findings include a large anterior fontanelle, cataracts, pigmented retinopathy, hearing loss, and vision loss. Liver function is abnormal, and jaundice occurs. Calcific stippling (discrete, precise calcifications) of the patella and epiphyses of the long bones is common. Most affected infants die before 1 year of age.

Confirm diagnosis by demonstrating elevated serum levels of very-long-chain fatty acids, phytanic acid, and pipecolic acid.

X-Linked Adrenoleukodystrophy (X-ALD)

There are multiple clinical presentations for boys with X-ALD; the most severe is the childhood cerebral form. It rapidly progresses with central demyelination and begins between 3 and 10 years of age. The childhood cerebral form occurs in > 33% of those affected and eventually progresses to death within 5–10 years of diagnosis. Almost all these boys have adrenal insufficiency. Another phenotype is adrenomyeloneuropathy. It does not show up until the 30s or 40s and presents with distal axonopathy of the spinal cord, causing gait disturbance and urinary sphincter dysfunction; ~ 66% have adrenal insufficiency, and nearly 40% have cerebral effects. Diagnosis is aided by looking for elevated plasma very-long-chain fatty acid levels, particularly C26:0.

Note: X-ALD has been added to the Recommended Uniform Screening Panel (RSUP). See if your state has added X-ALD disease to its newborn screening: babysfirsttest.org/newborn-screening/rusp-conditions#adrenoleukodystrophy.

METABOLIC DISORDERS

DISORDERS OF MINERAL ABSORPTION OR METABOLISM

Menkes Disease (Kinky Hair Disease)

Menkes disease is a very rare X-linked recessive disease (therefore, only present in males) due to a mutation in the Menkes gene (*ATP7A*), which causes impaired uptake of copper. It occurs in ~ 1/50,000 to 1/250,000 births.

Males usually present in the neonatal period with premature delivery, temperature instability, hypothermia, hypotonia, and hypoglycemia. They have characteristic facies: pudgy cheeks and sagging jowls and lips. Hair and eyebrows are sparse with little pigment and are easily broken. It is called kinky hair disease because of the characteristic look of the hair. Under the microscope, the hair has pili torti—a flattened shaft with clusters of narrow twists at irregular intervals. By 2–3 months of age, infants have progressive neurologic deterioration, along with seizures and loss of milestones; that is, if they ever made any developmental gains. Collagen and bone formation are abnormal. This is one of the few genetic diseases (glutaric acidemia Type 1 is another) that can have **subdural hematomas** and **retinal hemorrhages** not due to child abuse. It usually progresses, with death at ~ 2 years of age.

Copper measurements are high in intestinal biopsies but low in liver biopsies. When considering the diagnosis in an infant, you cannot rely on copper and ceruloplasmin levels because they are normally low. You need to measure dopamine-β-hydroxylase; partial deficiency of this enzyme is a hallmark of Menkes disease.

Wilson Disease

Wilson disease is an AR disorder of copper metabolism that results in excessive copper accumulation in tissues. (See the Gastroenterology section.)

Hereditary Hemochromatosis

Hereditary hemochromatosis is most commonly due to a mutation in the *HFE* gene that causes increased iron absorption from the intestines. (See the Gastroenterology section.)

PURINE DISORDERS

Purines, made up of carbon and nitrogen, are major components of cellular energy (e.g., adenosine triphosphate [ATP]), cellular signaling (e.g., cyclic adenosine monophosphate [cAMP]), and DNA/RNA production. Defects in the enzymes used to metabolize purines can lead to clinical disorders.

Lesch-Nyhan Syndrome

Lesch-Nyhan syndrome is an X-linked recessive disorder caused by deficiency of hypoxanthine guanine phosphoribosyltransferase (HGPRT). This enzyme preserves hypoxanthine and guanine and then converts them to nucleotides.

These males are normal at birth but have FTT, hypotonia, emesis, and irritability by 3–6 months of age. Most patients exhibit abnormal posturing by 18 months of age. By 2–3 years of age, **self-mutilation**, the most disturbing manifestation, develops. The children bite their lips and fingers. Renal stones and gout occur because of the huge increase in uric acid production.

Diagnose by finding HGPRT deficiency in RBCs and cultured skin fibroblasts.

DISORDERS OF LIPIDS AND LIPOPROTEINS

Screening guidelines are discussed in the Cardiology section.

Hyperlipoproteinemia Disorders

Familial Combined Hyperlipidemia

Familial combined hyperlipidemia is a syndrome in which low-density lipoprotein (LDL) is usually elevated but LDL receptor activity is normal. The increased LDL is due to overproduction of very-low-density lipoprotein (VLDL) and apolipoprotein B (apoB) in the liver. It occurs in ~ 1/100 births. These children can have elevated LDL alone (Type 2a), elevated LDL and triglycerides (Type 2b), or normal LDL and elevated triglycerides (Type 4). This presents in adults with early coronary artery disease, so ask about the child's family history of early heart disease. Corneal arcus (i.e., deposition of lipid in the peripheral corneal stroma) can occur, but xanthomas do not. Management consists of lifestyle changes in diet and exercise and statin drugs to lower LDL cholesterol.

Familial Hypercholesterolemia (FH)

FH occurs in 1/200 to 1/500 births. This AD disorder is caused by mutations at the gene locus for LDL receptor protein, resulting in reduced clearance of LDL. Homozygotes (HoHF) are more severely affected than heterozygotes (HeHF); HoHF is much rarer than HeHF.

Children with HeFH are usually asymptomatic in the 1st decade, but by the 2nd decade, nearly 10–15% develop xanthomas of the Achilles or extensor hand tendons. Achilles tendonitis or tenosynovitis can be the 1st clue in a teenage patient. HeFH is diagnosed by high levels of total cholesterol and LDL, in addition to at least one of the following:

- Family history of FH or hypercholesterolemia
- Personal or family history of premature coronary heart disease
- Physical signs of abnormal cholesterol deposition (e.g., tendon xanthomas)

Untreated FH male heterozygotes have a 100% risk of developing coronary heart disease by 70 years of age, whereas untreated females have a 75% risk. Treatment reduces this risk by normalizing cholesterol.

Children with HoHF develop planar xanthomas (flat, orange-colored skin lesions) from birth to 5 years of age. Serum cholesterol is usually 600–1,000 mg/dL. Tendon and tuberous **xanthomas** occur between 5 and 15 years of age. Angina and symptomatic coronary disease occur in the 2nd decade and have been documented in children < 10 years of age.

When considering a diagnosis of FH, look for a child with parents who have tendon xanthomas or with many 1st degree relatives with highly elevated LDL-cholesterol levels. Be aware that other conditions (e.g., biliary cirrhosis, congenital biliary atresia, myelomas) can cause lipid deposition, but other findings are also apparent to help you differentiate among them.

Treatment consists of a combination of lifestyle (diet and exercise) changes, cholesterol-lowering statins, and, in severe cases, LDL apheresis.

Be on the lookout for **sitosterolemia**, a rare inherited plant sterol storage disease. This disorder has tendon xanthomas in the 1st decade but only moderate hypercholesterolemia.

Lipoprotein-Lipase Deficiency

Lipoprotein-lipase enzyme deficiency/defectiveness results in huge increases of chylomicrons with marked hypertriglyceridemia (up to 10,000 mg/dL). Marked chylomicronemia usually indicates that the body cannot clear dietary fat. You can demonstrate this by leaving an affected individual's plasma in a test tube overnight—in the morning, a thick, creamy layer is apparent. VLDL is normal, and LDL and high-density lipoprotein (HDL) are low.

It usually presents before 10 years of age with abdominal pain as the initial complaint; colic, in particular, occurs in infants < 1 year of age. Eruptive xanthomas, hepatosplenomegaly, and retinal deposits can occur; atherosclerosis usually does not.

Hypolipoproteinemia Disorders

Abetalipoproteinemia

Abetalipoproteinemia is a rare AR disorder that presents in children with fat malabsorption, hypolipidemia, retinitis pigmentosa, cerebellar ataxia, and acanthocytosis. Chylomicrons, VLDL, and LDL are absent from plasma. Cholesterol and triglycerides are low. Clinically, this is important because the fat-soluble vitamins (A, D, E, and K) are dependent and cannot be absorbed or transported properly. However, only **vitamin E deficiency** is clinically apparent because of other available transport mechanisms. The retinal and nervous system effects are due to vitamin E deficiency.

Diagnosis is by jejunal biopsy, failure to form chylomicrons after a fatty meal, or demonstration of the absence of apoB in plasma.

Smith-Lemli-Opitz Syndrome

Smith-Lemli-Opitz is an AR disorder due to a defect in cholesterol biosynthesis resulting from deficient activity of 7-dehydrocholesterol reductase. It occurs in ~ 1/20,000 to 1/40,000 births. Remember: Cholesterol is very important in embryogenesis. Therefore, if abnormalities occur during this time, expect marked dysmorphology. The clinical findings range from an isolated partial 2/3-toe syndactyly (Figure 23-8) with developmental delay to severely malformed fetuses that die in utero.

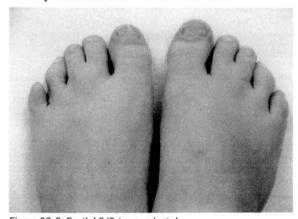

Figure 23-8: Partial 2/3-toe syndactyly

The characteristic facial features of the severe form include:

- Microcephaly
- Narrow bifrontal diameter
- Hypertelorism
- Ptosis
- Broad nasal tip
- Anteverted nostrils
- Cleft palate
- Micrognathia
- Low-set ears

In the severe form, the following additional findings are also typical:

- Postaxial polydactyly
- Overlapping fingers
- Abnormal thumbs
- Partial 2/3-toe syndactyly
- Hypospadias
- Ambiguous genitalia

All organ systems can be affected, and intellectual disability is standard. Congenital heart defects are common and should be investigated.

Serum levels of 7-dehydrocholesterol will be elevated, and cholesterol will be normal to low. Remember: The enzyme is deficient, so you get a backup of 7-dehydrocholesterol, and the cholesterol level inversely correlates with severity of disease.

No treatment has proven effective. Treatment with dietary cholesterol and bile-acid supplements to correct serum cholesterol levels may be helpful.

Tangier Disease

Tangier disease is a rare disorder in which plasma HDL is abnormal and deficient. Cholesterol ester is deposited in tissues, resulting in enlarged, orange-yellow tonsils; splenomegaly; and peripheral neuropathy.

NEWBORN SCREENING (NBS)

PREVIEW | REVIEW

- What is the purpose of the newborn screening?

Since its inception, NBS has detected progressively more inborn errors of metabolism. What was once known as the PKU test has now expanded to cover ~ 36 disorders in most U.S. states. It is important to know which disorders can be detected on NBS. NBS is accomplished in most states by tandem mass spectroscopy in newborn screening laboratories.

The goal of the NBS is to detect life-threatening and/or potentially serious disorders that can be treated effectively.

Currently, NBS tests primarily for IEMs that cause intoxications and/or energy metabolism defects:

- Amino acid defects
- β-Oxidation defects
- Galactosemia
- Biotinidase deficiency

Complex-molecule disorders that have recently been added to the Recommended Uniform Screening Panel (RSUP) include:

- X-linked adrenoleukodystrophy
- Pompe disease
- MPS 1

Nonmetabolic disorders on NBS are:

- Hemoglobinopathies
- Endocrine disorders such as congenital adrenal hyperplasia and congenital hypothyroidism
- Cystic fibrosis
- Immune deficiencies
- Neuromuscular disorders (spinal muscular atrophy)
- Congenital infections (toxoplasmosis)

Other disorders included on NBS that are not blood based include hearing impairments and congenital heart defects.

NBS does not screen for the liver forms of GSDs or mitochondrial defects.

Historically, NBS did not screen for lysosomal storage disorders. As this group of disorders has become treatable with enzyme replacement therapy or bone marrow transplants, there is a move to include them on the NBS. Some states have implemented screening for Fabry, Gaucher, and Niemann-Pick diseases, as well as MPS 2 and Krabbe disease (a.k.a. globoid cell leukodystrophy, a lysosomal storage disorder that results in globoid cell formation and decreased myelin in the central and peripheral nervous systems). Stay tuned—this list continues to grow!

Check out your state here: babysfirsttest.org/newborn-screening/rusp-conditions#all

THE MEDSTUDY HUB: YOUR GUIDELINES AND REVIEW ARTICLES RESOURCE

For both review articles and current pediatrics practice guidelines, visit the MedStudy Hub at

medstudy.com/hub

The Hub contains the only online consolidated list of all current guidelines focused on pediatrics. Guidelines on the Hub are easy to find, continually updated, and linked to the published source. MedStudy maintains the Hub as a service to the medical community and makes it available to anyone and everyone at no cost to users.

FIGURE SOURCES

Figure 23-1: MedStudy illustration
Figure 23-2: MedStudy illustration
Figure 23-3: MedStudy illustration
Figure 23-4: MedStudy illustration
Figure 23-5: MedStudy illustration
Figure 23-6: MedStudy illustration
Figure 23-8: AzaToth, CC BY-SA 3.0
The remaining figure is from the MedStudy archives.

METABOLIC DISORDERS

Hematology

SECTION EDITOR

Ewurabena A. Simpson, MD, MPH
Staff Physician
Children's Hospital of Eastern Ontario
Assistant Professor, Faculty of Medicine
University of Ottawa
Ottawa, Ontario, Canada

MEDICAL EDITOR

Lynn Bullock, MD
Colorado Springs, CO

Table of Contents

DEVELOPMENTAL CHANGES OF RED BLOOD CELLS (RBCs)

PREVIEW | REVIEW

- Describe the changes in location that take place in fetal red blood cell (RBC) production.
- What regulates the production of RBCs?
- Where is erythropoietin (EPO) produced in the fetus?
- Where is EPO produced after birth?
- What factors are responsible for the "physiologic anemia of infancy"?
- What is the difference between fetal hemoglobin and adult hemoglobin?
- What happens to the oxygen dissociation curve after birth?

SITES OF BLOOD FORMATION

The anatomic sites for RBC formation change during embryonic and fetal life. The 1st site of red blood cell formation in the fetus is the **yolk sac** at 2–3 weeks of gestation. By the 5–6th week of gestation, RBC formation shifts to the **liver**, increases, peaks at 5 months, and decreases thereafter. The **spleen** then takes over as the major site of activity until around 7 months of gestation, at which time the **bone marrow** takes over and remains the predominant site for RBC production (refer to Hemoglobin on page 24-2). In extraordinary circumstances, such as myelofibrosis or severe hemolytic anemia, RBC production occurs in extramedullary sites (e.g., liver, spleen).

RBC INDICES

The amount of oxygen delivered to tissues depends on cardiac output in combination with the supply and function of RBCs and hemoglobin. There are laboratory tests that demonstrate this.

The mean corpuscular volume (**MCV**) reflects the size of the RBCs, whereas the mean corpuscular hemoglobin (**MCH**) and the mean corpuscular hemoglobin concentration (**MCHC**) reflect the amount of hemoglobin in RBCs. MCH is the average mass of hemoglobin in each RBC. MCHC is a related value demonstrating the average concentration of hemoglobin per RBC.

Red blood cell distribution width (**RDW**) measures variability in RBC size (anisocytosis). An increased RDW means increased variation in RBC size.

Reticulocytes are immature RBCs. A reticulocyte count (**retic count**) is often reported as the percentage of reticulocytes to total number of RBCs in the blood and indicates if the bone marrow is producing an adequate number of RBCs. By early neonatal life, the normal range for retic count is approximately 0.5–2%, which is the same as that of an adult.

PRODUCTION RATES AND NORMAL VALUES

Production rates and normal values depend on age, sex, ethnicity, pubertal stage, altitude, and clinical conditions/factors.

The Fetus

In the fetus, the RBC count triples from 12 weeks of gestation to term. MCV decreases from 180 fL at 12 weeks to 108 fL at term (which is still macrocytic when compared to older children). Retic counts in term infants average ~ 5%, and it is common for nucleated RBCs to circulate freely for several days after birth.

The Newborn

In the first few days after birth, hemoglobin levels are much higher in capillaries than in venous blood due to a loss of plasma from the capillaries. Also, venous hemoglobin, hematocrit, and RBC counts increase between birth and the first 3 days of life due to a postnatal decrease in plasma volume.

The production of RBCs is regulated by erythropoietin (EPO), which is produced by the liver in the fetus. Production switches from the liver to the kidneys soon after birth. EPO production is regulated by tissue oxygenation. At birth, hemoglobin averages 17 g/dL; this relative polycythemia is due to the low arterial P_aO_2 in utero that stimulates EPO production and thus increases erythropoiesis. Arterial P_aO_2 rises acutely at birth, resulting in a decrease in EPO production. Nucleated RBCs disappear from the peripheral blood, and the retic count falls. Red cell lifespan during the first 6–8 weeks of life is around 90 days instead of the usual 120 days. This results in the "physiologic anemia of infancy," which reaches its nadir around 2–3 months of age, with an average hemoglobin level of 9–11 g/dL. If this is found on laboratory evaluation, no further biochemical follow-up is needed. After 6–8 weeks of life, RBC production resumes and retic counts increase, as does the hemoglobin.

The Preterm Infant

The preterm infant has an even more dramatic fall in hemoglobin concentration than the term newborn. By 2 months of age, hemoglobin falls to 9.5 g/dL in infants with birth weights between 1,500 and 2,000 g and to 9 g/dL for those infants weighing between 1,000 and 1,500 g at birth. Hemoglobin levels drop further for infants with a very low birth weight. Preterm infants have inappropriately low levels of EPO in response to their anemia and thus cannot stimulate production of RBCs.

Older Children and Adolescents

In preschool- and school-aged children, erythropoiesis keeps up with growth, and the mean hemoglobin increases. The values for boys and girls diverge at adolescence due to the erythroid-stimulating effects of androgens in adolescent males.

MCV falls during the first 6–12 months of life, during which time it reaches its nadir of 77 fL, and then rises throughout childhood and adolescence.

Retic counts are normally < 2% after 4 months of age, and nucleated RBCs disappear from the circulation after the first week of life.

Blood volume is fairly constant after 6 months of age and remains at 75–77 mL/kg.

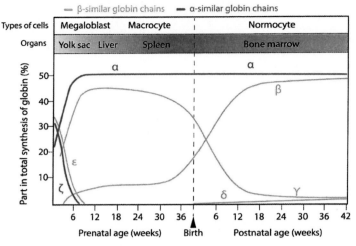

Figure 24-2: Developmental globin synthesis

HEMOGLOBIN

Hemoglobin is a tetramer made up of 2 pairs of globin chains, each attached to an iron-containing porphyrin ring (heme). The globin chain is designated by a Greek letter followed by a subscript that shows the number of chains per molecule. For example, normal adult hemoglobin (HbA) contains 2 pairs of alpha and beta chains and is designated $\alpha_2\beta_2$. See Figure 24-1.

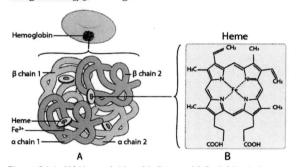

Figure 24-1: (A) Hemoglobin with 2 α- and 2 β-globin chains and 1 iron-containing heme group in each protein subunit; (B) the heme group with a porphyrin ring complexed with iron

In the embryo, hemoglobin is predominantly Gower-1, Gower-2, and Portland, and they contain zeta and epsilon (ζ and ε) chains. By 8–12 weeks of gestation, the Gower and Portland hemoglobins disappear and fetal hemoglobin (HbF) predominates. HbF contains alpha and gamma chains and is known as $\alpha_2\gamma_2$. It accounts for 90% of the circulating hemoglobin in a 24-week-old fetus, after which it begins to be replaced by adult hemoglobin. At birth, HbF makes up 50–80% of the total hemoglobin; by 4 months of age, HbF is less than 20% of the total; and by 1 year of age, it makes up less than 2% of hemoglobin. In patients with β-chain hemoglobinopathies, the amount of HbF remains elevated. HbA$_2$ ($\alpha_2\delta_2$), or minor adult hemoglobin, is produced in late gestation and accounts for about 2–3% of total hemoglobin after the first few months of life. HbA$_2$ is elevated in β-thalassemia and β-thalassemia trait (Figure 24-2).

OXYGEN TRANSPORT

Oxygen transport is tied to the intrinsic function of hemoglobin. In the fetus and newborn, the oxygen dissociation curve favors oxygen extraction from the maternal circulation. This limits the proportional release of oxygen to the tissues after birth. The oxygen dissociation curve shifts to the right after birth to allow better release of oxygen to the tissues; this is due mainly to the change from HbF to HbA and the effect of 2,3-diphosphoglycerate (2,3-DPG), which is found in RBCs and is a potent affinity modulator.

ANEMIA

PREVIEW | REVIEW

- Which tests are recommended in the initial workup of anemia?

- Know the significance of specific changes in the peripheral smear, as described in Table 24-1 on page 24-5.

- Know the defects, etiologies, and examples of the different classifications of anemia in Table 24-2 on page 24-7.

- What is the significance of elevated minor adult hemoglobin (HbA$_2$) in the evaluation of microcytic anemia?

- What is hemoglobin Bart? Under what conditions is Hb Bart seen?

- What is the most common type of hypoproliferative anemia?

- What infection is most commonly responsible for chronic gastrointestinal blood loss in children worldwide?

- How can you use red blood cell distribution width to differentiate iron deficiency anemia from β-thalassemia minor?

- Which animal's milk is low in folate and results in folate deficiency in infants exclusively given this type of milk?

- How do you differentiate between the congenital and juvenile forms of pernicious anemia?

- Which cause of macrocytic anemia can lead to neurologic problems?

- What is the genetic defect that results in hemoglobin S?

- What is the average lifespan of a sickle cell?

- How do you diagnose sickle cell disease (SCD)?

- What is the most common reason for hospital admission of a patient with SCD?

- What is the most common first crisis in children with SCD?

- What is the most common cause of death for adolescents with SCD?

- Which types of bacterial infection result in serious disease in children with SCD?

- At what age is penicillin prophylaxis started in patients with SCD?

- Which infection causes aplastic crisis in patients with SCD?

- What is the acute treatment for a stroke in a patient with SCD?

- What is priapism?

- What are the treatment options for priapism with SCD?

- When are people with sickle cell trait at risk for sickle cell–related complications?

- What is the genetic defect in hemoglobin C (HbC)?

- What clinical features are found with HbCC?

- What clinical features are found with HbC trait?

- Is G6PD testing reliable during a hemolytic crisis?

- How do you diagnose glucose-6-phosphate dehydrogenase (G6PD) deficiency?

- What is the underlying defect in hereditary spherocytosis?

- How are the direct and indirect Coombs tests performed, and when are they ordered?

- Which pathogens cause cold agglutinin disease in children?

NORMAL ERYTHROPOIESIS

Erythropoietin regulates RBC production. Normal erythropoiesis involves maturation of stem cells: proerythroblasts → erythroblasts of different stages → reticulocytes → mature cells (Figure 24-3). Reticulocytes have lost their nucleus but retain RNA. The mature RBCs in the peripheral blood have lost their RNA. A special stain is used to quantify reticulocytes, but they are easily recognized on a peripheral blood smear (polychromasia).

Mature RBCs have a lifespan of 120 days. The spleen removes old or damaged RBCs, which are then ingested by macrophages —part of the reticuloendothelial system. The hemoglobin (Hgb) is catabolized, and the porphyrin ring of heme is opened, forming unconjugated (indirect) bilirubin. Haptoglobin binds and transports free Hgb in serum.

Proerythroblast
↓
Basophilic erythroblast
↓
Polychromatic erythroblast
↓
Pyknotic erythroblast
↓
Reticulocyte
↓
Mature RBC

Figure 24-3: Erythropoiesis

Iron released from heme, or absorbed in the intestine from the diet, is transported by transferrin to the bone marrow and stored as ferritin. Therefore, ferritin typically reflects iron stores—but remember that it is also an acute phase reactant and does not accurately reflect iron stores if there is ongoing inflammation. (Transferrin saturation and total iron-binding capacity [TIBC] are indirect measures of iron levels as well.)

CLINICAL MANIFESTATIONS OF ANEMIA

Patients with chronic anemia are usually asymptomatic, even with significant anemia. Some symptomatic clues are:

- Pica, ice-eating (pagophagia), lethargy: iron deficiency
- Distal paresthesias: B_{12} deficiency
- Left upper quadrant abdominal pain: hereditary spherocytosis with splenomegaly
- Right upper quadrant pain or intolerance to fatty foods: cholelithiasis from chronic hemolysis
- Constipation and cold intolerance: hypothyroidism

LABORATORY RESULTS

The initial workup of anemia is often prompted by the clinical presentation, which can include pallor, jaundice, and decreased activity. The evaluation starts with a complete blood count (CBC), including red cell indices, retic count, and examination of the peripheral blood smear. See Figure 24-4 through Figure 24-9 on page 24-4 for different magnifications of normal peripheral smears and bone marrow aspirates.

One approach to classification of anemias is based on the red cell indices (Figure 24-10 on page 24-4). Mean corpuscular volume (MCV) is the average size of RBCs in a specimen, and anemias are characterized as microcytic (low MCV), normocytic (normal MCV), or macrocytic (high MCV):

- Microcytic anemia results from iron deficiency (Figure 24-11 on page 24-5), thalassemia traits, certain hemoglobinopathies, sideroblastic anemia, and, sometimes, anemia of chronic disease (ACD; a.k.a. anemia of chronic inflammation).
- Normocytic anemias result from acute blood loss, certain hemolytic anemias, and most cases of ACD.

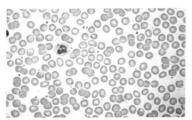

Figure 24-4: Normal peripheral smear: low-power view. RBCs, platelets, and segmented neutrophil

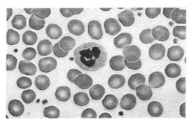

Figure 24-5: Normal peripheral smear: low-oil view. Normocytic, normochromic RBCs; platelets; and normal segmented neutrophil

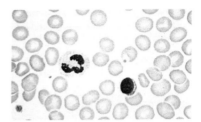

Figure 24-6: Normal peripheral smear: high-dry view. RBCs, platelets, normal segmented neutrophil, and normal lymphocyte

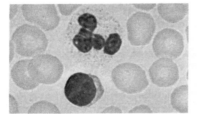

Figure 24-7: Normal peripheral smear: high-oil view. Normal RBCs, segmented neutrophil, and lymphocyte. No platelets are visible in this field.

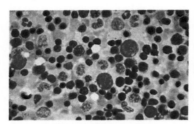

Figure 24-8: Normal bone marrow aspirate: low-power view. M:E (myeloid to erythroid) ratio is usually 3:1. This field has more than the normal number of erythroid precursors. Many of the erythroid precursors have dark, condensed nuclei.

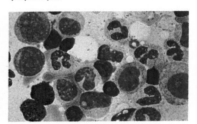

Figure 24-9: Normal bone marrow aspirate: low-oil view. 5 erythroid precursors (dark, condensed nuclei). Remaining cells are myeloid precursors/cells—from myeloblasts to segmented neutrophils.

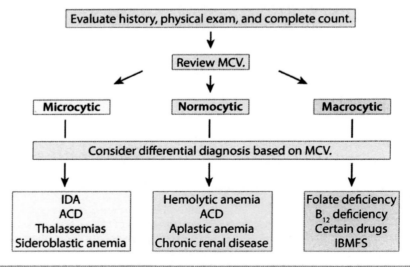

Evaluate history, physical exam, and complete count.

Review MCV.

Microcytic   Normocytic   Macrocytic

Consider differential diagnosis based on MCV.

Microcytic	Normocytic	Macrocytic
IDA ACD Thalassemias Sideroblastic anemia	Hemolytic anemia ACD Aplastic anemia Chronic renal disease	Folate deficiency B$_{12}$ deficiency Certain drugs IBMFS

Review blood smear for clues to the diagnosis.
Review history, physical exam, and red cell indices based on differential diagnosis.
Order additional diagnostic testing as indicated.

Make the diagnosis.

Figure 24-10: Diagnostic approach to anemia based on MCV

- Macrocytic anemias result from B$_{12}$ or folate deficiency (Figure 24-12), certain medications (e.g., valproic acid), reticulocytosis (e.g., with hemolytic anemia, recovery from bleeding), and inherited bone marrow failure syndromes (IBMFSs).

Other red cell indices can give clues to the diagnosis. For example, the red blood cell distribution width (RDW) is elevated in patients with iron deficiency, while the mean corpuscular hemoglobin concentration (MCHC) is elevated in hereditary spherocytosis.

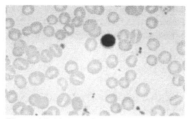

Figure 24-11: Iron deficiency. Thrombocytosis, microcytosis, and hypochromia

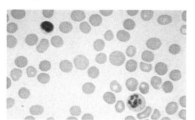

Figure 24-12: B₁₂ or folate deficiency with pernicious anemia. Low-power view shows hypersegmented neutrophil and macrocytosis.

Retic count is an important test in the evaluation of anemia. Low retic count is a key indicator for a hypoproliferative anemia caused by production or maturation defects. High retic counts are seen with hemorrhage, hemolysis, and as a response to therapy (e.g., after chemotherapy, after treatment for anemias caused by iron/folate/B₁₂ deficiency).

Reviewing RBC, platelet, and white blood cell (WBC) morphology provides important diagnostic clues. For example, crescent-shaped cells are diagnostic of sickle cell anemia. Spherocytes are seen in autoimmune hemolytic anemia and hereditary spherocytosis. Basophilic stippling indicates lead poisoning. Review the slide for platelets; low platelets in association with anemia can indicate Evans syndrome, hemolytic uremic syndrome (HUS), thrombocytopenic purpura (TTP), disseminated intravascular coagulation (DIC), aplastic anemia, or leukemia. Anemia can be a presenting sign of childhood leukemia. Review the WBC morphology for blasts. Table 24-1 lists specific findings seen on peripheral blood smear in different types of anemia.

Table 24-1: Significance of Specific Changes in the Peripheral Smear

Change	Finding	Meaning
Red blood cell fragments (schistocytes)		Microangiopathic hemolytic anemia (seen in TTP, HUS, HELLP syndrome, DIC, and occasionally vasculitis), severe burns, and valve hemolysis (Figure 24-13 on page 24-6)
Spherocytes		Autoimmune hemolytic anemia and hereditary spherocytosis (Figure 24-14 on page 24-6)
Target cells		Significant liver disease, thalassemia syndromes, sickle cell disease, homozygous hemoglobin C, and other hemoglobinopathies (Figure 24-15 on page 24-6)
Teardrop cells (dacrocytes)		Classic for myelofibrosis and other infiltrating bone marrow processes; also seen with thalassemia (Figure 24-16 on page 24-6)
Burr cells (echinocytes; top) vs. spur cells (acanthocytes; bottom)		Burr cells (Figure 24-17 on page 24-6) are seen in uremic patients. These are distinct and different from spur cells (Figure 24-18 on page 24-6), which are seen in liver diseases. Figure 24-19 on page 24-6 shows hepatorenal failure, with the presence of burr and spur cells.
Hypersegmented polymorphonuclear leukocytes (neutrophils)		Megaloblastic anemia, e.g., pernicious anemia/vitamin B₁₂ deficiency, folate deficiency (Figure 24-20 on page 24-6)
Elliptocytes		Hereditary elliptocytosis, severe iron-deficiency anemia (Figure 24-21 on page 24-6)
Sickle cells (crescent shaped)		Sickle cell disease (HbSS) and HbS β-thalassemia; less common in HbSC (Figure 24-22 on page 24-6)
Howell-Jolly bodies (nuclear remnants)		Splenectomy or functional asplenia (as seen in sickle cell disease). Howell-Jolly bodies (Figure 24-23 on page 24-6) are the result of nuclear remnants, causing the formation of small, round, black particles in erythrocytes. This is a normal occurrence, and the functioning spleen efficiently removes them.
Basophilic stippling (RNA)		Indicates ineffective erythropoiesis; lead poisoning, thalassemia, pyrimidine 5'-nucleotidase deficiency (Figure 24-24 on page 24-6)

DIC = disseminated intravascular coagulation
HELLP syndrome = hemolysis, elevated liver enzymes, low platelets syndrome
HUS = hemolytic uremic syndrome
TTP = thrombotic thrombocytopenic purpura

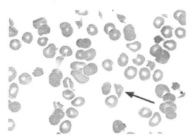

Figure 24-13: Hemolytic anemia with schistocytes

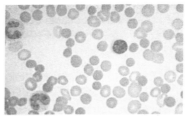

Figure 24-14: Hereditary spherocytosis. Note the lack of central pallor. The normal-sized lymphocyte shows that these are microcytic spherocytes.

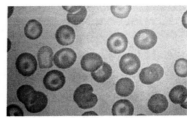

Figure 24-15: Target cells: low-oil view

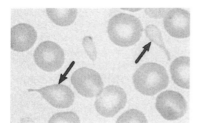

Figure 24-16: Teardrop cells. This patient has myeloid metaplasia, which is also seen in thalassemias and other hemoglobinopathies.

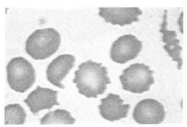

Figure 24-17: Burr cells (echinocytes) in uremia. These are RBCs with regularly spaced, short, spiny projections. These membrane changes disappear when uremia is corrected.

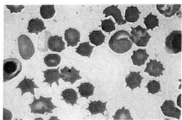

Figure 24-18: Spur cells (acanthocytes). Nucleated RBCs. Spur cells are RBCs with multiple irregular projections that vary in length, width, and regularity. The usual cause is hepatic failure.

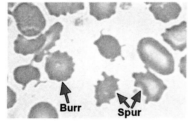

Figure 24-19: Hepatorenal failure. Burr cells as seen in uremia, and spur cells as seen in hepatic failure.

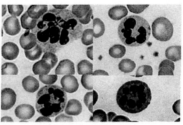

Figure 24-20: Various views of hypersegmented neutrophils

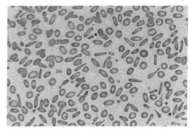

Figure 24-21: Hereditary elliptocytosis

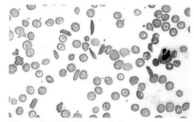

Figure 24-22: Sickle cell disease

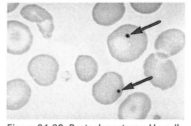

Figure 24-23: Postsplenectomy. Howell-Jolly bodies are the dense inclusion bodies in the RBCs. Also see target cells and a burr cell in this field.

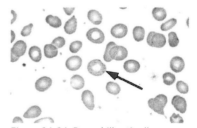

Figure 24-24: Basophilic stippling

ETIOLOGY OF ANEMIAS

The etiology of anemia can be classified as either a production defect or a survival defect. Production defects include problems producing sufficient numbers of RBC precursors in the bone marrow, or problems with the maturation of these precursors into fully formed RBCs. Survival defects are problems with the survival of the fully formed RBCs.

These can be intrinsic (due to a defect in the construction of the RBCs) or extrinsic (due to a destructive force acting on the normal RBCs). All survival defects result in hemolytic anemia. Table 24-2 summarizes the production and survival defects that cause anemia.

Production defects include the following:

- Inherited
  - Thalassemias (also survival defect secondary to hemolysis)
  - Inherited bone marrow failure syndromes (IBMFSs; see Aplastic Anemia on page 24-15)
- Acquired
  - Acquired bone marrow failure
  - Decreased erythropoietin (renal disease)
  - Iron deficiency anemia
  - Anemia of chronic disease
  - Folate deficiency
  - B$_{12}$ deficiency (also inherited)
  - Sideroblastic anemia (also inherited)

Survival defects can be inherited or acquired. Most inherited survival defects are due to a problem intrinsic to the RBC membrane, hemoglobin, or machinery. Most acquired survival defects are due to external forces acting on the RBCs.

Survival defects include the following:

- Inherited
  - Hereditary spherocytosis
  - Hereditary elliptocytosis
  - Paroxysmal nocturnal hemoglobinuria (PNH)
  - Glucose-6-phosphate dehydrogenase (G6PD) deficiency
  - Sickle cell disease
  - Other hemoglobinopathies (e.g., HbC disease, HbE disease)
- Acquired
  - Immune-mediated hemolytic anemia

RBC lifespan is shortened, resulting in hemolytic anemia. The body tries to compensate for this by increasing the bone marrow output, resulting in bony changes if the hemolytic process is long-term. The presence of reticulocytosis points to a hemolytic cause. Symptoms include pallor (especially noticeable in the conjunctiva, palm, and nail beds), scleral icterus, jaundice, and hepatosplenomegaly.

Inherited Production Defects

Normal adult hemoglobin has 2 α- and 2 β-globin chains (Figure 24-1 on page 24-2). Thalassemias are inherited disorders in which there is unbalanced globin chain synthesis due to absent or decreased production of either the beta chain (β-thalassemia) or the alpha chain (α-thalassemia). Each chromosome 16 contains 2 alleles coding for the α-globin chain (4 alleles total), and each chromosome 11 contains 1 allele for the β-globin chain (2 alleles total).

Table 24-2: Classification of Anemia — Production and Survival Defects			
Defects		**Etiology**	**Examples**
Production Defects	Fewer RBC precursors formed in bone marrow	• Decreased erythropoietin • Bone marrow failure	• Chronic kidney disease • Aplastic anemia
	Maturation defects: Cytoplasmic	• Impaired Hgb synthesis • Abnormalities in heme synthesis • Decreased globin synthesis	• Iron deficiency anemia • Sideroblastic anemia • Thalassemias
	Maturation defects: Nuclear	• DNA synthesis defects	• Vitamin B$_{12}$, folate deficiencies
Survival Defects	Intrinsic	• Membrane cytoskeleton protein • Membrane protein deficiency • Metabolic enzymes • Hemoglobinopathies	• Spherocytosis, elliptocytosis • PNH • G6PD deficiency • HbSS disease, HbC, HbE
	Extrinsic	• Immune-mediated hemolytic anemias • Drug-induced hemolysis • Other causes	• Autoimmune hemolytic anemia, HDFN • Penicillin, quinine • DIC, mechanical trauma, oxidative injury, hypersplenism

DIC = disseminated intravascular coagulation
G6PD = glucose-6-phosphate dehydrogenase
HbC = hemoglobin C
HbE = hemoglobin E

HDFN = hemolytic disease of the fetus and newborn (a.k.a. erythroblastosis fetalis)
HbSS = hemoglobin SS
PNH = paroxysmal nocturnal hemoglobinuria
RBC = red blood cell

β-Thalassemias

There are 3 categories of β-thalassemias: minor, intermedia, and major. A more recent classification of thalassemia groups these subtypes into non-transfusion-dependent thalassemia and transfusion-dependent thalassemia, depending on the clinical phenotype and need for chronic red cell transfusions.

In β-thalassemia, gene variants are classified as β^0 with no β-globin production, or β^+ with very reduced β-globin production. Details on the 3 categories follow:

1) β-Thalassemia minor (heterozygous; i.e., 1 normal β-globin allele [β] and 1 thalassemic allele [β^0 or β^+]): mild anemia, with a disproportionate degree of microcytosis. These patients are asymptomatic. Hypochromia, microcytosis, target cells, elliptocytes, and basophilic stippling occur. RDW is normal. Finding minor adult hemoglobin (HbA_2) > 3.5% is diagnostic for β-thalassemia minor.

2) β-Thalassemia intermedia (homozygous β^+/β^+): some normal β-globin production and, therefore, milder symptoms than with β-thalassemia major. These patients usually do not require transfusions. Decreased production of β-globin leads to increased delta and gamma chains; therefore, HbA_2 ($\alpha_2\delta_2$) and HbF ($\alpha_2\gamma_2$; fetal hemoglobin) are increased. This is of use diagnostically because quantitative hemoglobin electrophoresis measures the levels of these hemoglobins.

3) β-Thalassemia major (Cooley anemia; homozygous β^0/β^0-thalassemia or compound heterozygous β^0/β^+-thalassemia): homozygosity for impaired gene synthesis with essentially no β-globin production. The remaining highly insoluble α-globin precipitates into inclusion bodies (Heinz bodies, seen with special staining of the blood smear), causing severe clinical symptoms. Most erythroblasts die in the bone marrow (intramedullary hemolysis), resulting in erythroid hyperplasia in the bone marrow. By 6–12 months of age, most infants show pallor, irritability, growth restriction, hepatosplenomegaly, profound anemia, and jaundice. Expansion of the bone marrow space in facial bones leads to characteristic changes such as frontal bossing and prominent malar eminences (i.e., "chipmunk facies" in children). Mature RBCs that are produced have a shortened lifespan. On blood smear, RBCs are hypochromatic and microcytic. In addition, the RBCs are abnormally shaped and include target cells, teardrop cells, echinocytes, and fragmented cells. Nucleated red cells are present. Hemoglobin electrophoresis shows almost all HbF. HbA is absent in homozygous β^0/β^0-thalassemia and is present in very small amounts in compound heterozygous β^0/β^+-thalassemia. Patients with β-thalassemia major are **transfusion dependent** and often develop iron overload, requiring chelation therapy. Iron overload can cause endocrine abnormalities, heart failure, and arrhythmias due to deposition of iron in the organs. Splenectomy is beneficial in some cases, and bone marrow transplant can be curative.

On newborn screening, β-thalassemia major (β^0/β^0) is diagnosed by a demonstration of HbF only. Other β-thalassemias have the normal newborn hemoglobin pattern of fetal hemoglobin and adult hemoglobin A (abbreviated FA) (Table 24-3).

α-Thalassemias

There are 4 categories of α-thalassemias, each of which involves the deletion or dysfunction of 1 or more of the 4 alleles (Table 24-3). The more loci affected, the worse the symptoms:

1) α-Thalassemia trait: 1 locus, asymptomatic, no hematologic abnormalities (the "silent carrier")
2) α-Thalassemia minor: 2 loci, asymptomatic, MCV low, mild anemia
3) Hemoglobin H (HbH) disease: 3 loci, moderate-to-severe hemolysis
4) Hydrops fetalis: 4 loci, death in utero

Table 24-3: Newborn Screening and Hemoglobinopathies		
Condition	**Hemoglobin Electrophoresis: Newborn***	**Hemoglobin Electrophoresis: Children and Adults***
Sickle Cell Disease		
HbSS	FS	S, may have elevated F
HbSC	FSC	SC
HbS β^0-thalassemia	FS	S
HbS β^+-thalassemia	FSA or FS	SA
Sickle cell trait (HbAS)	FAS	AS
Thalassemias		
β-Thalassemia minor	FA	A, elevated HbA_2, elevated HbF
β-Thalassemia intermedia	FA or F	A, elevated HbA_2, elevated HbF
β-Thalassemia major (β^0/β^0)	F	F
β-Thalassemia major (β^0/β^+)	FA	FA
α-Thalassemia trait, silent carrier (single α-gene deletion)	FA, may have elevated Hb Bart†	A
α-Thalassemia minor (2 α-gene deletions)	FA, elevated Hb Bart†	A
HbH disease (3 α-gene deletions)	FA, elevated Hb Bart†	A, elevated HbH‡
Hydrops fetalis (4 α-gene deletions)	Mainly Hb Bart†	Death in utero

* Hemoglobin order is dictated by quantity, high to lower.
† Hb Bart = 4 gamma chains
‡ HbH = 4 beta chains

Note that hemoglobin electrophoresis can identify HbH and Hb Bart, which gives clues about α-thalassemia, but is not sensitive enough to make the diagnosis of the type of α-thalassemia. In patients with α-thalassemia trait and α-thalassemia minor, electrophoresis often shows normal amount of HbA, which is the same as in people without hematologic dysfunction. In Iron Deficiency, we discuss how to differentiate the thalassemia traits from iron deficiency anemia (the other major condition that causes a low MCV).

Patients with α-thalassemia have FA with differing levels of hemoglobin Bart (a tetramer of gamma chains) on their newborn screen, depending on the number of alleles affected.

Acquired Production Defects

Iron Deficiency

The major nutritional deficit in youth is iron deficiency, which can result in iron deficiency anemia (IDA)—the most common hypoproliferative anemia. Iron is essential for the production of hemoglobin. An adult has up to 5 g of body iron, whereas a newborn has as little as 0.25 g. Thus, during childhood and adolescence, a total of 4.75 g of iron must be absorbed. During times of maximal growth, such as infancy or adolescence, the iron requirements exceed the actual iron accrual rate. Only about 5% of dietary iron is absorbed, and most children require 10–15 mg of iron per day to maintain a positive iron balance. During infancy, this requires the use of iron-fortified foods beyond 4 months of age.

Iron deficiency is caused by poor intake, poor absorption, or excess blood loss. Inadequate iron intake is the most common cause of IDA in the pediatric population. In infants and young children, excess intake of cow's milk is a typical factor. In a child with a normal diet, remember to consider bleeding as a cause of iron deficiency. Menstrual loss is an obvious contributor in the adolescent girl. In all age groups, chronic blood loss from the gastrointestinal (GI) tract is a common cause of iron deficiency; GI blood loss results from Meckel diverticulum, *Helicobacter pylori* with gastric ulcer, and inflammatory bowel disease. Children with celiac disease often have concomitant IDA. Worldwide, hookworm infection (*Necator americanus* or *Ancylostoma duodenale*) is the most common cause of chronic GI blood loss. See the Infectious Disease section for more information. Consider testing all children with IDA for occult GI blood loss.

Most patients with IDA are asymptomatic. Sometimes, there is a history of pica (repeated ingestion of nonnutritive substances). In severe cases, the patient can present with pallor, irritability, poor feeding, tachycardia, tachypnea, or exercise intolerance. In addition to anemia, iron deficiency also causes nonhematologic effects, such as atrophic glossitis, behavior and learning disturbances, and impaired growth. Spoon-shaped (concave) nails, called koilonychia, is a manifestation of chronic iron deficiency.

MCV varies with age and ethnicity: Table 24-4 gives normal MCV values. The RBCs in iron deficiency are often microcytic (low MCV) and hypochromic (decreased MCHC = hemoglobin/hematocrit × 100). The retic count is low, as are serum iron and ferritin (iron stores). Remember that ferritin is an acute phase reactant and can be high in the setting of iron deficiency if there is ongoing inflammation. Serum iron-binding capacity is increased because transferrin iron saturation is low. RBC count is usually low. Reactive thrombocytosis often occurs.

Table 24-4: Normal Mean Corpuscular Volume by Age and Ethnicity		
Age (years)	Ethnicity	Mean Corpuscular Volume (fL)
1	Caucasian	71–89
	African American	63–88
2–3	Caucasian	74–89
	African American	64–89
4–6	Caucasian	77–91
	African American	67–91
7–10	Caucasian	78–91
	African American	72–92
11–14	Caucasian	80–94
	African American	71–95
15	Caucasian	81–96
	African American	71–96

Adapted from Brugnara C, et al. Diagnostic approach to the anemic patient. In: Nathan and Oski's *Hematology and Oncology of Infancy and Childhood*, 8th ed, Orkin SH, Fisher DE, Ginsburg D, et al (Eds), WB Saunders, Philadelphia 2015. p. 293.

It is important to distinguish IDA from β- and α-thalassemia trait because microcytosis is present in all of these conditions. To differentiate these traits from iron deficiency, first look at the CBC results. There are 2 indices that will give you a hint. The Mentzer index is MCV/RBC. This index is ≥ 13 in iron deficiency and < 13 in thalassemia, which is explained by the fact that the RBC count is generally low in iron deficiency but normal or increased in both β- and α-thalassemia trait. The RDW is normal in patients with β- and α-thalassemia trait but is increased in early iron-deficient patients. Checking the ferritin level gives the 3rd clue. Ferritin is normal in thalassemia trait and low in iron deficiency. Ferritin is often elevated with β-thalassemia intermedia or major and with HbH disease (3 α-gene deletions). Basophilic stippling and target cells can also be seen in thalassemia trait.

It is also important to distinguish IDA from **anemia of chronic disease** (ACD).

ACD occurs in patients with a chronic malignant, infectious, or inflammatory disorder. Treatment is aimed at management of the underlying disorder.

Understanding the role of hepcidin can be helpful in distinguishing these 2 types of anemia. Hepcidin is a small protein (i.e., a peptide) released from hepatocytes that block iron absorption from the gut and iron release by hepatocytes and macrophages. When hepcidin levels are high, iron absorption is low and there is less iron released from storage. In IDA, hepcidin levels decrease in response to low iron stores and iron absorption increases. In contrast, with ACD, iron stores are normal to high, but the cytokine-mediated production of hepcidin inhibits their use and causes anemia. See Table 24-5 for a comparison of lab values in IDA vs. ACD.

Table 24-5: Iron Deficiency Anemia vs. Anemia of Chronic Disease		
Lab Parameter	Iron Deficiency Anemia	Anemia of Chronic Disease
Iron	Low	Low
TIBC	High	Low
Transferrin saturation	Low	Low to normal
Ferritin	Often low	Normal to high
TIBC = total iron-binding capacity		

Pica is the link between lead poisoning and IDA. Pica involves eating clay and other nonnutritional substances and is a symptom—not a cause—of IDA. Iron deficiency increases the absorption of lead. Peripheral smear in patients with lead poisoning demonstrates coarse basophilic stippling, and labs show elevated levels of blood erythrocyte protoporphyrin. Lead level ≥ 45 μg/dL requires chelation therapy.

Treatment of IDA is aimed at correcting the underlying cause (e.g., limiting cow's milk, looking for GI bleeding). Oral iron therapy is almost always sufficient to correct anemia and replace iron stores. Give oral iron as 3–6 mg/kg of elemental ferrous sulfate per day divided on a schedule from 1–4× daily. Most children can handle the iron without GI upset or constipation (unlike adults). Look for reticulocytosis to begin 3–5 days after starting therapy and peak at 7–10 days. If the retic count does not rise in response to iron therapy, you must consider patient nonadherence or an alternative diagnosis. Give packed red blood cell transfusion only in cases of severe anemia with hemodynamic instability.

Expect the hemoglobin to increase 1–2 g/dL in the 1st month. It is critical to continue ferrous sulfate therapy, even after the hemoglobin concentration has returned to normal, in order to ensure correction of total body iron deficit. Parenteral iron is rarely indicated. Red cell indices are not accurate in measuring the iron status of patients with α- or β-thalassemia because the MCV is low in patients with thalassemia regardless; serum iron studies are required. Children with α- or β-thalassemia trait do not require iron supplementation unless they have a concomitant iron deficiency.

To prevent iron deficiency, the 2010 American Academy of Pediatrics recommendations include the following:

- Breast milk is recommended for at least the first 5–6 months of life. Provide elemental iron supplementation of 1 mg/kg/day for infants who are exclusively breastfed beyond 4 months of age. (Premature infants require supplementation by 1–2 months of age.)
- Iron-supplemented formula is recommended for the 1st year of life in infants who are not breastfed.
- Include iron-enriched cereals among the first foods introduced.
- Do not give cow's milk during the 1st year of life to prevent occult GI bleeding. (Iron in cow's milk is poorly absorbed; infants with iron deficiency often have a history of consuming large amounts of cow's milk.)

Bone Marrow Failure

Profound endocrine failure due to deficiencies in thyroid hormone, glucocorticoids, testosterone, or growth hormone can lead to anemia. Therefore, hypoproliferative anemia often complicates hypothyroidism, primary adrenal insufficiency (a.k.a. Addison disease), hypogonadism, and/or panhypopituitarism. These are rare in children.

See Aplastic Anemia on page 24-15.

Decreased Erythropoietin

Patients with renal failure have anemia due to decreased erythropoietin production, and the anemia is usually responsive to recombinant erythropoietin.

Folate and Vitamin B$_{12}$ Deficiencies

Folate and B$_{12}$ deficiencies cause slowing of DNA (deoxyribonucleic acid) synthesis and delayed maturation of the entire erythrocyte cell line, resulting in large, immature erythrocytes called megaloblasts. This, in turn, causes anemia with macrocytosis. Additionally, abnormalities of neutrophils can occur—especially nuclear hypersegmentation.

Folate is absorbed in the jejunum and deficiency can result from inadequate dietary intake, increased metabolic demand (e.g., infancy, pregnancy, lactation), malabsorption, or metabolic interference (e.g., methotrexate, sulfonamide). Little folate is stored, so deficiency states can occur quickly. Folic acid supplementation is recommended for sickle cell disease and other hemolytic disorders, but efficacy has not been well established in pediatric patients.

Folic acid taken before and during pregnancy can help prevent neural tube defects in the fetus. All females of childbearing age capable of becoming pregnant need to take folic acid supplementation.

Infants require 3–5 mcg/kg/day. Breast milk and cow's milk are sufficient to provide daily allowances. Goat's milk is a poor source of folate and results in megaloblastic anemia in unsupplemented infants if used as the sole food.

Folate deficiency in infancy can follow chronic diarrhea and malabsorptive states. Initially in folate deficiency, homocysteine levels increase, followed by a fall of RBC folate levels to the lower limit of normal. At this point, hypersegmented neutrophils appear, and then RBC folate levels fall below normal. Finally, megaloblastic anemia occurs. In folate-deficient patients, macroovalocytes (large oval RBCs), neutropenia, and thrombocytopenia are common.

Treat with folic acid at a dose of 1–5 mg daily. If the patient has concomitant vitamin B_{12} deficiency, use of high-dose folate can correct RBC problems but worsen neurologic manifestations of B_{12} deficiency. Therefore, it is important to determine if B_{12} deficiency is also present.

Vitamin B_{12} (cobalamin) deficiency in children occurs most commonly because of abnormalities in the absorption of vitamin B_{12}. The absorption of vitamin B_{12} is dependent on its forming a complex with intrinsic factor (IF), which is produced by the parietal cells of the stomach. The B_{12}-IF complex is then absorbed in the terminal ileum. After absorption, vitamin B_{12} separates from the complex and is released into circulation. In the plasma, vitamin B_{12} is bound to transcobalamin I and II proteins. Cobalamin is metabolized to adenosylcobalamin, which is required for the metabolism of methylmalonic acid (MMA)—helpful in diagnosis. Risk factors for vitamin B_{12} deficiency are small bowel resection and maternal vegan diet in a child who is exclusively breastfed.

Pernicious anemia is a specific form of B_{12} deficiency. There are 2 types of pernicious anemia in children:

1) Congenital pernicious anemia occurs before 3 years of age and is associated with consanguinity with autosomal recessive (AR) inheritance. Gastric histology and acid secretion are normal, but IF is absent. There are no antibodies to IF and no endocrinopathies.

2) Juvenile pernicious anemia occurs in older children and is similar to the adult form. This is due to an autoimmune-mediated decrease in gastric IF. In this case, gastric atrophy and decreased secretion of acid and pepsin are commonly found. There are often other autoimmune manifestations, including vitiligo or thyroiditis.

B_{12} deficiency, in contrast to folate deficiency, leads to neurologic symptoms and eventually to irreversible neurologic damage, including bilateral paresthesias, decreased proprioception and vibration sense (dorsolateral column "dropout"), spastic ataxia, central scotomata, and dementia. These neurologic deficits can occur even in the absence of anemia or macrocytosis. B_{12} deficiency can also cause skeletal changes, including osteoporosis and hip/spine fractures.

The diagnostic workup includes measurement of vitamin B_{12} and folate levels. Peripheral smear reveals macroovalocytosis, anisocytosis, and poikilocytosis. The retic count can be normal or low. Thrombocytopenia is present in half of patients, and often the platelets have bizarre shapes.

Pernicious anemia is commonly diagnosed by assessing the presence of anti-IF antibodies in association with low B_{12} levels and high serum MMA.

Treatment usually requires parenteral vitamin B_{12} for life: monthly subcutaneous injections of 1 mg cyanocobalamin or hydroxocobalamin. However, high-dose oral supplementation has been effective for the treatment of B_{12} deficiency in adults.

Inherited and Acquired Production Defects — Sideroblastic Anemias

Sideroblastic anemias are unusual anemias characterized by ringed sideroblasts in the bone marrow; these are normoblasts with iron-laden mitochondria surrounding the nucleus. Normoblasts are normal-sized erythroblasts that are the nucleated immediate precursors to normal erythrocytes.

There are a variety of causes for sideroblastic anemia (both acquired and inherited). The blood smear shows **Pappenheimer bodies,** which are often at the periphery of the cell; these are dark blue cytoplasmic inclusions of iron occurring as small single or multiple blue granules.

The peripheral blood smear usually has 2 populations of erythrocytes, including normal-appearing cells along with hypochromic microcytic cells (low MCV; low MCH [mean corpuscular hemoglobin]). This variation in size and shape is reflected in the CBC with a large RDW. Again, bone marrow shows ringed sideroblasts.

Less common causes can produce normo- to macrocytic erythrocytes.

Inherited Survival Defects

Sickle Cell Disease (SCD)

SCD is a group of inherited RBC disorders characterized by the presence of hemoglobin S (HbS). HbS is caused by a point mutation in the 6th codon of the β-globin gene, which is located on the short arm of chromosome 11. Adenine is replaced by thymidine, which results in valine being encoded instead of glutamic acid. Upon deoxygenation, HbS polymerizes, leading to sickled RBCs and hemolytic anemia.

4 common types of SCD occur (listed in decreasing order of severity):

- **HbSS**
- **HbS/β⁰-thalassemia** (hemoglobin S from one parent and β⁰-thalassemia from the other parent)
- **HbSC** (hemoglobin S from one parent and hemoglobin C from the other parent)
- **HbS/β⁺-thalassemia** (hemoglobin S from one parent and β⁺-thalassemia from the other parent)

The type of SCD can be distinguished on the basis of hemoglobin electrophoresis pattern, red cell indices, and genetic testing.

SCD affects 1/375 African American newborns. The disease also affects many other ethnic groups, including Mediterranean, Middle Eastern, and Asiatic Indian.

HbS forms polymers that damage the RBC and decrease its lifespan. The average lifespan of an RBC in HbSS disease is only 15–50 days (normal = 120 days). Sickled RBCs adhere to and damage endothelial layers of small and large blood vessels, resulting in vasoocclusion. Vasoocclusion with ischemia and tissue damage results in acute complications, including pain, acute chest syndrome (ACS), splenic sequestration, priapism, and stroke. Chronic hemolysis results in hyperbilirubinemia and cholelithiasis. Chronic organ damage affects the kidneys, spleen, lungs, and brain. Chronic complications of SCD include delays in growth and sexual maturation. Median life expectancy for patients with SCD in the U.S. is approximately 50 years.

In the U.S., SCD is diagnosed through newborn screening programs (Table 24-3 on page 24-8). Prenatal diagnosis is useful when both parents are known to have either SCD or trait. Amniotic fluid, fetal erythrocytes, or chorionic villi can be sampled for testing. At birth, infants have high levels of HbF, which interferes with sickling; therefore, newborns are not anemic. Symptoms generally occur starting at 6 months of age, as HbF decreases.

Hydroxyurea (Droxia, Hydrea) is the only disease-modifying medication shown to reduce acute and chronic complications. Side effects of the drug include neutropenia and, less commonly, thrombocytopenia and/or leukopenia. These cytopenias often resolve after hydroxyurea is held and restarted after blood cell count recovery. Hematopoietic stem cell transplant is increasingly utilized as a curative therapy for high-risk patients. Best outcomes are seen with matched related donors.

Pain (vasoocclusive) crisis is the most common complication of SCD and the most common reason for hospitalization. The first pain crisis in about 1/3 of patients is sickle cell **dactylitis**, a symmetric painful swelling of the hands and feet. As the child ages, the crises usually affect the long bones, vertebrae, sternum, ribs, lower back, and abdomen. Infarction leads to bone and joint destruction and compensatory bone marrow hyperplasia. Repeated infarction of a long bone leads to sclerosis, which often gives the appearance of a bone within a bone, reflecting old cortex within new cortex. Additional examples of skeletal findings in SCD include avascular necrosis of the femoral head; an expanded medullary space on a radiograph of the skull due to the shortened lifespan of erythrocytes; angular depression of the central portion of vertebral endplates; and irregular sclerosis, narrowing, and lucency of the joints reflecting numerous prior infarcts. Clinically, some children have very few crises, while others have frequent, debilitating crises. Treatment is aimed at relieving pain and providing hydration. IV hydration, nonsteroidal antiinflammatory drugs (NSAIDs), and opioid analgesics are typically used for hospitalized children.

Acute chest syndrome is defined as the development of a new pulmonary infiltrate with fever, chest pain, tachypnea, and/or hypoxia. Etiology of ACS includes infection, infarction, atelectasis, and/or fat embolism from the bone marrow. ACS can progress rapidly to respiratory failure. ACS is the leading cause of death in children and adults with SCD. Treatment includes respiratory support, hydration (if necessary), and antibiotics that cover pneumococcus, *Mycoplasma*, and *Chlamydia*. Exchange transfusions are administered to patients with significant hypoxia and respiratory distress and to those who do not improve with appropriate respiratory support, hydration, and antibiotic therapy. Exchange transfusion can rapidly decrease HbS and improve symptoms. If a patient with sickle cell anemia is undergoing surgery, preoperative transfusion to Hgb of ~ 10 g/dL is the standard of care to reduce the risk of postoperative complications, including ACS. Clinicians may consider a preoperative exchange transfusion for patients with SCD and a baseline hemoglobin > 9–10 g/dL.

Splenic sequestration is a life-threatening condition that occurs most often in young children with SCD. Children with splenic sequestration of sickled RBCs have massively enlarged and engorged spleens, resulting in abdominal pain, hypovolemia, severe anemia, and shock. Splenomegaly and thrombocytopenia suggest the diagnosis of acute splenic sequestration. Intravenous (IV) hydration and RBC transfusion decrease sequestration in the spleen and alleviate symptoms. Splenic sequestration often recurs; children with life-threatening sequestration or recurrent events undergo splenectomy.

Risk of infection with encapsulated organisms (*Streptococcus pneumoniae*, *Neisseria meningitidis*, and *Haemophilus influenzae*) is high due to functional asplenia, which is a result of autoinfarction from repeated sickling of RBCs within the spleen. Patients are also at higher risk of infection with *Salmonella*, including bacteremia and osteomyelitis. *Staphylococcus aureus*, the most common cause of osteomyelitis in normal hosts, accounts for only 25% of all cases in patients with SCD. Prescribe penicillin prophylaxis to infants diagnosed with SCD by newborn screening because it dramatically decreases invasive pneumococcal infections in children < 5 years of age with SCD. Children with SCD require immunizations against encapsulated organisms. Pneumococcal conjugate and polysaccharide vaccines are recommended for all children with SCD.

Aplastic crisis (red cell aplasia) occurs most commonly because of infection with parvovirus B19. Parvovirus B19 destroys early red cell precursors in the bone marrow and causes an abrupt cessation of RBC production. In the patient with SCD, in which RBC lifespan is only 15–50 days and maintaining RBC numbers is predicated on rapid bone marrow production, parvovirus B19 infection can quickly cause a life-threatening anemia. Presenting symptoms can vary and include fever, fatigue, pallor, coryza, and headache. The aplastic crisis is characterized by a falling hemoglobin (over 1–3 days) and reticulocytopenia. The low retic count differentiates aplastic crisis from other causes of worsening anemia. Diagnosis of parvovirus B19 is made using parvovirus DNA polymerase chain reaction (PCR) and/or serology. Elevated IgM indicates acute infection. Acute red cell aplasia is typically short and self-limited, and rapid production of IgM antibodies against parvovirus B19 quickly curbs the infection. Usually, reticulocytosis returns in 1–2 weeks. During this time, periodic transfusions are frequently required.

Stroke risk is high for children with sickle cell anemia (HbSS and HbSβ⁰-thalassemia). The peak incidence occurs in children between 2 and 5 years of age. Children are more likely to have infarctive stroke secondary to occlusion of the large intracerebral blood vessels. Symptoms include weakness, changes in speech, headache, and seizures. If a stroke is suspected or confirmed on physical examination, imaging with computed tomograph (CT) and/or magnetic resonance imaging (MRI) is done to evaluate for areas of ischemia and vasculopathy. Acute treatment is emergent exchange transfusion, which should be done even before an MRI in patients with sickle cell who are diagnosed with a stroke on the basis of the physical examination. In addition, patients with SCD who have had a stroke require chronic RBC transfusion therapy to keep the HbS < 30% to reduce the risk of recurrence.

Use transcranial Doppler ultrasound (TCD) to screen children with HbSS and HbSβ⁰-thalassemia starting at 2 years of age. To prevent strokes, chronic RBC transfusions are recommended for children with abnormally high TCD velocities.

Cerebral vasculopathy is a risk factor for stroke. **Moyamoya disease** occurs in some patients with SCD and is the collateral formation of vessels due to vascular occlusion. "Moyamoya" is a Japanese word meaning "puff of smoke"; the vessels on angiography appear to be a cluster of vessels with a smoky appearance. More information about Moyamoya disease is found in the Neurology section.

Priapism is a prolonged, painful erection, and it occurs in up to 10% of older boys and adolescents with SCD. It requires rapid intervention to prevent damage to the penis. Consult a hematologist and a urologist. Management includes hydration and pain control. In many cases, aspiration of the corpora cavernosa and irrigation with a dilute solution of epinephrine rapidly alleviates the condition. Rarely, surgical intervention (i.e., glans-cavernosum shunt) is indicated.

Other Hemoglobinopathies

Sickle cell trait (HbAS): People with sickle cell trait have normal hemoglobin, peripheral blood smears, and red cell indices. Their life expectancy is normal. It is unusual for a person with sickle cell trait to have any sickle cell–related complications, except in cases of extreme physical exertion or low oxygen tension (e.g., unpressurized aircraft, high altitude). Hyposthenuria (inability to concentrate urine) and renal papillary necrosis with gross hematuria are the most common complications. The incidence of renal medullary carcinoma, a rare kidney tumor, is higher in patients with sickle cell trait. Screening is not necessary due to the rarity of this tumor.

Hemoglobin SC disease (HbSC): Patients with HbSC are usually less anemic and have less severe hemolysis than those with HbSS. These patients have equal amounts of HbS and hemoglobin C (HbC), and there is no HbA. HbC occurs because of the substitution of a lysine for the glutamic acid residue in the 6th position of the β-globin chain. Peripheral smears show microcytosis, target cells, and irreversibly sickled cells. Splenomegaly remains throughout adolescence and adulthood. Adolescents are at risk for retinal disease and avascular necrosis of the hips.

Hemoglobin C disease (HbCC): Homozygotes for HbC have a mild hemolytic anemia and splenomegaly but do not have vasoocclusive problems. RBCs are microcytic with a large number of target cells on peripheral smear. Heterozygotes (HbAC) have no symptoms and only a large number of target cells as the hematologic manifestation.

Hemoglobin E disease (HbEE): Patients homozygous for HbE have mild hemolytic anemia with significant microcytosis, hypochromia, and target cells. Heterozygotes have minimal findings. HbEE is very common in the populations of south and southeast Asia (~ 30%) and in northeast India (up to 60%). It is thought that this is because RBCs with HbEE are resistant to infection by *Plasmodium falciparum*, the protozoan that causes malaria in humans.

Glucose-6-Phosphate Dehydrogenase (G6PD) Deficiency

All 250 variants of X-linked recessive G6PD deficiency result in decreased amounts of reduced glutathione. This disorder is more common in males, as well as among individuals of African, Mediterranean, Asian, and Middle Eastern ethnicity. Reduced glutathione is an antioxidant required to protect RBCs from oxidative stress. When an oxidant stress is present (e.g., systemic infection, dapsone, primaquine, fava beans), there is an inadequate reserve of reduced glutathione, and RBCs hemolyze. Consider G6PD deficiency as a possible cause for unexplained neonatal jaundice. Symptoms of a hemolytic crisis include sudden onset of pallor, fatigue, and dark urine. Except during an acute hemolytic crisis (when all the affected RBCs have hemolyzed and the remaining RBCs have normal or near-normal G6PD levels), measurement of G6PD level is diagnostic. Peripheral blood with supravital staining shows **Heinz bodies**, which consist of denatured globin (Figure 24-25 on page 24-14). Removal of Heinz bodies by splenic microphages can produce bite cells, while cross-binding of oxidized hemoglobin leads to the formation of blister cells. Bite and blister cells are visible on peripheral blood films without supravital staining.

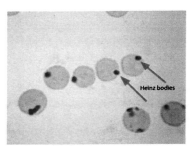

Figure 24-25: Heinz bodies in G6PD

Hereditary Spherocytosis (HS)

HS is the most common congenital hemolytic anemia in northern European populations (but also less commonly affects nonwhite populations). The incidence in the U.S. is about 1/5,000 births. A majority of cases are autosomal dominant (AD); however, for 10–25% of patients, no family history is found.

HS is due to a structural or functional abnormality of cytoskeletal proteins, spectrin, ankyrin, and, less commonly, band 3 or protein 4.2. Newly produced RBCs entering the circulation are not spherocytic, but the spherocytic shape gradually occurs due to splenic effects. Spherocytes are more rigid than normal cells and cannot easily pass through pores of the splenic sinusoids. Loss of RBC membrane occurs without a reduction in RBC volume, and the cell becomes more spherical. This cell becomes even less deformable and at greater risk for lysis in the spleen.

Diagnosis is made by finding the presence of anemia (of varying degrees), reticulocytosis, increased MCHC, spherocytes in the peripheral blood smear, and a positive osmotic fragility test (i.e., increased susceptibility of erythrocytes to osmotic lysis in a hypotonic solution).

Some children with HS have a chronic hemolytic anemia, jaundice, reticulocytosis, and splenomegaly. Other children have compensated anemia with few symptoms at baseline. Increasing pallor in a child with HS is a sign of an aplastic crisis, with decreased hemoglobin and retic count typically caused by parvovirus B19 infection. Close monitoring of hemoglobin and retic count is imperative. In contrast, a sudden increase in jaundice is a sign of increasing hemolysis, which also can result in worsening anemia and the need for RBC transfusion. HS can be a life-threatening cause of hyperbilirubinemia/kernicterus in the neonatal period. Chronic complications include cholelithiasis due to bilirubin stones.

Splenectomy is sometimes required to prolong RBC survival. Prior to splenectomy, administer pneumococcal, *H. influenzae*, and meningococcal vaccinations to minimize the risk of postsplenectomy sepsis. Postsplenectomy penicillin prophylaxis is also required, and urgent medical evaluation is necessary for splenectomized children with fever.

Hereditary Elliptocytosis (HE)

HE occurs at a rate of 1/2,500 births in the U.S. The most common cause of HE is abnormal spectrin, which is critical for cytoskeletal lateral interactions. There are 2 forms of the disorder:

1) **Common HE**, which is asymptomatic and has uniformly elliptical RBCs without other hematologic abnormalities
2) **Hemolytic HE**, which causes splenomegaly with mild-to-moderate anemia and hemolysis and has both spherocytes and elliptocytes

Splenectomy is generally curative.

Acquired Survival Defects

Immune-Mediated Hemolytic Anemias

The most common form of acquired hemolytic anemia is immune-mediated destruction of RBCs by antibodies. Symptoms include pallor, fatigue, jaundice, and dark urine.

There are 2 broad groups of immune-mediated hemolytic anemias:

- Autoimmune hemolytic anemia (warm, cold, or paroxysmal)
- Hemolytic disease of the fetus and newborn (a.k.a. erythroblastosis fetalis)

Autoimmune Hemolytic Anemia (AIHA)

In **warm AIHA**, IgG antibodies specific for the Rh group of RBC antigens can bind to these antigens at body temperature. Macrophages and monocytes are attracted to these IgG-coated cells and start attacking them, converting them to spherocytes and causing them to hemolyze. IgG-coated RBCs and spherocytes are sequestered by the spleen. AIHA is either primary or secondary. Secondary AIHA is seen with infection, certain medications (e.g., penicillins, cephalosporins, NSAIDs), and lymphoproliferative and collagen vascular disorders (e.g., systemic lupus erythematosus). Clinical history includes acute onset of pallor, jaundice, and sometimes dark urine. Investigate the patient's history for a new medication or recent febrile illness. Physical exam findings are significant for pallor, jaundice, and splenomegaly.

The direct Coombs test is a necessary evaluation tool in a child with acute onset anemia. In AIHA, the direct Coombs test is positive. Table 24-6 explains the Coombs tests. Briefly, the direct Coombs test reveals what components (IgG or C3) are "directly" attached to the patient's RBCs, suggesting an autoimmune reaction. The indirect Coombs test reveals antibodies in the patient's serum that have the potential to bind to RBCs.

AIHA can be life-threatening. Treat warm AIHA with corticosteroids. If necessary, transfuse the most compatible RBCs. Splenectomy or immunosuppressive agents are used in refractory cases.

Table 24-6: Coombs Tests			
Coombs Test	**Description of Test**	**Positive Test**	**Possible Indications**
Direct	Antibodies against IgG or C3 are prepared in an animal and then mixed with the patient's blood.	Patient's RBCs agglutinate— which means there is IgG (or C3) on the surface of the patient's RBCs.	Autoimmune hemolytic anemia Infectious mononucleosis *Mycoplasma* infection
Indirect	The Rh- and ABO-compatible RBCs are mixed with the patient's serum. Testing is done to see if the patient's serum contains antibodies that can cause agglutination of other RBCs.	Patient's RBCs agglutinate.	Incompatible blood match with transfusion Erythroblastosis fetalis

Cold agglutinin disease can occur with *Mycoplasma* and Epstein-Barr virus. IgM-RBC complexes activate complement and cause intravascular hemolysis. IgM disease is positive for C3 but negative for IgG on Coombs testing.

Paroxysmal cold hemoglobinuria (PCH) is caused by a cold-reacting IgG (Donath-Landsteiner antibody). This antibody binds at cold temperatures and causes RBC lysis at warm temperatures. PCH is common after viral illness, and treatment is supportive. Keep the patient warm and use a blood warmer for transfusions. Consider plasmapheresis for severe disease. Steroids are less helpful than with warm AIHA.

Hemolytic Disease of the Fetus and Newborn (HDFN)

A distinctive form of immune hemolytic anemia is **HDFN** (a.k.a. erythroblastosis fetalis), which presents in infancy due to maternal production of antibodies against fetal RBC antigens that cross the placenta during pregnancy. This can be due to ABO antibodies (ABO incompatibility) or to Rh antibodies (Rh hemolytic disease of the newborn). Classification as Rh positive or negative is based upon whether or not the major D antigen is expressed on erythrocytes. The direct Coombs test is positive, as with most AIHAs. Classically, Rh hemolytic disease of the newborn does not occur with the first pregnancy. In contrast, ABO hemolysis can occur with the first pregnancy due to the natural production of isohemagglutinins. Anemia and hyperbilirubinemia resolve as maternal antibodies are cleared.

See the Neonatology section for more information on hemolytic disease of the fetus and newborn.

Drug-Induced Hemolysis

Many drugs cause hemolysis. Penicillin bound to RBCs elicits an antibody response that can cause hemolysis. Quinine, methyldopa, and certain cephalosporin antibiotics are also known culprits.

The other causes of extrinsic survival defects:

• DIC
• Mechanical trauma to RBCs
• Oxidative injury
• Hypersplenism

STEM CELL DISORDERS

PREVIEW | REVIEW

• What are the treatment options for children with severe aplastic anemia?

• Why should blood products be leukoreduced and irradiated in patients with aplastic anemia?

• Describe congenital anomalies seen in children with Fanconi anemia.

• Children with Fanconi anemia are at risk for which malignancies?

• Which virus infects red blood cells and results in aplastic crisis in children with congenital hemolytic anemias?

• How do you differentiate among the 3 most common causes of red cell aplasia?

APLASTIC ANEMIA

Aplastic anemia is a condition in which there are reduced numbers of RBCs, WBCs, and platelets due to bone marrow aplasia/hypoplasia caused by damage to the hematopoietic stem cells (Figure 24-26 on page 24-16). Aplastic anemia is a stem cell disorder with the clinical presentation of **pancytopenia**, rather than an isolated anemia—and, therefore, is a misnomer. Aplastic anemia involves all cell lines, whereas aplastic crisis involves the red cell line only. Aplastic crises occur most commonly in individuals with primary red cell disorders.

Bone marrow examination is necessary in the evaluation of any child with pancytopenia and is required to make the diagnosis of aplastic anemia. Patients with aplastic anemia have hypocellular or acellular bone marrow.

A diagnosis of severe aplastic anemia requires a bone marrow cellularity < 25% and at least 2 of the following: peripheral blood platelet count < 20,000/µL ($< 20 \times 10^9$/L), peripheral blood absolute neutrophil count (ANC) < 500/µL ($< 0.5 \times 10^9$/L), and/or peripheral blood reticulocyte count < 20,000/µL ($< 20 \times 10^9$/L).

The cause of aplastic anemia is unknown in > 50% of cases, with the remainder due to certain drugs, toxins, infections, or radiation exposure. The dose-related causes

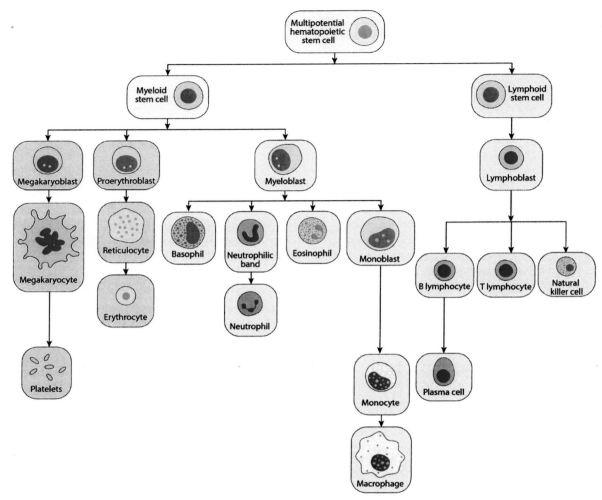

Figure 24-26: Blood cell development

include benzene and radiation. Idiosyncratic causes are sulfa drugs, gold, chloramphenicol, and insecticides. In the initial evaluation of aplastic anemia, include testing for hepatitis A, B, and C; cytomegalovirus (CMV); Epstein-Barr virus (EBV); human immunodeficiency virus (HIV); and parvovirus. In addition, evaluate children with aplastic anemia for inherited bone marrow failure syndromes (IBMFSs). Other causes of pancytopenia include fibrosis or infiltration with neoplastic cells (such as in neuroblastoma), B_{12} or folic acid deficiency, primary hematologic malignancies, and hemophagocytic lymphohistiocytosis.

The combination of bruising and pallor suggests a marrow disorder affecting > 1 cell line. Typically, these patients present with recurrent infections, mucosal bleeding, and increased menstrual flow in premenopausal females. They can also present with fatigue and petechiae.

Treatment of severe aplastic anemia:

• Matched sibling hematopoietic stem cell transplant (HSCT), if available, is the treatment of choice and has a 10-year survival rate of > 80%.

• Immunosuppressive therapy with antithymocyte globulin (ATG), cyclosporine, and prednisone offers a complete response rate of 65%, although relapses are common.

A patient treated medically is at risk for a secondary malignancy if the patient has an underlying IBMFS.

Patients with severe aplastic anemia receiving immunosuppressive therapy should be transfused with leukocyte-reduced, irradiated blood products to decrease the risk of transfusion-associated graft-versus-host disease. To prevent pretransplant alloimmunization, minimize the number of transfusions if possible. If transfusions are required before transplant:

• Do not use family members as donors.

• Use leukocyte-filtered, irradiated blood components.

• Use single-donor platelets.

FANCONI ANEMIA

Fanconi anemia is an AR disorder involving **poor DNA repair** mechanisms. It most commonly presents with pancytopenia that occurs at a mean age of 8–9 years. Note: The anemia can begin at birth or be delayed to as late as 48 years of age. Only 3% are diagnosed before 1 year of age and only 10% after 16 years of age; so, the majority fall close to the mean age of 8–9 years. In some cases, patients can present with an isolated thrombocytopenia or neutropenia. In other cases, cytopenias may be mild early in the disease course, or cytopenias may develop later in life. Bone marrow aspiration will reveal a hypocellular marrow with fatty replacement.

Classically, patients present with short stature, skeletal abnormalities (including absent or abnormal thumbs, abnormal radii, microcephaly, and vertebral abnormalities), café au lait spots, hyperpigmentation or hypopigmentation, and renal anomalies—although congenital anomalies are not required for the diagnosis. Hypogonadism, hypothyroidism, dyslipidemia, adrenal dysfunction, and other endocrine disorders may also be associated with Fanconi anemia. There are at least 17 different mutations, and *FANCA* and *FANCC* are the 2 most commonly affected genes.

Fanconi anemia can present in children as macrocytic anemia with or without other cytopenias. The diagnostic test of choice is the identification of DNA repair abnormalities in cultured peripheral blood lymphocytes, including a high number of metaphases with breaks, gaps, rearrangements, and other abnormalities. A screening laboratory test is done with diepoxybutane or mitomycin C, which induces chromosomal damage in cells with defective DNA repair.

On average, patients with Fanconi anemia live into their mid-30s. In developed countries, there has been a significant improvement in the survival of patients with Fanconi anemia due to a reduction in severe infections and bleeding complications.

Patients with Fanconi anemia have a 40–50% risk of myelodysplastic syndrome and a 15% risk of developing acute myelogenous leukemia by 50 years of age. Allogenic HSCT is the only known cure for the aplasia, but it does not decrease the risks of nonhematologic cancers. Because the defect is in DNA repair, use of chemotherapy requires dose reductions. Hepatic malignancy and squamous cell carcinoma are also more common in patients with Fanconi anemia than in the general population. Do not confuse this with Fanconi syndrome, which is a renal condition characterized by generalized proximal tubular dysfunction.

RED CELL APLASIA

Red cell aplasia is defined by anemia in the setting of reticulocytopenia. The most common known causes of red cell aplasia in the pediatric population are parvovirus B19-associated red cell aplasia, transient erythroblastopenia of childhood (TEC), and congenital hypoplastic anemia (a.k.a. Diamond-Blackfan anemia).

Red cell aplasia can also be idiopathic, or secondary to drugs (particularly phenytoin and chloramphenicol) or immune disorders (e.g., thymoma, systemic lupus erythematosus, chronic lymphocytic leukemia).

Parvovirus B19

Parvovirus B19 can infect erythroid progenitors and cause an acute or chronic red cell aplasia. In an otherwise healthy patient, this is a transient phenomenon and is often asymptomatic; however, chronic infection with red cell aplasia can be seen in the immunocompromised.

Remember: In patients with hemolytic anemias such as sickle cell disease, parvovirus B19 infection can cause an **aplastic crisis**. (See more on aplastic crisis in sickle cell disease under Sickle Cell Disease (SCD) on page 24-11.)

Suspect parvovirus B19 infection in patients presenting with red cell aplasia in the setting of fever, rash, and/or arthropathy. The rash can have the "slapped cheek" presentation of erythema infectiosum (one of the presentations of parvovirus B19 seen in otherwise healthy children).

Diagnose by finding parvovirus B19 DNA and/or parvovirus-specific IgM in serum, blood, or bone marrow cells. Viral studies for CMV, parvovirus B19, and EBV are usually done during workup for any case of red cell aplasia. Lab confirmation is typically not needed if the signs and symptoms are characteristic. Treatment is supportive. Intravenous immunoglobulin (IVIG) is prescribed for complicated cases in immunocompromised patients.

Transient Erythroblastopenia of Childhood (TEC)

TEC is an acquired, self-limited condition seen in previously healthy children between 1 and 3 years of age. Affected children exhibit pallor and decreased activity. There is no organomegaly or petechiae on exam.

Laboratory evaluation shows normocytic anemia with reticulocytopenia but without other cytopenias. Parvovirus is not responsible.

Treatment includes supportive care with transfusion for symptomatic anemia. In most cases, the anemia resolves in 1–2 months without transfusions. Children with TEC are not at increased risk of developing additional hematologic problems.

Congenital Hypoplastic Anemia (Diamond-Blackfan Anemia)

Diamond-Blackfan anemia presents in infancy with macrocytic anemia, reticulocytopenia without other cytopenias, and absence or marked deficiency of RBC precursors. Most children are diagnosed at < 1 year of age. About 1/3 of patients have various congenital deformities, including thumb anomalies; dysmorphic features (e.g., "snub nose," thickened upper lip, wide-set eyes); short stature; glaucoma; renal anomalies; hypogonadism; short, webbed neck; congenital heart disease; and intellectual disability.

Manage these children with transfusions until 6–12 months of age, then try corticosteroids. Because corticosteroids affect bone growth, many wait until 12 months of age. The anemia responds to corticosteroids in up to 80% of patients. Spontaneous remission occurs in about 25% of cases. Chronic RBC transfusions are indicated for those who are steroid refractory or steroid dependent. Consider bone marrow transplant for patients requiring chronic red cell transfusion therapy.

Differentiating the Pure Red Cell Aplasias

If a child comes in with anemia and low reticulocytes, consider the aforementioned disorders: parvovirus B19, TEC, and Diamond-Blackfan anemia (DBA). During the history and physical exam, keep in mind that you are still ruling out drugs and autoimmune disorders as causes.

Consider the following findings to differentiate among these 3 disorders:

- Parvovirus B19 usually occurs in school-aged children and has associated fever, rash, and arthropathy.
- TEC typically occurs in children between 1 and 4 years of age, has normocytic RBCs, and has no rash, fever, or arthropathy.
- DBA is most often diagnosed in children < 1 year of age and has macrocytic RBCs. Patients also often have congenital deformities.

WHITE BLOOD CELL (WBC) DISORDERS

PREVIEW | REVIEW

- Define severe neutropenia.
- Why should patients with severe neutropenia be evaluated immediately for any fever?
- Differentiate cyclic neutropenia from chronic benign neutropenia.
- What is Kostmann syndrome?
- What is Shwachman-Diamond syndrome?
- Describe neonatal isoimmune neutropenia.

NEUTROPENIA

Severe neutropenia is generally defined as having an absolute neutrophil count (ANC) of < 500/μL (< 0.5 × 10⁹/L). (The ANC is obtained by multiplying the total WBC count by the percentage of neutrophils + band forms.) Moderate neutropenia is generally considered between 500 and 1,000/μL (0.5–1 × 10⁹/L), whereas mild neutropenia is defined by neutrophil counts between 1,000 and 1,500/μL (1–1.5 × 10⁹/L). Patients with severe neutropenia are at

marked risk for developing serious bacterial infections. Those with less severe neutropenia frequently develop skin infections, otitis media, or stomatitis. Recurrent bacterial infection is a manifestation of all WBC disorders (neutropenia, as well as qualitative defects). Children with severe neutropenia are often infected with their own skin and bowel flora. Children are at risk for overwhelming bacterial infection; febrile and ill-appearing children with neutropenia require immediate evaluation, blood cultures, and parenteral broad-spectrum antibiotics.

Neutropenias include the following:

- Inherited
  - Cyclic neutropenia
  - Severe congenital neutropenia (Kostmann syndrome)
  - Shwachman-Diamond syndrome
- Acquired
  - Neonatal isoimmune neutropenia
  - Chronic benign neutropenia (autoimmune)
  - Virus- or drug-induced neutropenia

The severity of neutropenia increases as 3 factors increase:

- Duration
- Bone marrow deficit
- Number of immunologic impairments

A child who presents with all 3 of these factors is in greater danger than one who has only 1 or 2 of these findings.

Inherited Neutropenias

Cyclic Neutropenia

In cyclic neutropenia, the neutropenia occurs at a regular interval of every 21 +/− 3 days. It is characterized by defective maturation of uncommitted stem cells. During 3- to 7-day periods of neutropenia, which usually have an ANC < 200/μL (< 0.2 × 10⁹/L), the patient often presents with fever, aphthous stomatitis, pharyngitis, cervical lymphadenitis, and/or rectal and vaginal ulcers. In ~ 10% of cases, infections can be severe or even fatal. Patients with cyclic neutropenia are at particular risk of sepsis caused by *Clostridium septicum*. In about 1/3 of patients, the disorder is inherited in an AD (autosomal dominant) pattern. Mutations involve the *ELA2* gene. Management includes granulocyte colony-stimulating factor (G-CSF) and antibiotics for infections. Oral hygiene is important.

Severe Congenital Neutropenia (Kostmann Syndrome)

Kostmann syndrome is a rare AR disorder. Mutations can involve multiple genes, including *ELA2* and *HAX1*. The ANC is typically < 200/μL (< 0.2 × 10⁹/L), and there is also monocytosis and eosinophilia. Children are at risk for severe bacterial infections and early death. Management includes G-CSF (often at a high dose). Bone marrow transplant (BMT) is curative. There is a national registry for patients. Note: Some patients acquire a mutation in the

G-CSF receptor, followed by a transformation to myelodysplasia and acute myelogenous leukemia; however, malignancy is not attributed to G-CSF therapy.

Shwachman-Diamond Syndrome

Shwachman-Diamond syndrome is an AR disorder resulting from mutations in the *SBDS* gene. Children present with features similar to those of children with cystic fibrosis, including failure to thrive, steatorrhea due to pancreatic exocrine insufficiency, and recurrent infections. Unique features of Shwachman-Diamond syndrome include neutropenia and metaphyseal dysostoses.

A sweat test will be normal. Diagnostic evaluation includes complete blood count, bone marrow aspirate and biopsy, serum isoamylase, serum pancreatic trypsinogen, and fecal elastase levels. Genetic testing is available for *SBDS* gene analysis.

Treatment options include supportive care with pancreatic enzyme replacement and, depending on frequency and severity of infections, G-CSF administration or BMT. Patients are predisposed to myelodysplastic syndrome and acute myeloid leukemia (AML).

Acquired Neutropenias

Neonatal Isoimmune Neutropenia (NIN)

NIN is a self-limited disease that occurs in ~ 1/1,000 newborns. NIN is similar to Rh disease—except with NIN, the mother becomes sensitized to fetal neutrophil antigens of paternal origin. These antigens are absent from the mother's neutrophils, causing production of maternal antibodies. Maternal IgG antineutrophil antibodies cross the placenta and result in destruction of fetal neutrophils, with a resultant neutropenia. The infant's neutrophil count recovers in 6–12 weeks. Any infection requires quick, appropriate antibiotic therapy. Subsequent siblings are at risk for the same condition.

Chronic Benign Neutropenia

Chronic benign neutropenia is characterized by a persistently low ANC of < 1,000/μL (1×10^9/L); patients usually have an ANC of 0–500/μL (0–0.5×10^9/L), which is caused by autoantibodies to granulocytes. It is also called autoimmune neutropenia. It is the most common cause of neutropenia in "healthy" children and must be differentiated from more serious forms of neutropenia. It can be AD or sporadic. Chronic benign neutropenia has a median age of diagnosis of 8–11 months and typically lasts about 2 years.

The disease is mild and usually does not require treatment. G-CSF is given for severe infections.

Virus- or Drug-Induced Neutropenia

The most common etiology of neutropenia in children is viral infection resulting in transient bone marrow suppression. Viral infection can also induce immune-mediated neutropenia. In this case, either an antiviral antibody cross-reacts with a neutrophil, or a drug attaches to the neutrophil and acts as a hapten, stimulating antibody production. Viral-induced neutropenia is very common and does not require specific treatment.

Drugs that can cause mild-to-moderate neutropenia include antiseizure medications, antithyroids, NSAIDs, antihistamines, sulfas, and synthetic penicillins. The neutrophil count is usually not in the severely low range, and significant secondary infections are unusual. If a drug is the suspected cause of neutropenia, discontinue the drug if possible.

Chemotherapeutic agents induce neutropenia that is often severe. It is important to remember that even though signs and symptoms of infection (including erythema, swelling, and pain) may be mild and blunted, the neutropenic patient can still have an acute infection. Treatment for fever in a child on immunosuppressive chemotherapy is urgent administration of parenteral broad-spectrum antibiotics and subsequent tailoring of treatment after causal organisms are known. A patient with a concerning physical exam should be admitted to the hospital. However, per a 2017 update from the Journal of Clinical Oncology, low-risk febrile oncology patients (e.g., no oxygen requirement, no severe pain, no neutropenia) can be treated on an outpatient basis.

DISORDERS OF NEUTROPHIL FUNCTION

Neutrophil function disorders are inherited conditions that frequently present with recurrent infections and a normal neutrophil count. Symptoms include aphthous ulcers, stomatitis, otitis media, cervical lymphadenopathy, and skin abscesses in the first few months of life. Initial workup includes neutrophil count, neutrophil morphology, and either a test for respiratory burst (usually a nitroblue tetrazolium dye test if chronic granulomatous disease is a concern) or flow cytometry for other disorders (e.g., leukocyte adhesion deficiency Type 1 [LAD1]). Figure 24-26 on page 24-16 describes normal blood cell development.

The major disorders of neutrophil function are covered in the Allergy & Immunology section and include:

- LAD1
- Hyper-IgE syndrome (Job syndrome)
- Chédiak-Higashi syndrome
- Chronic granulomatous disease

DISORDERS OF EOSINOPHILS

Occurrence

In the U.S. and other developed countries, eosinophilia is most commonly caused by allergens; worldwide, the most common cause is parasites. Eosinophilia can also be seen in Hodgkin disease, leukemias, dermatitis, and gastrointestinal disorders.

Hypereosinophilic Syndrome

Hypereosinophilic syndrome is an acquired, chronic syndrome whereby an overabundance of eosinophils creates tissue damage. It has no known etiology and is distinct from eosinophilic leukemia, a subtype of AML. Treat with corticosteroids, vinca alkaloids, hydroxyurea, and, if necessary, BMT.

DISORDERS OF BASOPHILS

Basophils are the least numerous WBCs and normally make up < 1% of the total circulating WBC pool. Basophils contain histamine and heparin and are the bloodborne equivalent of tissue-bound mast cells. Excess numbers of basophils occur in chronic myelogenous leukemia, ulcerative colitis, and myxedema.

HEMOSTASIS

PREVIEW | REVIEW

- Describe primary hemostasis.
- At the bedside, how can you differentiate between a primary hemostatic problem and a coagulation problem?
- Which 5 tests are commonly done in the initial evaluation of a bleeding disorder?
- What does the thrombin time measure?
- What does it mean if the prothrombin time (PT) is prolonged but the partial thromboplastin time (PTT) is normal?
- What does it mean if the PTT is prolonged but the PT is normal?
- What does a mixing study show?
- What is the normal platelet lifespan?
- What is Wiskott-Aldrich syndrome?
- What is TAR syndrome?
- What is the next diagnostic step if a patient has an unexpectedly very low platelet count after previously having normal counts?
- What preceding medical history is commonly reported in children diagnosed with immune thrombocytopenia (ITP)?
- Describe the peripheral blood smear findings in ITP. What diagnosis should be considered in a child with giant platelets (the size of red blood cells)?
- What are the typical blood counts in children with acute ITP?
- What is the role of bone marrow aspiration and biopsy in the evaluation of a child with thrombocytopenia?
- What bone marrow findings are consistent with a diagnosis of ITP?
- How soon do platelet counts normalize in children with ITP?
- What are the laboratory and clinical indications for treatment of ITP? What is the typical platelet count trigger for treatment of ITP?
- What are the 1st line treatments for ITP?
- Describe the clinical presentation and management of infants of women with maternal autoimmune neonatal thrombocytopenia.
- What are the clinical features of von Willebrand disease (vWD)?
- What tests are included in the laboratory evaluation of vWD?
- What are the treatment options for children with vWD?
- Giant, abnormal platelets and decreased platelet aggregation in response to ristocetin are seen in which inherited platelet disorder?
- What does aspirin do to platelets? How long does it last?
- What treatment does reactive thrombocytosis require?
- Which clotting factor is low in children with hemophilia A?
- What will the PT and PTT be in hemophilia A?
- Which clotting factor deficiencies have X-linked inheritance?
- What medication can you give to a child with mild hemophilia A (> 5% Factor 8) before a tooth extraction? Which test should be done prior to relying on this medication for treatment?
- What is hemophilia B?
- How is hemophilia B treated?
- Which clotting factor deficiencies have autosomal inheritance?
- What can cause disseminated intravascular coagulation (DIC)?
- What are the lab abnormalities seen in DIC?
- Name the vitamin K–dependent coagulation factors.
- Why are individuals with protein C deficiency at risk for warfarin-related skin necrosis?
- Which congenital thrombophilias result in neonatal purpura fulminans in infancy?

HEMOSTATIC PROCESS

Clotting after a vascular injury must be quick to initiate, localized to the area of injury, and durable enough for the healing process to occur.

The entire hemostatic process occurs in 4 overlapping phases:

1) **Primary hemostasis**—local vasoconstriction and formation of a loose platelet plug

2) **Secondary hemostasis**—circulating coagulation factors, via the clotting cascade, form fibrin that stabilizes the platelet plug.

3) **Clot limitation**

4) **Clot dissolution** (fibrinolysis)

The green-colored text in the following description of the clotting sequence highlights certain key elements in the process.

NORMAL CLOTTING SEQUENCE

Primary Hemostasis — Platelet Plug Formation

Primary hemostasis consists mainly of platelet plug formation, although vasoconstriction and capillary endothelial adhesion (where capillaries collapse and stick closed when empty) also play a part. The fix from the loose platelet plug is temporary and lasts only 12–24 hours—which is why hemophiliacs often do not have a deep bleed until 12–24 hours after trauma occurs. Glycoprotein (GP), either alone or in complexes, acts as a receptor on the platelet surface. Consult Figure 24-27 (Steps A–G) as you read through the following descriptions.

Platelet plug formation has 4 processes:

1) **Adhesion** of platelets to subendothelium (Step A)— Platelets bind immediately to exposed collagen with GP1a/2a platelet surface receptors. Platelet binding is further reinforced by vWF, a constituent of the subendothelial matrix, which binds platelet surface receptors GP1b/9/5 and GP2b/3a.

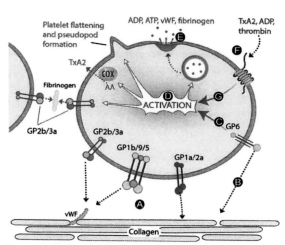

ADP, ATP, vWF, fibrinogen

Platelet flattening and pseudopod formation

TxA2, ADP, thrombin

TxA2

COX

AA

Fibrinogen

ACTIVATION

GP2b/3a   GP2b/3a   GP6

GP1b/9/5

GP1a/2a

vWF

Collagen

Figure 24-27: Primary hemostasis

2) **Activation**—As the platelets bind to the collagen, the collagen is then able to bind to the platelet GP6 signaling receptor (Step B), which initiates a signaling cascade (Step C) that results in platelet activation (Step D) with the following results:

- Dramatic flattening and spreading out of the platelet, with pseudopod formation allowing better coverage and more collagen-receptor interaction.

- Secretion of a host of products by the platelets, including adenosine diphosphate (ADP), adenosine triphosphate (ATP), von Willebrand factor (vWF), and fibrinogen (Step E).

- Configurational change to GP2b/3a receptors on the platelet surface, allowing binding to fibrinogen—which will result in platelet-to-platelet aggregation. Remember there are about 50,000 GP2b/3a receptors on the surface of each platelet!

- Arachidonic acid (AA) is converted by cyclooxygenase (COX) into other precursors of thromboxane A_2 (TxA_2). TxA_2 strongly induces more platelet activation and more thrombogenesis. TxA_2 is also a potent vasoconstrictor (Steps F and G).

- ADP has a similar effect as TxA_2 on activating platelets (Steps F and G).

3) **Aggregation** by platelet-to-platelet cohesion occurs when circulating fibrinogen binds to the newly exposed GP2b/3a receptors on adjacent platelets.

4) **Thrombin**, produced in secondary hemostasis (see Secondary Hemostasis — Coagulation), causes a spiraling increase in platelet activation and coagulation (Steps F and G).

See Disorders of Primary Hemostasis on page 24-24.

Secondary Hemostasis — Coagulation

Follow along in Figure 24-28 on page 24-22 as you review secondary hemostasis. Most of the inactivated coagulation factors float freely in the plasma—basically waiting for an injury to occur. While the platelets are aggregating (process 3 in Primary Hemostasis — Platelet Plug Formation), the clotting pathway is activated. The **intrinsic pathway** is comprised of Factors 12, 11, 9, and 8, while the **extrinsic pathway** is made up of 7a-tissue factor complex. Both pathways converge to activate Factor 10, which in turn converts prothrombin to thrombin.

Stop for a minute to look at Figure 24-28 again, and appreciate what an important substance thrombin is. Thrombin is critical in both the conversion of fibrinogen to fibrin in the platelet plug (that was formed in primary hemostasis) and in activating Factor 13; the resulting Factor 13a interacts with the fibrin to make a covalently bonded, stabilized, cross-linked fibrin clot. Thrombin is an important platelet activator and also stimulates self-regeneration by activating Factors 5, 8, and 11.

Additionally, thrombin activates platelets in primary hemostasis (see Figure 24-27).

See Disorders of Secondary Hemostasis on page 24-28.

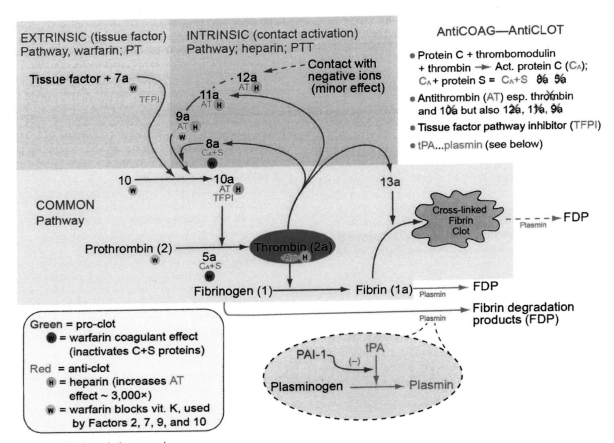

Figure 24-28: Coagulation cascade

CLOT LIMITATION AND DISSOLUTION

Clot size limitation occurs because thrombin also modulates its own production by combining with an endothelial cell surface protein, thrombomodulin, to activate protein C. Activated protein C, combined with protein S, deactivates Factors 5a and 8a, thereby limiting thrombin production.

Clot dissolution (fibrinolysis) is initiated by tissue plasminogen activator (tPA) released from endothelial cells. tPA is an enzyme that catalyzes the conversion of plasminogen to plasmin, which breaks down fibrin and fibrinogen and dissolves the clot.

Protein C also blocks the inhibitor of tPA (platelet activating factor [PAF]).

Clinical correlations quick review:

- Protein C or protein S deficiency causes a thrombogenic tendency. If mild, either deficiency predisposes the patient to deep vein thrombosis (DVT).
- tPA, as a drug, is used for thrombolysis in acute ischemic conditions (e.g., cardiac, limb, pulmonary, stroke).

CLINICAL EVALUATION OF BLEEDING DISORDERS

At the bedside, you can use family history, patient history, and physical examination to establish a differential diagnosis for a patient with a suspected bleeding disorder:

- Primary hemostatic problems (90% involve low platelets or platelet dysfunction) result in multiple, tiny, superficial hemorrhages. Patients present with petechiae, ecchymosis, and mucocutaneous bleeding. Remember that vasculitic disorders are a cause of bruising or palpable purpura in a child with a normal platelet count.
- Factor disorders are problems with secondary hemostasis. Patients with a coagulation disorder, such as hemophilia, develop deep tissue bleeding, including hematomas or hemarthroses.
- Menorrhagia is classic for von Willebrand disease.

LAB TESTS IN BLEEDING DISORDERS

Know these 5 tests, which are used to assess coagulation and platelet status:

1) **Prothrombin time** (PT) measures the time it takes plasma to clot when exposed to tissue factor, thus assessing the function of extrinsic and common pathways. (Think Factor 7.)

2) **Activated partial thromboplastin time** (PTT; a.k.a. aPTT) measures the time it takes plasma to clot when mixed with substances that activate intrinsic factors, thereby assessing function of the intrinsic and the common pathways.

3) **Thrombin time** measures the time it takes to convert fibrinogen to fibrin. A prolonged thrombin time reflects decreased or defective fibrinogen, elevated fibrin degradation products (FDPs), or the presence of heparin or heparin-like anticoagulants.

4) **Platelet count**

5) **Rapid platelet function anaylsis** (PFA) measures both platelet adhesion and aggregation (i.e., qualitative platelet defects). **Bleeding time** (< 10 minutes is normal) is used to measure the effectiveness of platelet aggregation; however, because it is technically difficult, bleeding time is infrequently used.

Most clotting factors are synthesized primarily in the liver, except for tissue factor (which is expressed on the surface of various cell types), von Willebrand factor (which is produced in endothelial cells and megakaryocytes), and Factor 8 (which is mainly produced by endothelial cells).

Review Figure 24-29 and Table 24-7 for an approach to diagnosis based on the PT, PTT, and mixing studies.

Table 24-7: Lab Results of Inherited and Acquired Bleeding Disorders	
Lab Results	**Etiology**
Prolonged PT and PTT	Congenital Factor 1, 2, 5, or 10 deficiency Acquired deficiency of vitamin K–dependent Factors 2, 7, 9, and 10 Liver disease Disseminated intravascular coagulation Vitamin K deficiency Warfarin, supratherapeutic Antiprothrombin antibody (rare)
Prolonged PT, normal PTT	Congenital Factor 7 deficiency Acquired Factor 7 deficiency Mild liver disease Mild vitamin K deficiency Warfarin, therapeutic
Prolonged PTT, normal PT—corrected by addition of normal plasma	Factor deficiency (e.g., Factor 8, 9, 11, 12* deficiency; von Willebrand disease with low Factor 8)
Prolonged PTT, normal PT—not corrected by addition of plasma	Circulating factor inhibitor (e.g., lupus anticoagulant [does not cause bleeding], acquired Factor 8 inhibitor [does cause bleeding], heparin contamination)
Normal PT and PTT	von Willebrand disease Thrombocytopenia Platelet function disorder Dense granule deficiency; storage pool defect Bernard-Soulier (giant platelet) syndrome (absent GP1b) Glanzmann thrombasthenia (absent GP2b/3a)

* Factor 12 deficiency does not cause bleeding.

PT = prothrombin time
PTT = partial thromboplastin time

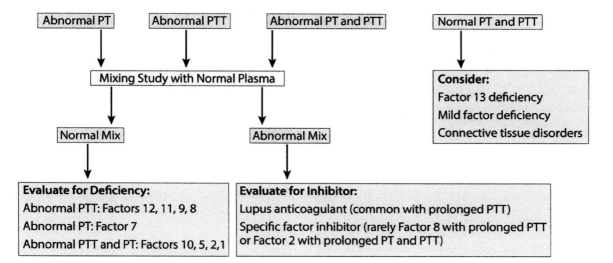

Figure 24-29: Diagnostic approach to bleeding disorders based on PT, PTT, and mixing study

Know: If initial lab tests demonstrate a greatly increased PTT, but a normal PT and normal platelet count, mix the patient's plasma 1:1 with normal plasma (a "**mixing study**"). If the PTT normalizes, the patient has a clotting factor deficiency; if it does not correct, the patient has developed an inhibitor to a clotting factor protein, usually a lupus anticoagulant or Factor 8 inhibitor. When there are Factor 8–specific antibodies, the PTT may initially correct; however, after incubation with normal plasma for 2 hours, it remains prolonged. Factor 8 inhibitors occur in some patients with congenital hemophilia A in response to clotting factor or in older patients with acquired hemophilia A.

DISORDERS OF PRIMARY HEMOSTASIS

Most disorders of primary hemostasis are due to abnormal platelet count or abnormal platelet function.

Normal Platelet Production

Platelets normally live 7–10 days in the blood. Megakaryocytes in the bone marrow undergo cytoplasmic fragmentation to form platelets. See Figure 24-26 on page 24-16. The production and maturation of megakaryocytes is regulated by thrombopoietin.

Platelets are involved in primary hemostasis, which is the forming of a platelet plug. See Primary Hemostasis – Platelet Plug Formation on page 24-21 for a detailed review of the mechanisms involved with platelet adhesion and aggregation during primary hemostasis.

Thrombocytopenia

Thrombocytopenia can be caused by immune thrombocytopenia (ITP; formerly known as immune thrombocytopenic purpura), disseminated intravascular coagulation (DIC), thrombotic thrombocytopenic purpura (TTP), hemolytic uremic syndrome (HUS), **HELLP** (hemolysis, elevated liver enzymes, low platelets) syndrome, dilution, transfusion, or amniotic fluid embolism (during childbirth). Medications/drugs causing thrombocytopenia include heparin, quinine, quinidine, phenytoin, gold salts, and alcohol. Beware that pseudothrombocytopenia may occur due to platelet clumping; for more information, see Pseudothrombocytopenia.

Children with thrombocytopenia have symptoms that include bruising, petechiae, and mucosal bleeding. Severity of bruising and bleeding depends on the degree and etiology of thrombocytopenia.

The first step in the diagnostic evaluation of thrombocytopenia is to confirm the platelet count and to exclude pseudothrombocytopenia or laboratory error. Once thrombocytopenia has been confirmed, obtain a careful history to clarify the presence, frequency, and severity of bleeding symptoms, as well as potential causes for the thrombocytopenia (e.g., systemic symptoms, medications, recent infection, immunizations, dietary history, family history, travel history).

A complete physical examination reveals signs (if present) of thrombocytopenia (e.g., bruising, bleeding, petechiae), concurrent infection or sepsis (e.g., fever, tachycardia, hypotension), stigmata for inherited causes of thrombocytopenia (e.g., short stature, thumb and/or radial ray abnormalities, café au lait macules), and findings that could suggest chronic or lymphoproliferative diseases (e.g., hepatomegaly, splenomegaly, lymphadenopathy).

The CBC and peripheral blood smear provide important diagnostic clues, depending on whether or not there is an isolated thrombocytopenia and if there are morphological features that are associated with specific causes of thrombocytopenia (e.g., megathrombocytes, microthrombocytes, leukocyte inclusion bodies). An isolated thrombocytopenia in the absence of splenomegaly is suggestive of ITP.

A combined cytopenia may represent a condition with decreased blood cell production (i.e., bone marrow suppression or bone marrow infiltration) or a peripherally destructive process where blood cells are being consumed through splenic sequestration, autoimmune destruction, or a microvascular process. Bone marrow evaluation is indicated for a combined cytopenia, presence of systemic symptoms, or presence of lymphadenopathy or organomegaly.

We'll cover a few causes of thrombocytopenia:

- Inherited
  - Wiskott-Aldrich syndrome
  - Myosin heavy chain 9 gene (*MYH9*)–related disorders
  - Thrombocytopenia-absent radius (TAR) syndrome
- Acquired
  - Pseudothrombocytopenia
  - ITP
  - TTP
  - Maternal autoimmune neonatal thrombocytopenia (maternal ITP)
  - Kasabach-Merritt phenomenon

Inherited Thrombocytopenia

Thrombocytopenia may be inherited. Consider inherited thrombocytopenia if it occurs at a very young age and is chronic or if the patient has family history of thrombocytopenia. Inherited thrombocytopenia can be mistaken for ITP; consider it if the patient does not respond to ITP therapy. Look at the blood smear for morphological clues.

4 inherited platelet disorders cause abnormal platelet morphology:

1) Bernard-Soulier syndrome (uniformly large platelets)
2) Wiskott-Aldrich syndrome (uniformly small platelets)
3) *MYH9*-related disorders, including May-Hegglin anomaly (large platelets; white cell inclusions called Döhle bodies)
4) Gray platelet syndrome (pale platelets)

Wiskott-Aldrich Syndrome

Wiskott-Aldrich syndrome is an extremely rare X-linked disorder characterized by severe thrombocytopenia and microthrombocytes (in contrast to ITP, in which platelets are mostly large but of variable sizes) that can present in the neonatal period. Affected boys develop eczema and immunodeficiency. Individuals are at risk for lymphoma later in life. See the Allergy & Immunology section for more information.

MYH9-Related Disorders

This group of *MYH9*-related disorders is characterized by AD (autosomal dominant) mutations in the gene for nonmuscle myosin heavy chain 2A. This defect leads to defective megakaryocyte maturation. Characteristics on the blood smear include macrothrombocytes and Döhle bodies in WBCs. Clinical characteristics include bleeding tendency and nephritis, sensorineural hearing loss, and/or cataracts.

Thrombocytopenia-Absent Radius (TAR) Syndrome

TAR syndrome is an inherited disorder that presents with bleeding in the neonate. Thrombocytopenia is severe, and there is an increased risk of death during the neonatal period and early infancy as a result of intracranial bleeds associated with platelet counts of < 30,000/μL ($< 30 \times 10^9$/L). TAR syndrome has an AR (autosomal recessive) inheritance pattern. Half of all affected infants are symptomatic in the 1st week of life, and 90% are symptomatic by 4 months of age. Thrombocytopenic episodes are most frequent during the first 2 years of life and then decrease in frequency. Thrombocytopenia can fluctuate, and levels can even be normal at times. Infection and dietary factors, especially cow's milk allergy, sometimes precipitate episodes. Leukocytosis can occur. There is a decrease or absence of megakaryocytes in the bone marrow.

These patients also have no radii (Figure 24-30), but their thumbs are normal (as opposed to Fanconi anemia and trisomy 18, in which thumbs are abnormal).

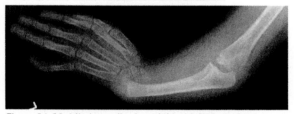

Figure 24-30: Missing radius in a child with TAR syndrome

In addition to absent radii, upper extremity abnormalities include hypoplastic carpals and phalanges, syndactyly, clinodactyly, and phocomelia. Lower extremity abnormalities are also common and can include hip dysplasia, femoral and/or tibial torsion, and deformities of the knees and/or feet. Dysmorphic features of the face include micrognathia; hypertelorism with a broad forehead; and low-set, posteriorly rotated ears. Congenital heart disease (most often atrial septal defect, isolated ventricular septal defect, or tetralogy of Fallot) occurs in 30–35% of patients with TAR syndrome.

Most patients survive, and platelet counts improve spontaneously over time. Treatment, if necessary for clinically significant bleeding, is best accomplished with platelet transfusion.

Acquired Thrombocytopenia

Thrombocytopenia is most often an acquired condition and is caused by 1 or more of the following processes:

- Decreased production of platelets (e.g., leukemia, aplastic anemia, viral infection, medications)
- Increased destruction of platelets (e.g., ITP, medications, DIC)
- Sequestration (pooling) of platelets in an enlarged spleen

If there are normal or increased numbers of megakaryocytes in the bone marrow, you do not have a production problem!

Know:

- Many children with sepsis have thrombocytopenia due to DIC.
- Neonates with CMV (cytomegalovirus) present with thrombocytopenia, microcephaly, and/or other congenital anomalies.
- Always review the medication history when evaluating a child with thrombocytopenia.

Pseudothrombocytopenia

If a patient has unexpected thrombocytopenia, then review the blood smear. In some cases, platelet clumping results in a factitiously low platelet count on the automated reader. Platelet clumping results from naturally occurring antibodies that interact with EDTA (ethylenediaminetetraacetic acid) in the blood collection tube. Platelets do not clump in a light-blue-topped tube (sodium citrate); so, redraw the sample in this type of tube.

Immune Thrombocytopenia (ITP)

ITP (formerly known as immune thrombocytopenic purpura) is a common cause of true thrombocytopenia in children. There are between 1 and 6 cases per 100,000 children per year in the U.S. In this condition, thrombocytopenia results from an immune-mediated destruction of circulating platelets. It is usually acute in onset and self-limited, but it can become chronic or recurrent. ITP is a diagnosis of exclusion, so other causes must be ruled out.

Acute ITP affects boys and girls equally and has a peak between 2 and 5 years of age. Chronic ITP more commonly occurs in adolescents or adults. A history of recent (in the preceding 1–6 weeks) viral infection or immunization is found in a large percentage of those affected. Acute bruising, petechiae, or bleeding is usually the 1st sign.

Petechiae and purpuric lesions occur spontaneously or with minor trauma. No hepatosplenomegaly is noted. In menstruating girls, a platelet count < 10,000/μL (< 10 × 10⁹/L) can result in severe blood loss. Intracranial hemorrhage occurs in < 1% of children with ITP and is fatal in 1/3 of these cases.

The major laboratory finding is a low platelet count of varying severity. The few platelets seen on the smear are megathrombocytes—large, but not as large as red blood cells. In ITP, there will be megathrombocytes as well as normal sized platelets that are seen in a blood film. A predominance of giant platelets indicates an inherited platelet disorder (e.g., Bernard-Soulier syndrome). The platelets, recently released in response to the low numbers (which, remember, is due to destruction and not to a production problem), are "reticulated"; that is, they still contain RNA. Bottom line: The bone marrow is cranking out the platelets as fast as it can, but the destructive process is eliminating them just as fast. Unless significant bleeding has occurred, hemoglobin is usually normal in ITP, which helps differentiate it from TTP, HUS, and DIC. In ITP, the WBC count is also usually normal.

A bone marrow study is necessary in patients with ITP if:

• features are not classic for ITP and/or
• the platelet count does not increase with initial therapy.

If performed, the bone marrow study shows normal-to-increased megakaryocytes.

Platelet counts normalize in nearly 80% of children with ITP within 12 months of diagnosis. Risk factors for chronic ITP are > 10 years of age, female gender, and insidious onset of original symptoms. In rare instances, ITP is recurrent.

Decision to treat depends on bleeding symptoms. Treatment is not indicated if the platelet count is > 10,000–20,000/μL (> 10 × 10⁹ to 20 × 10⁹/L) and there are no substantial bleeding symptoms. If there is significant skin or mucosal bleeding, initiate treatment. The American Society of Hematology's 2019 evidence-based practice guidelines for ITP suggest observation rather than treatment for children with no bleeding or mild bleeding, irrespective of the platelet count. In all patients with ITP, NSAIDs and aspirin are contraindicated because these interfere with platelet function. Patients should also be counseled to avoid activities that are associated with a risk of traumatic injury.

There are 3 first-line treatments available for acute ITP—corticosteroids, IVIG (intravenous immunoglobulin), and anti-Rh (D) immunoglobulin:

1) Corticosteroids have a rapid action that reduces reticuloendothelial destruction of antibody-coated platelets and also slows down antibody production. Various treatment regimens have been used. Corticosteroids are recommended over IVIG and anti-Rh(D) as first-line treatments for ITP. Note: Corticosteroids can mask a diagnosis of acute leukemia. Consider evaluation for leukemia if clinical presentation includes lymphadenopathy, bone pain, weight loss, anemia, or neutropenia.

2) IVIG blocks the Fc receptors of the reticuloendothelial phagocytes and prevents them from binding and destroying the IgG antibody–coated platelets.

3) Anti-Rh (D) immunoglobulin causes a mild hemolytic anemia that saturates the Fc receptors of the reticuloendothelial phagocytes and results in increased survival of antibody-coated platelets. There is a black box warning about acute renal insufficiency due to severe hemolysis, and close monitoring is required. Note: Anti-Rh can be used only in Rh+ patients who are Coombs negative and not splenectomized.

IVIG yields a response rate of 94–97%, followed by anti-Rh (D) immunoglobulin (82–90%) and corticosteroids (79%). Duration of response is variable. Some patients with acute ITP require multiple treatments until thrombocytopenia and bleeding symptoms resolve. Platelet transfusions are not generally recommended because they are destroyed by the same antibodies as the native platelets. In the case of intracranial bleeding, platelets are given with IVIG, high-dose IV steroids, and (rarely) splenectomy.

If ITP becomes chronic, splenectomy, immunosuppressive agents, or thrombopoietin mimetics are treatment options. Splenectomy can be "curative" by eliminating the site of destruction of platelets, but the antibody can remain.

Thrombotic Thrombocytopenic Purpura (TTP)

TTP is a thrombotic microangiopathic hemolytic anemia typically caused by antibodies against ADAMTS13—a protease that breaks down ultralarge von Willebrand factor (vWF) multimers. Persistence of ultralarge vWF multimers leads to platelet agglutination, microvascular thrombi formation, and multiorgan dysfunction. In addition to the anemia, previously healthy patients present with thrombocytopenia. Characteristic lab findings include an elevated lactate dehydrogenase, hyperbilirubinemia, and azotemia. The condition is life-threatening because of the risk of thrombosis in small arteries supplying the heart and central nervous system. The treatment of TTP includes emergent plasma pheresis and corticosteroids.

Maternal Autoimmune Neonatal Thrombocytopenia (Maternal ITP)

Maternal ITP is a fairly common disorder in pregnant women (about 5%). The infants of these mothers are not affected. However, infants whose mothers have maternal ITP may develop thrombocytopenia because of the transplacental passage of maternal IgG antiplatelet antibodies. The condition lasts about 1–2 months after birth.

IVIG is given during the 3rd trimester to mothers who have maternal ITP, especially if there is maternal bleeding. IVIG is given to the newborn if the platelet count is < 20,000/μL (< 20 × 10⁹/L). If the affected newborn has evidence of bleeding, including intracranial hemorrhage (< 1% risk), give steroids and platelet transfusions in addition to IVIG.

Kasabach-Merritt Phenomenon

The Kasabach-Merritt phenomenon is due to the destruction of platelets in certain vascular tumors of the skin, liver, or spleen. These tumors include tufted angiomas and kaposiform hemangioendotheliomas. This disorder usually presents early in life. Some patients have evidence of a consumptive coagulopathy with low fibrinogen and elevated D-dimers with microangiopathic hemolytic anemia. Management includes medications (e.g., corticosteroids, propranolol, vincristine, interferon-α) and supportive care. The tumors often cannot be surgically excised or embolized if they are too large or inaccessible.

Platelet Function Abnormalities

Etiology of platelet function abnormalities includes:

- Inherited
  - von Willebrand disease
  - Bernard-Soulier syndrome
- Acquired
  - Drug-induced
  - Uremia

Children with platelet function abnormalities most often have normal or near-normal platelet counts with reduced platelet function. Symptoms include bruising, petechiae, and mucosal bleeding.

Inherited Abnormalities

von Willebrand Disease (vWD)

von Willebrand factor (vWF) helps platelets stick to exposed subendothelium and to other platelets; it is also the carrier protein for Factor 8.

vWF multimers in the bloodstream have little affinity for platelets. But this affinity increases dramatically when vWF attaches to an altered vascular surface, thereby causing an increased aggregation of platelets at that spot. vWF multimers in the bloodstream are various sizes, ranging from small to ultralarge. The larger the multimer, the more hemostatic potential.

von Willebrand disease (vWD) is usually AD and affects up to 1% of the population. Expression is variable—patients can have mild symptoms (e.g., bleeding with dental extractions, lifelong easy bruising) to more severe symptoms (e.g., frequent recurrent bleeding: nasal, oral, GI, genitourinary [including recurrent menorrhagia]). A frequent 1st manifestation of vWD in girls is heavy menstrual bleeding. vWD Type 2N and Type 3 are inherited in an AR pattern.

PTT is usually normal, although it is prolonged in severe subtypes (due to decreased Factor 8); in contrast, PT is always normal. Rapid PFA (platelet function analysis) and bleeding time are typically prolonged.

Individuals with Type O blood normally have lower vWF levels. Levels increase during pregnancy and with estrogen therapy.

There are 3 types of vWD:

- Type 1 vWD is the most common (90%) and is due to a decrease in the amount of vWF (i.e., a quantitative problem).
- Type 2 vWD results from a qualitative problem with vWF. All Type 2 vWD subtypes cause increased bleeding.
  - Type 2A—decreased binding of vWF to platelets
  - Type 2B—increased binding of vWF to platelets, but it is a bleeding disorder. This seems counterintuitive, but what is thought to happen is that the largest vWF multimers bind to platelets while still in the plasma, making these multimers unavailable for the hemostatic process. The largest multimers have the most hemostatic potential, so the result is a bleeding disorder.
  - Type 2M—decreased binding of vWF to platelets and a decreased quantity of vWF multimers
  - Type 2N—decreased binding of vWF to Factor 8
- Type 3 vWD is rare (1/1,000,000 in the general population). Patients have undetectable vWF levels and low Factor 8 levels. The bleeding symptoms are similar to those seen in severe hemophilia.

When decreased activity is tied to decreased amount of vWF, it is always a quantity problem—never a binding problem. Hence, diagnosis of Type 1 vWD is confirmed with the combination of all of the following:

- Decreased vWF antigen
- Proportional decrease in Factor 8 activity (vWF protein is a cofactor of Factor 8). With Type 1 vWD, Factor 8 activity remains within the normal range.
- Proportional decrease in biologic activity, as measured by the ristocetin cofactor (rCoF) assay

Diagnosis of Type 2 vWD (A, B, M, and N) requires specialized testing.

Diagnosis of Type 3 vWD is based on finding absent vWF antigen and activity, and very low Factor 8 activity.

Diagnostic testing is complicated by patient stress and delayed processing times. Stress temporarily increases vWF levels (a blood draw can be stressful for many patients), and delayed processing yields falsely low vWF levels.

Treatment options for children with vWD:

- Desmopressin (DDAVP) causes a release of stored vWF and Factor 8 from endothelial cells. DDAVP may be used to treat and prevent bleeding in most patients with Type 1 vWD and some patients with Type 2A vWD.
- Patients with Type 1 or Type 2A vWD who do not respond to DDAVP (or have major bleeding or surgery) are treated with vWF/Factor 8 concentrates.
- Treatment with vWF/Factor 8 concentrates is required for patients with Type 2B, Type 2M, Type 2N, and Type 3 vWD.

- Cryoprecipitate contains vWF and Factor 8, but it has been replaced by the concentrates that have less risk of viral contamination. These concentrates are preferred over cryoprecipitate because cryoprecipitate contains fibrinogen, Factor 8, vWF, and Factor 13 (which has a higher risk of viral contamination).
- The antifibrinolytic agents, ε-aminocaproic acid and tranexamic acid, are useful for minor mucosal bleeding and can be given as an oral rinse to prevent local fibrinolysis.

Menorrhagia is a common symptom of vWD. Treatment options include ε-aminocaproic acid, tranexamic acid, and oral contraceptives.

Bernard-Soulier Syndrome

Bernard-Soulier syndrome is an AR disorder with mild thrombocytopenia and giant, abnormal platelets that do not aggregate in response to ristocetin but do aggregate in response to ADP (adenosine diphosphate), epinephrine, or collagen. There is a prolonged rapid PFA and bleeding time with this disorder. The abnormality is a deficiency of platelet GP1b (glycoprotein 1b) in the platelet membrane, which results in the inability of the platelets to aggregate properly. There is severe mucocutaneous bleeding starting in infancy.

Acquired Abnormalities

Drug-Induced Platelet Dysfunction

Drug-induced platelet dysfunction can be reversible or irreversible. NSAIDs reversibly bind with COX (cyclo-oxygenase), inhibiting platelet function. Serotonin reuptake inhibitors also inhibit platelet function by depleting platelet serotonin and thus inhibiting serotonin-induced platelet aggregation amplification. In contrast to NSAIDs, aspirin (acetylsalicylic acid [ASA]) irreversibly inactivates platelet COX, preventing the conversion of AA to TxA_2 (see Figure 24-27 on page 24-21) and thereby altering platelet function for the entire lifespan of the platelet. Chronic ASA use of as little as 40 mg/day causes suppression of 95% of the TxA_2.

Uremic Platelet Dysfunction

The major cause of bleeding in patients with renal disease is platelet dysfunction that results from impaired platelet adhesiveness and decreased platelet aggregation.

Most commonly, this condition manifests as GI bleeding, but it can also involve the skin, mucous membranes, urinary tract, and respiratory system.

Treatment of platelet dysfunction is needed in symptomatic patients or in those about to undergo a surgical procedure. Options include correction of anemia, desmopressin, dialysis, or administration of conjugated estrogens.

Thrombocytosis

Thrombocytosis (or excess platelets) is defined as $> 450,000/\mu L$ ($> 450 \times 10^9$/L). Platelets are an acute phase reactant (i.e., increase with inflammation and tissue injury). Thrombocytosis in children is usually due to a reaction to some secondary cause: acute or chronic infection, iron deficiency anemia, inflammatory disorders, or acute blood loss. It is a benign condition and does not require specific therapy. Thrombocytosis is also common in mucocutaneous lymph node syndrome (Kawasaki syndrome) and in patients who are hyposplenic or asplenic.

Essential Thrombocythemia

Based on the World Health Organization (WHO) diagnostic criteria, essential thrombocythemia is a rare myeloproliferative disorder that meets the following 4 major criteria or the first 3 major criteria and the minor criterion.

Major criteria:

1) Persistent platelet counts $> 450,000/\mu L$ ($> 450 \times 10^9$/L)

2) Bone marrow morphology showing proliferation, mainly of the megakaryocyte lineage

3) WHO criteria for other myeloid neoplasm are not met.

4) Presence of *JAK2*, *MPL*, or *CALR* mutations

Minor criterion:

- Absence of identifiable cause of thrombocytosis (e.g., iron deficiency anemia, infection, inflammation) or identification of another clonal marker (*ASXL1*, *EZH2*, *TET2*, *IDH1*/*IDH2*, *SRSF2*, or *SR3B1* mutation)

Thrombosis and bleeding commonly occur because platelet function is abnormal. Patients who are not bleeding are treated with a platelet aggregation inhibitor, such as aspirin. In addition, a platelet-lowering drug (such as hydroxyurea or anagrelide) is prescribed.

DISORDERS OF SECONDARY HEMOSTASIS

We will discuss some of the most common coagulation factor disorders here. These include Factor 8, 9, and 11 deficiencies, DIC, vitamin K deficiency, and lupus anticoagulants.

Factor 8 Deficiency (Hemophilia A)

Hemophilia A is due to a deficiency of Factor 8. In the intrinsic pathway, activated Factor 8 serves as cofactor to activated Factor 9, greatly accelerating the production of Factor 10 (1,000-fold).

With either Factor 8 or 9 deficiency, the PTT is increased and the PT is normal.

Factor 8 deficiency is X-linked recessive; i.e., the patient is virtually always male, and the family history might be positive for bleeding in males on the maternal side of the family. Female carriers have one normal Factor 8–producing gene (*F8*) but may still have lower Factor 8 levels due to skewed X-inactivation and bleeding symptoms.

There are a few additional facts to know about inheritance of hemophilia:

- A female carrier of hemophilia has:
  - a 50% chance that a male offspring will inherit that bleeding disorder, and
  - a 50% chance that a female offspring will also be a carrier.
- Test children born to the daughters of patients with hemophilia for the relevant bleeding disorder (e.g., Factor 8 deficiency, Factor 9 deficiency).
- Approximately 30–50% of children with hemophilia have a negative family history.
- Both Factor 8 and 9 deficiencies can be diagnosed prenatally.

Presentation

The presentation is similar in Factor 8 and 9 deficiencies, with easy bruising, muscle and joint hemorrhages, and prolonged hemorrhage after surgery or trauma—but typically no mucosal bleeding or excessive bleeding after minor cuts.

Excessive bleeding following neonatal elective circumcision is a classic presentation of hemophilia. Infants can also present with bleeding from heel stick, intramuscular hematoma from hepatitis B immunization, or caput succedaneum with traumatic delivery. In ambulatory patients, hemarthrosis is the most common site for bleeding and presents with pain and reduced mobility. See Table 24-7 on page 24-23 for a summary of test results in the factor deficiencies.

With Factor 8 deficiency, the risk of bleeding correlates with the plasma levels of Factor 8. Patients with < 1% of normal activity have severe disease. Patients with 1–5% activity have moderate disease, and patients with 6–40% Factor 8 activity have mild disease.

It is important to know when to suspect intracranial hemorrhage and how to manage it. A new or worsening headache in a patient with hemophilia is very concerning for a possible intracranial bleed. Symptoms of intracranial bleeding in infants include lethargy and poor feeding. Start factor therapy immediately for hemophilia patients with serious head trauma, even in the absence of loss of consciousness or an abnormal neurologic exam. Consider emergent CT of the head without contrast after factor is administered.

It is important to recognize and aggressively treat bleeding into the forearm. Bleeding in the forearm of a person with hemophilia is an emergency because of the risk of compartment syndrome, nerve damage, and long-term risk of contractures. This type of bleeding requires aggressive factor replacement and frequent neurovascular assessment. Patients with compartment syndrome require urgent surgical intervention.

Treatment

DDAVP is a treatment option for some patients with mild Factor 8 deficiency. DDAVP causes a release of vWF and Factor 8 stores from endothelial cells. A DDAVP challenge is done to prove response. If a patient has an adequate response to DDAVP, it can be used as treatment for an acute bleed and prophylactically for a tooth extraction in patients with mild disease (i.e., Factor 8 levels > 5%). DDAVP is not effective in patients with moderate or severe hemophilia.

Patients with moderate or severe Factor 8 deficiency who have acute bleeding are treated with **Factor 8 concentrate**.

The most serious side effect of current factor products is development of a neutralizing inhibitor, an antibody that inactivates or causes increased clearance of the "foreign" product. This occurs in ~ 25% of patients with severe hemophilia A. If a patient does not respond to clotting factor replacement, suspect the presence of an inhibitor. The presence of an inhibitor can be confirmed with a Factor 8 inhibitor assay. If positive, **bypassing agents** (i.e., rF7a, Feiba, Autoplex) must be used to treat bleeding. Immune tolerance induction (frequent, high doses of Factor 8) is done to provide immune tolerance and eradicate the inhibitor.

It is important to begin the treatment of a bleeding episode with the onset of symptoms and not wait until it is clinically established. Early treatment delays or prevents the hemophilic arthropathy and subsequent severe joint deformity. Prophylactic use of Factor 8 reduces arthropathy.

Factor 9 Deficiency (Hemophilia B)

Factor 9 deficiency is called hemophilia B or Christmas disease and is X-linked recessive. It is one-tenth as common as hemophilia A. Presentation is similar to Factor 8 deficiency and is dependent on severity. Treat an acute bleed with a Factor 9 concentrate.

Inhibitors are much less common in hemophilia B. Factor 9 inhibitors can present with anaphylaxis and nephrotic syndrome.

Factor 11 Deficiency (Hemophilia C)

Factor 11 deficiency and other rare clotting factor deficiencies (including deficiencies of fibrinogen and Factors 5, 7, 10 and 13) have an AR pattern of inheritance. Hemophilia C is found equally in men and women and is most common in certain ethnic groups—especially Ashkenazi Jews (occurs in up to 8%). Most patients with hemophilia C have less severe bleeding problems than those with Factor 8 or 9 deficiency and do not get hemarthroses. Bleeding in these patients is most commonly surgery or trauma related, and they tend to have more mucosal bleeding (e.g., epistaxis, menorrhagia). The risk of bleeding does not correlate with the level of Factor 11. Tranexamic acid and ε-aminocaproic acid are useful for mucosal bleeding. For severe bleeding episodes, use fresh frozen plasma (FFP).

Disseminated Intravascular Coagulation (DIC)

DIC is the most common acquired coagulopathy. It is always a secondary condition, so the underlying disease must be treated for the DIC to resolve. DIC occurs in diseases that promote tissue-factor release. These include:

- Massive direct tissue trauma
- Production of tumor necrosis factor (especially seen in solid tumors)
- Sepsis
- Endotoxin production in certain infections
- Placental tissue substances in obstetric patients with placental abruption, dead fetus, or amniotic fluid embolism
- Acute promyelocytic leukemia
- Rattlesnake or viper envenomation

In DIC, large amounts of released tissue factor interact with Factor 7 and initiate coagulation. There is excessive thrombin and plasmin production, resulting in both increased clot formation (via thrombin cleaving fibrinogen to fibrin) and clot breakdown (via plasmin degradation of fibrin clots). The plasmin breaks down fibrinogen and fibrin into fibrinogen/fibrin degradation products (FDPs; a.k.a. fibrin split products [FSPs]).

Lab results in DIC reflect these described abnormalities with:

- Prolonged PT and PTT
- Thrombocytopenia
- Decreased fibrinogen
- Elevated D-dimer (This is an FDP specifically produced by the action of plasmin on fibrin.)
- Increased thrombin time (due to both decreased fibrinogen and increased FDPs)
- RBC fragments (i.e., schistocytes, characteristic of microangiopathic hemolytic anemia) seen in the peripheral smear in up to 50% of patients (The fibrin strands span the small blood vessels and shear the RBCs.)

The massive depletion of coagulation factors and platelets and the increased FSPs result in bleeding. Symptoms in DIC result from bleeding or microvascular thrombosis as well as the underlying disorder. Some symptoms can include petechiae, ecchymosis, hemorrhage, hypotension, tachycardia, altered consciousness, and GI bleeding.

Treatment of DIC: Treat the underlying disorder! With severe bleeding, give FFP and platelets. Give cryoprecipitate if fibrinogen is low.

Vitamin K Deficiency

Vitamin K deficiency results in decreased production of Factors 2, 7, 9, and 10, and of proteins C and S. Causes of vitamin K deficiency are low stores (e.g., neonates), liver disease, decreased dietary absorption (e.g., no dietary intake of leafy greens, malabsorption, taking broad-spectrum antibiotics), and antagonists (e.g., warfarin).

Newborn infants are functionally vitamin K deficient and require vitamin K supplements soon after birth. Newborns who do not receive vitamin K at birth are at risk for vitamin K deficiency bleeding (VKDB; previously known as hemorrhagic disease of the newborn). Other risk factors for VKDB include antibiotics, gastrointestinal malabsorption, and a breastfeeding mother treated with vitamin K antagonists (warfarin, hydantoins, and phenobarbital). Infants can present with bruising, gastrointestinal hemorrhage, or intracranial hemorrhage. See the Neonatology section for more on VKDB.

Because the vitamin K–dependent coagulation factors are synthesized in the liver, severe liver disease can result in deficiency of these factors.

Vitamin K is a fat-soluble vitamin, so any condition that causes fat malabsorption can also result in vitamin K deficiency. Some of these conditions include cystic fibrosis, biliary cholangitis, inflammatory bowel disease, and short bowel syndrome.

Warfarin causes an effective vitamin K deficiency. When warfarin treatment is initiated, if the patient has increased thrombosis (e.g., DVT, pulmonary embolism [PE]), it is due to the negative effect of warfarin on protein C, which has anticoagulant effects. Initially, warfarin therapy causes a prothrombotic effect, which outweighs its antithrombotic effect on Factor 7. This is especially likely to happen if the patient is protein C deficient (patients should be on heparin or low molecular weight heparin until a therapeutic dose of warfarin is achieved). 1/3 of patients who develop warfarin-related skin necrosis have a protein C deficiency.

Administer vitamin K to patients with vitamin K deficiency if the patient is bleeding. FFP or nonactivated prothrombin complex concentrate can be used while waiting for the vitamin K to take effect (8 hours). Likewise, the effect of warfarin can be reversed with vitamin K; however, if a patient on warfarin has significant bleeding, give FFP or nonactivated prothrombin complex concentrate for immediate factor replacement.

Lupus Anticoagulants (LACs)

LACs result in a prolonged PTT. In most cases, a patient with LAC does not present with bleeding. It is associated with thrombosis.

LACs are common in young children in the setting of viral infection. They are not pathogenic and resolve spontaneously.

Use a PTT mixing study to differentiate a congenital factor deficiency from an LAC. The patient's plasma is mixed with an equal amount of pooled normal plasma, and the clotting test is repeated immediately after an established incubation period.

Because only ~ 30–40% of an individual factor is necessary to yield a normal PTT, a patient with a deficiency of a clotting factor corrects completely when mixed with normal plasma (i.e., with normal factor levels). On the other hand, the PTT of patients with inhibitors remains abnormally prolonged after the mix. In these cases, a 1:1 dilution of the patient's plasma is not sufficient to eliminate the full effect of the inhibitor on the PTT.

THROMBOTIC DISORDERS

Thrombotic disorders are rare in infants and children, but they are extremely important clinically. Venous thrombosis is more common than arterial thrombosis. Venous thrombosis can occur in upper and lower extremity veins, presenting with extremity pain, swelling, and color change. Cerebral sinovenous thrombosis presents with seizures, altered mental status, stroke, and/or headache. Portal vein thrombosis occurs in newborns with umbilical vein catheters.

Infants with a history of birth asphyxia, shock, and/or sepsis are at increased risk of developing endothelial cell injury leading to **renal vein thrombus** formation. It is also more common in infants of diabetic mothers and in those with congenital hypercoagulable states. This disorder presents with the sudden onset of gross hematuria and a unilateral or bilateral flank mass. On ultrasound, many infants are found to have a thrombus that extends into the inferior vena cava. Doppler flow studies of the inferior vena cava and renal veins confirm the diagnosis. Microangiopathic hemolytic anemia and adrenal hemorrhage can also occur. Although all 3 signs are not present in every patient with renal vein thrombosis, almost all patients have at least 1 of the following: gross hematuria, unilateral or bilateral flank mass, and/or thrombocytopenia.

Most children with thrombosis have multiple risk factors. The most common cause of DVT in children is a central venous catheter. Other acquired risk factors include trauma, immobilization, smoking, and estrogen-based oral contraceptives. LAC and antiphospholipid antibodies (anticardiolipin and anti-β_2-glycoprotein-1) are acquired risk factors for thrombosis and are associated with higher risk for recurrence.

A strong family history of PE or DVT suggests a congenital hypercoagulable disorder. Antithrombin and proteins C and S are naturally occurring anticoagulants. These proteins help to oppose thrombin's procoagulant activity. Activated protein C (APC), in conjunction with its cofactor, protein S, cleaves activated Factors 5 and 8, rendering them inactive. (Recall that activated Factors 5 and 8 are necessary cofactors in the clotting cascade, helping to promote clotting.) Antithrombin inhibits thrombin. (Heparin functions as an anticoagulant by accentuating the effect of antithrombin.)

Deficiencies of natural anticoagulants are either acquired (e.g., nephrotic syndrome, asparaginase treatment) or inherited in an AD fashion. Infants who are homozygous for protein S or C deficiency have **neonatal purpura fulminans** with life-threatening thrombosis.

Other inherited thrombophilias include **Factor 5 Leiden** (APC resistance) and prothrombin gene mutations. 5% of the Caucasian population is heterozygous for the Factor 5 Leiden gene (*F5*), which increases the risk of venous thrombosis 5- to 8-fold. 1% of the Caucasian population is heterozygous for prothrombin gene mutation, which increases the risk of venous thrombosis 3- to 6-fold. The absolute risk of thrombosis depends on the baseline risk of an individual. Screening for acquired and inherited thrombophilia may be considered for all young patients with thrombosis.

See the Neurology section for more information on prothrombotic disorders.

ANTICOAGULATION TREATMENT

The most common anticoagulants used in children are unfractionated heparin, low molecular weight heparin, and warfarin. Thrombolytic therapy such as tPA is usually reserved for children with life- or limb-threatening arterial or venous thrombosis. tPA increases the conversion of plasminogen to plasmin in the presence of fibrin, so most of the plasmin made is localized to the fibrin clot. However, tPA also results in systemic lysis and, therefore, can cause serious bleeding.

TRANSFUSION TREATMENT

RBC transfusions: Packed RBCs (PRBCs) are the primary product used; whole blood is rarely used. Exceptions include major hemorrhage from trauma and pediatric cardiac surgery. A donated unit of whole blood is usually separated into packed RBCs, platelets, and plasma. PRBCs are the product of choice and are ordered according to blood type. A unit is typically a total volume of 250–350 mL of PRBCs reconstituted in plasma. A transfusion of 10 mL/kg typically raises the hemoglobin by 2.5–3 g/dL. Complications of RBC transfusions include hemolytic reaction (life-threatening with fever, chills, flank pain, and oozing from IV sites), febrile nonhemolytic reaction (fever and chills only), or urticarial reaction (hives without other allergic symptoms). A unit of PRBCs has 250 mg of elemental iron. Chronic transfusions result in iron overload.

Platelet transfusions: Alloimmunization can be a problem in patients who receive multiple transfusions. Transfusions can be ordered as random-donor or single-donor (pheresis) products. 1 unit of random-donor platelets/kg raises the platelet count by ~ 50,000/μL (~ 50 × 10^9/L). 1 single donor unit is the equivalent of 6–8 random donor units, but this is variable.

The actual platelet transfusion thresholds can be quite low in patients without bleeding who are undergoing chemotherapy. This is a pretty controversial area because all recommendations are from expert consensus statements, as virtually all studies have been done only in adults.

Patients with ITP are an exception because these patients almost never require platelet transfusions—even with very low platelet counts (their platelets seem to work better); also, transfusion of platelets is usually ineffective due to destruction. Platelet transfusion in TTP is usually avoided.

WBC transfusions are only rarely done. G-CSF or granulocyte-macrophage colony-stimulating factor (GM-CSF) is used in select circumstances to increase WBCs—most commonly in patients receiving myelosuppressive chemotherapy with active, life-threatening infections or in children with severe congenital neutropenia.

THE MEDSTUDY HUB: YOUR GUIDELINES AND REVIEW ARTICLES RESOURCE

For both review articles and current pediatrics practice guidelines, visit the MedStudy Hub at

medstudy.com/hub

The Hub contains the only online consolidated list of all current guidelines focused on pediatrics. Guidelines on the Hub are easy to find, continually updated, and linked to the published source. MedStudy maintains the Hub as a service to the medical community and makes it available to anyone and everyone at no cost to users.

FIGURE SOURCES

Figure 24-1: MedStudy illustration
Figure 24-2: MedStudy illustration
Figure 24-3: MedStudy illustration
Figure 24-10: MedStudy illustration
Figure 24-21: Dr Erhabor Osaro, CC BY-SA 3.0
Figure 24-26: MedStudy illustration
Figure 24-27: MedStudy illustration
Figure 24-28: MedStudy illustration
Figure 24-29: MedStudy illustration
Figure 24-30: Riaz Ahmad, CC BY 2.0
The remaining figures are from the MedStudy archives.

Oncology

SECTION EDITORS

Jeffrey Deyo, MD, PhD
Medical Director, Pediatric Hematology & Oncology
Our Lady af the Lake Children's Hospital
St. Jude Baton Rouge Affiliate Clinic
Baton Rouge, LA

Osman Farooq, MD
Clinical Associate Professor
John R. Oishei Children's Hospital
Buffalo, NY

MEDICAL EDITOR

Lynn Bullock, MD
Colorado Springs, CO

Table of Contents

CANCER INCIDENCE

PREVIEW | REVIEW

- What is the most common type of cancer in the first 15 years of life?

The annual incidence of childhood cancer in the U.S. is approximately 125/1,000,000 for children < 15 years of age. The following chart demonstrates the breakdown of the types of cancer by percentage in the 0- to 15-year age range (Table 25-1).

Table 25-1: Types of Cancer in the 0- to 15-Year Age Range	
Type	**% of Total Childhood Cancers**
Leukemias	25
Central nervous system tumors	17
Neuroblastoma	7
Non-Hodgkin lymphoma	6
Wilms tumor	6
Hodgkin lymphoma	5
Rhabdomyosarcoma	3
Retinoblastoma	3
Osteosarcoma	3
Ewing sarcoma	2

HEMATOLOGIC MALIGNANCIES

LEUKEMIA

PREVIEW | REVIEW

- What is the single most common childhood malignancy?
- Which disorders correlate with increased risk of acute lymphoblastic leukemia (ALL)?
- What diagnosis should you consider in a child with pallor and a limp?
- True or false? Splenomegaly is common in ALL.
- Which cytopenias are seen in children with ALL?
- What test is required to diagnose ALL?
- What must the test show to be diagnostic for ALL?
- What is the most important predictive factor for achieving a 2nd remission in ALL?
- What disorders have an increased risk of acute myeloid leukemia (AML)?
- What procedure is required for the diagnosis of AML?
- What peripheral blood cell finding is pathognomonic for AML?

Leukemia is the most common cancer in childhood, accounting for ~ 25% of all pediatric cancers. Leukemia is cancer of the white blood cells (WBCs) resulting in abnormally functioning cells that crowd out other healthy cells in the bone marrow. The type of leukemia that develops depends on the type of blood cell affected and the stage of development during which the cell becomes malignant. The stem cell differentiates into either lymphoid cells that mature into B or T lymphocytes or myeloid cells that mature into granulocytes (Figure 25-1). There are 2 main types of leukemia in children:

1) Acute lymphoblastic leukemia—cancer that develops in the lymphoid precursor cells

2) Acute myeloid leukemia—cancer that develops in the myeloid precursor cells

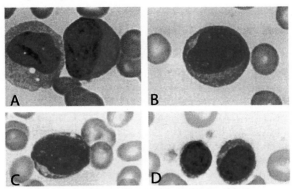

Figure 25-1: Myeloblast vs. lymphoblast. A) Monoblast and myeloblast. B) Myeloblast. C) Lymphoblast. D) Normal lymphocytes are smaller than myeloblasts and have few cytoplasmic granules and several nucleoli.

Symptoms of leukemia include anemia, fatigue, bruising, bleeding, bone pain, lymphadenopathy, and recurrent infections. Complete blood count (CBC) is the initial test if leukemia is suspected. If abnormal, a bone marrow biopsy is performed as well as a lumbar puncture to determine if the central nervous system is affected. Treatment depends on the type of leukemia.

Acute Lymphoblastic Leukemia (ALL)

Occurrence of ALL

ALL is the single most common childhood malignancy and one of the most curable (90%) cancers today. Its incidence peaks between 2 and 5 years of age. Annual incidence is ~ 3/100,000. ALL accounts for ~ 75% of all pediatric leukemia cases.

Although most patients do not have any known risk factors, there are a few accepted risk factors for ALL. These include the following:

- Prenatal radiation exposure
- Postnatal exposure to high doses of radiation
- Down syndrome
- Ataxia telangiectasia
- Bloom syndrome
- Fanconi anemia
- Neurofibromatosis

Clinical Findings in ALL

Signs and symptoms of ALL:

- The "4 **P**s"—**p**allor, **p**yrexia, **p**urpura, and **p**ain. This is the most common presentation of ALL.
- Fatigue and anorexia in the weeks to months before the diagnosis is made
- Petechiae or purpura in ~50% (due to thrombocytopenia)
- Bone pain with refusal to bear weight
- Lymphadenopathy (> 50%)
- Hepatomegaly (> 50%)
- Splenomegaly (frequently causes early satiety)

Be aware of the limping 2- to 5-year-old with pallor! The presence of bone pain can distinguish the pancytopenia of leukemia from the pancytopenia of aplastic anemia. Many children with leukemia present with bone pain and refuse to bear weight. Also, watch for the child with persistent oral candidiasis or infiltrated gums.

In addition to fever, bleeding, and bone pain, lymphadenopathy is typical. Generalized lymphadenopathy and hepatosplenomegaly are seen in > 50% of patients.

The lymph nodes, liver, and spleen are the most commonly affected organs, followed by the central nervous system (CNS), testes, and kidneys. Involvement of the CNS or testes is known as extramedullary disease. CNS disease occurs in < 5% of patients and frequently is asymptomatic. If symptoms do occur in CNS disease, they most commonly are headache, nausea, vomiting, lethargy, and/or irritability. Nuchal rigidity and papilledema also can be found but are uncommon. Cranial nerve involvement is rare but has a poor prognosis. Kidney enlargement is common at diagnosis but is not a prognostic indicator.

Laboratory Findings in ALL

Almost 90% of patients with ALL have an abnormal CBC at the time of diagnosis. Normocytic normochromic anemia and reticulocytopenia occur frequently. The WBC count can be very low to very high, with lymphoblasts visible on the peripheral smear. Most have an elevated WBC count: 50% have a count > 10,000/μL, and 20% have a count > 50,000/μL. However, it is important to remember that the WBC count can be normal or low.

Despite typically high WBC counts at presentation, a number of patients have severe neutropenia, putting them at an increased risk for infection. Thrombocytopenia is also very common (~ 50% have < 100,000 platelets/μL); thus, many patients have petechiae and purpura. Electrolyte abnormalities are common, and uric acid, phosphorus, potassium, and lactate dehydrogenase (LDH) levels can be high. Renal dysfunction can occur in those with hyperuricemia secondary to tumor lysis.

Definitive diagnosis requires a bone marrow evaluation. The marrow is classically hypercellular and infiltrated with leukemic lymphoblasts (Figure 25-2). Diagnosis of acute leukemia requires that at least 25% of the marrow must be involved. A lack of blasts on a peripheral blood smear in a pancytopenic patient does not rule out the diagnosis of leukemia. To evaluate for CNS involvement, a lumbar puncture is performed looking for leukemic cells in the cerebrospinal fluid (CSF) or evidence of cranial nerve involvement.

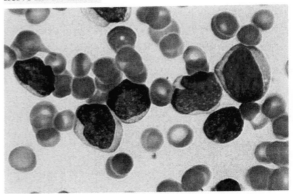

Figure 25-2: ALL: Many lymphoblasts. Note how large the blasts are compared to red blood cells.

Almost 85% of ALL cases develop from monoclonal proliferation of B-cell precursors, 14% have T-cell lineage, and the remaining 1% are mature B-cell ALL.

Treatment of ALL

Treatment for ALL consists of sophisticated multidrug, multiphase regimens divided into 4 categories:

1) Induction therapy
2) Consolidation therapy
3) Maintenance therapy
4) CNS preventive therapy

Most children receive 30–36 months of therapy, depending on prognosis and risk factors. The overall approach to therapy is one of risk stratification, which offers more intensive therapy for the highest-risk groups and less therapy and potentially less toxicity for the lowest-risk groups.

More than 95% of patients with standard-risk ALL enter remission following induction therapy. The rapidity of clearance of leukemic blasts during the induction month is an important predictor of overall outcome. Mortality rates during induction therapy are 3%, often due to infectious complications.

Every patient with ALL receives CNS chemoprophylaxis or preventive therapy, regardless of the initial CNS findings. Usually, a series of lumbar punctures with single-agent intrathecal methotrexate or triple-agent intrathecal therapy is given, reducing the occurrence of CNS leukemia to < 5–10%. CNS preventive therapy begins during the induction phase and continues throughout the treatment program. CNS radiation is primarily used in the setting of CNS relapse.

Outcomes of ALL

Overall cure rates for pediatric ALL are ~ 90% and are dependent on risk stratification.

Good prognostic indicators for ALL:

- Rapid response to treatment
- Hyperdiploidy (> 50 chromosomes or DNA index > 1.16)
- Trisomies of chromosomes 4 and 10
- t(12;21) translocation (*ETV6-RUNX1*)

Poorer prognostic indicators for ALL:

- Age < 1 year or > 10 years at diagnosis
- Presence of the Philadelphia chromosome t(9;22)
- WBC count > 50,000 cells/μL on presentation
- Abnormalities of the *MLL* gene; i.e., t(4;11)
- Mature B-cell leukemia
- T-cell leukemia
- Measurable residual disease at the end of induction (> 0.01% blasts)

Expected 5-year event-free survival:

- > 95% for patients with low-risk disease
- 90–95% for patients with standard-risk disease
- 75–90% for patients with high-risk disease
- < 75% for patients with very high-risk disease

The Philadelphia chromosome is present in < 5% of pediatric ALL; however, it is found in all chronic myelogenous leukemia (CML). The presence of the Philadelphia chromosome requires treatment with a tyrosine kinase inhibitor in addition to chemotherapy.

For response to treatment and 1st indication of relapse, the bone marrow is the best site to evaluate. The bone marrow is usually checked after induction and consolidation phases of treatment and later for relapse. The most important predictive factor for achieving a 2nd remission is the length of time the 1st remission lasted (i.e., the longer the 1st remission lasted, the better the survival rate). Salvage therapies to induce another remission can be very intense. BMT (blood and bone marrow transplant; a.k.a., hematopoietic stem cell transplant [HCT]) has become standard for treatment of the 1st relapse if it occurs early in the course (< 36 months from initial diagnosis), whereas patients with a late relapse may be salvageable with chemotherapy alone. Isolated CNS and testicular relapses are much less common, each accounting for < 10% of relapses. These extramedullary relapses can potentially be cured by treatment with chemotherapy and site-directed radiation therapy.

Side Effects of Therapy in ALL

Early and late CNS toxicities have been noted in patients receiving intrathecal and radiation therapy. Seizures occur in 5–15% of children with standard CNS therapy. Cerebral atrophy, necrotizing encephalopathy, and microangiopathy can occur over time in survivors. Cranial radiation results in neurodevelopmental and neuroendocrine abnormalities (including growth hormone deficiency), and spinal radiation can cause growth restriction. L-asparaginase treatment may cause acute pancreatitis in pediatric ALL patients. Prolonged corticosteroid use causes osteonecrosis.

Hepatotoxicity occurs with antimetabolite therapy (e.g., methotrexate, 6-mercaptopurine [6-MP]). Cardiomyopathy is seen with anthracyclines (doxorubicin and daunorubicin). Infertility is also an issue for those undergoing chemotherapy during or after puberty. Epipodophyllotoxins (most notably etoposide [VP-16]) have been reported to increase the risk of secondary malignancies, specifically acute myeloid leukemia.

Acute Myeloid Leukemia (AML)

AML accounts for ~ 20% of leukemia in children but makes up > 80% of adult acute leukemias. It is due to the proliferation of myeloid precursors. With AML, the World Health Organization (WHO) published a new classification system:

- **AML with recurrent genetic abnormalities**–e.g., AML with t(8;21)(q22;q22), RUNX1-RUNX1T1 (previously AML1-ETO); APL with PML/RARa, AML with t(9;11) (p21.3;q23.3)
- **AML with myelodysplasia-related changes**—i.e., following myelodysplastic syndrome (MDS) or MDS/myeloproliferative disease
- **Therapy-related myeloid neoplasms**—e.g., after alkylating agent or radiation
- **AML, not otherwise classified**—e.g., AML with minimal differentiation, acute myelomonocytic leukemia

The older French-American-British (FAB) classification system may still be used to differentiate, by morphology, the different subtypes (M0 through M7). AML survival rates are much lower than those for ALL—about 60–70% with current chemotherapy and transplant regimens.

Some conditions predispose to AML:

- Trisomy 21
- Diamond-Blackfan anemia
- Fanconi anemia
- Bloom syndrome
- Kostmann syndrome
- Paroxysmal nocturnal hemoglobinuria
- Neurofibromatosis

Previous exposure to VP-16 and ionizing radiation also predisposes to AML.

Clinical Manifestations of AML

Signs and symptoms of AML (note similarity to those of ALL):

- Fatigue, anorexia in the weeks to months before the diagnosis is made
- Bleeding, petechiae, purpura
- Lymphadenopathy, hepatomegaly, splenomegaly

- Fever is typical at presentation.
- Chloromas may be the 1st indication of AML (incidence is 2–9% in AML). These are localized leukemic infiltrations of the skin that present as a green-hued lesion (chloro = green).

AML frequently presents with signs and symptoms related to the different cytopenias encountered:

- Fatigue and pallor due to anemia
- Bruising, petechiae, epistaxis, or gum bleeding due to thrombocytopenia
- Infection due to neutropenia

Laboratory findings for AML are similar to ALL with high, low, or normal WBCs, anemia, and thrombocytopenia. Anemia and thrombocytopenia are nearly universal. The median hemoglobin at presentation is 7 g/dL. The WBC count can vary from low to extremely high.

Diagnosis of AML

Oncologists use bone marrow evaluation to diagnose AML. Bone marrow morphology, flow cytometry, cytogenetics, and molecular testing are used to classify AML. Finding **Auer rods** inside peripheral blood blast cells is pathognomonic for AML (Figure 25-3 and Figure 25-4).

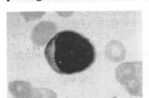
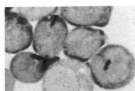

Figure 25-3: High-oil view of a normal myeloblast. Few cytoplasmic granules. Several nucleoli.

Figure 25-4: AML: Bone marrow aspirate with peroxidase-positive blasts and 2 peroxidase-positive Auer rods.

Treatment of AML

Risk stratification is primarily based on cytogenetics and molecular lesions and directs treatment offered to the patient:

- Favorable findings include t(8;21), inv(16), and CEBPA mutations.
- Unfavorable findings include monosomy 7, monosomy 5, and FLT3/ITD (duplications), among others.

These patients receive intensive chemotherapy +/– bone marrow transplant, depending on the risk stratification. Although the incidence of CNS disease is low, CNS prophylaxis is necessary for AML.

Children with acute promyelocytic leukemia (APML) represent a unique subset of AML patients who have excellent cure rates without undergoing transplant. Also, children with Down syndrome have a 10- to 20-fold greater risk for developing AML than children without Down syndrome. They do very well with chemotherapy alone, but are at higher risk for side effects.

For those who respond rapidly to initial therapy, the prognosis is better. For those who do not respond or who have a relapse, the prognosis is very poor. Overall, survival with favorable findings can be as high as 80% while unfavorable findings are associated with survival of 30 to 40% (or less).

LYMPHOMA

PREVIEW | REVIEW

- Why are steroids contraindicated as primary therapy for lymphadenopathy?
- What is the classic histologic hallmark of Hodgkin lymphoma?
- True or false? Hodgkin lymphoma is mostly of B-cell lineage.
- What is the most common presentation for Hodgkin lymphoma?
- What are B symptoms in Hodgkin lymphoma?
- How do you definitively diagnose Hodgkin lymphoma?
- In general, how are patients treated for Hodgkin lymphoma?
- What is the most common type of lymphoma in pediatrics?
- What is the most common form of non-Hodgkin lymphoma in pediatrics in the U.S.?
- How do most children with Burkitt lymphoma present?
- In children, lymphoma in the anterior mediastinum must be distinguished from what normal structure?
- Describe the staging system for non-Hodgkin lymphoma.
- True or false? Radiation therapy is a major component of most therapy for non-Hodgkin lymphoma.

Lymphoma refers to cancer of the lymphatic system, which includes lymph nodes, spleen, thymus, and bone marrow. Lymphomas are divided into 2 categories, **Hodgkin lymphoma** and **non-Hodgkin lymphoma**, depending on the microscopic appearance and characteristics of the malignant cells. Hodgkin lymphoma is defined by the presence of Reed-Sternberg cells, which are large multinucleated cells that divide rapidly and live longer than normal cells. Non-Hodgkin lymphomas do not have Reed-Sternberg cells and, in children, are commonly subdivided into Burkitt lymphoma, lymphoblastic lymphoma, and large cell lymphoma. Common symptoms of lymphoma include lymphadenopathy, fever, fatigue, night sweats, weight loss, and difficulty breathing (if chest mass). Worrisome features of lymphadenopathy are:

- Systemic symptoms (a.k.a. B symptoms; e.g., fever, night sweats, weight loss)
- Fixed, nontender nodes

- Supraclavicular nodes
- Lymph nodes > 2 cm with no response to a 2-week course of antibiotics

Do not treat lymphadenopathy with steroids until cleared by the oncologist. If the lymph nodes are infectious, steroids will inhibit the body's ability to fight infection. If the lymph nodes are leukemia or lymphoma, steroids will compromise the histopathologic diagnosis.

Diagnosis is made by lymph node biopsy. Treatment depends on the type of lymphoma and involves chemotherapy with or without radiation therapy, depending on risk features and response to treatment with chemotherapy.

Hodgkin Lymphoma

Occurrence

Lymphoma is the 3rd most common childhood cancer, and 40% of these are Hodgkin lymphoma. The highest incidence is seen in adolescents between 15 and 19 years of age.

Epidemiology

There are 3 typical age ranges for Hodgkin lymphoma:

1) Childhood (≤ 14 years of age)
2) Young adult (15–34 years of age)—most common form
3) Older adult (55–74 years of age)

Under the age of 10, boys are more commonly affected than girls. In adolescence, boys and girls are affected equally. Infectious etiologies, including Epstein-Barr virus (EBV), have been postulated; however, to date, none have been explicitly implicated. Genetic factors seem to come into play, with increased risk noted in twins and 1st degree relatives, but the specific link is unknown.

Pathology

There are many pathologic subtypes but nodular sclerosing is the most common type in children.

The classic histologic hallmark of Hodgkin lymphoma (though not always present) is the **Reed-Sternberg cell**, a large cell with multiple or multilobulated nuclei (looks like "owl's eyes"; Figure 25-5). Most cases are of B-cell lineage, but those of T-cell lineage are occasionally noted.

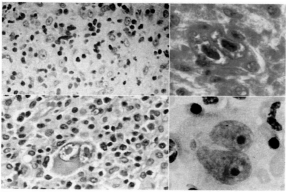

Figure 25-5: Hodgkin lymphoma: Views of Reed-Sternberg cell

Clinical Manifestations

The most common presentation for Hodgkin lymphoma is asymptomatic lymphadenopathy, which often involves the cervical or supraclavicular region. Supraclavicular lymphadenopathy is uncommon in inflammatory or infectious conditions and requires further evaluation with chest radiograph to rule out malignancy. Approximately 2/3 of patients have a mediastinal mass, which, on occasion, produces cough or tracheal/bronchial compression. < 10% of children have primary nodal disease below the diaphragm.

1/3 of children have B symptoms (constitutional symptoms), which include fever, drenching night sweats, and unexplained weight loss. These B symptoms usually indicate a more advanced disease and a worse prognosis.

Fevers are periodic in character: Febrile episodes last several days and are then followed by afebrile periods.

Additionally, cellular immunity is impaired in these patients, so tuberculosis, varicella zoster, and fungal infections are more common.

Clinical Diagnosis and Staging

Diagnosis of Hodgkin lymphoma is confirmed by excisional biopsy of an accessible lymph node.

Lab work can show nonspecific findings (although it is often normal), but some findings are helpful with staging and as prognostic indicators:

- CBC
- Erythrocyte sedimentation rate
- Serum ferritin
- Liver function tests
- Chest x-ray (CXR; to rapidly evaluate for mediastinal mass)
- Chest/abdomen/pelvis computed tomography (CT) with contrast
- Positron emission tomography (PET) scan
- Bone marrow aspiration and biopsy

The above staging tests help guide treatment and determine prognosis. The following are unfavorable features as adapted from the International Prognostic Score for Hodgkin lymphoma:

- Albumin < 4 g/dL
- Hemoglobin < 10.5 g/dL
- Male gender
- Stage IV disease
- WBC count ≥ 15,000 cells/μL
- Absolute lymphocyte count < 600 cells/μL or < 8% of total WBC count

The Ann Arbor staging classification is the international standard for staging of Hodgkin lymphoma (Table 25-2 on page 25-6).

ONCOLOGY

Table 25-2: Ann Arbor Staging of Hodgkin Lymphoma with Cotswolds Modifications

Stage	Definition
I	Involvement of a single lymph node region or localized involvement of a single extralymphatic organ or site
II	Involvement of ≥ 2 lymph node regions on the same side of the diaphragm
III	Involvement of lymph node regions on both sides of the diaphragm
IV	Disseminated involvement of ≥ 1 or more extralymphatic organs or tissues

A symptoms = absence of B symptoms
B symptoms = at least 1 of the following:
• Unexplained weight loss of > 10%
• Unexplained recurrent fevers
• Drenching night sweats
The designation "E" refers to extranodal contiguous extension.
The description bulky disease refers to a single nodal mass of ≥ 10 cm or > 1/3 the transthoracic diameter at the level of disease.

Therapy

Treatment consists of multiagent chemotherapy and radiation. Therapy for Hodgkin lymphoma is risk adapted and response based. Patients are assigned to low-, intermediate-, or high-risk groups based on clinical stage and the presence or absence of B symptoms and bulk disease. It has also been shown that rapid responders to therapy have better prognoses than slow responders. Some low- and intermediate-risk patients have good long-term disease control with chemotherapy alone, whereas high-risk patients still receive radiation therapy to maximize the chance of a long-term cure.

Prognosis

Hodgkin lymphoma is a very treatable disease with cure rates > 90% in patients with early-stage disease, and > 85% in those with late-stage disease. However, treatment-related morbidity can be substantial and includes infertility, cardiomyopathy (doxorubicin), and pulmonary toxicity (bleomycin). Second malignancies—the most common being non-Hodgkin lymphoma, breast, lung, and colon cancer—are the leading cause of death in long-term survivors of Hodgkin lymphoma.

Non-Hodgkin Lymphoma (NHL)

NHL is the most common type of lymphoma to occur in pediatrics (NHL 60% vs. Hodgkin lymphoma 40%). There are no distinct age groups for NHL; infants can even be affected. Males outnumber females 3:1.

There is a high rate of NHL in children with:

• Ataxia telangiectasia
• Wiskott-Aldrich syndrome
• Human immunodeficiency virus
• Other immunosuppressive diseases

EBV DNA (Epstein-Barr virus deoxyribonucleic acid) is present in the tumor cells of 95% of endemic cases of Burkitt NHL in equatorial Africa, but it is found in only 15–20% of U.S. cases. NHL can arise from B-cell, T-cell, or indeterminate-cell origin.

Classification

Most pediatric cases are high-grade, diffuse neoplasms. There are 3 main histologic subtypes:

1) Small, noncleaved cell lymphoma (Burkitt and non-Burkitt subtypes, B-cell origin)
2) Lymphoblastic (80% T-cell origin, 20% early B-cell origin)
3) Large cell (T-cell, B-cell, or indeterminate-cell origin)

The most common form of childhood NHL in the U.S. is the sporadic form of Burkitt lymphoma, which makes up ~ 50% of pediatric NHLs. This is followed by lymphoblastic lymphoma (30–40%) and large cell lymphoma (15–25%).

Burkitt Lymphoma (BL)

BL is the most common form of NHL in the U.S., with 90% of Burkitt-type lymphomas originating from relatively mature B cells in gastrointestinal (GI) tract Peyer patches, most commonly at the ileocecal junction. In this way, BL can serve as the lead point for intussusception in children. Only about 10% of U.S. cases begin in the B lymphocytes within the Waldeyer ring (adenoids/tonsils). These U.S. cases are the so-called sporadic form of BL and are rarely associated with EBV infection; however, African or endemic BL is strongly associated with EBV, with > 90% of cases positive for EBV DNA at the time of diagnosis.

A majority of patients with BL present with an abdominal mass or pain with nausea and vomiting. Jaw involvement is very common in the African form but occurs in only ~ 15% of U.S. cases. BL is the fastest-growing malignant tumor—it can double in 2–3 days—so tumor lysis syndrome is common. (See more under Supportive Care During Cancer Treatment on page 25-19.)

Lymphoblastic Lymphoma

Lymphoblastic lymphoma represents approximately 33% of NHLs. The cells of this tumor are biologically indistinguishable from lymphoblastic leukemia. Around 80% are of thymic T-cell origin. Symptoms develop quickly over several weeks. The clinical presentation includes respiratory distress from tracheal and bronchial compression by an anterior mediastinal mass; nontender cervical, supraclavicular, or axillary nodes; and involvement of the liver, spleen, and kidneys. These are typically seen in adolescent males. The other 20% of lymphoblastic lymphomas are of B-cell lineage and present in unusual locations such as skin or bone.

Large Cell NHL

Large cell NHLs contain cells with large nuclei and can manifest anywhere, including abdominal disease (e.g., Burkitt lymphoma) and mediastinal disease (e.g., lymphoblastic lymphoma). Large cell lymphomas can also go to unusual sites (e.g., skin, bone, lung). CNS disease is rare, and bone marrow disease is less likely.

Lymphoma in the anterior mediastinum must be distinguished from the thymus. This is another reason children with suspected lymphoma should be referred to a children's hospital—pediatric radiologists are familiar with this common pitfall.

Also, constitutional symptoms (e.g., fever, night sweats, weight loss; B symptoms, but this has nothing to do with histopathology or cell of origin) are much more common in large cell disease. Most large cell lymphomas are of B-cell origin, but T-cell and null-cell types are also seen.

Diagnosis and Staging

CBC is often normal. Biopsy of an enlarged lymph node is usually required for diagnosis but can be dangerous, depending upon the location of the tumor. If airway obstruction is a problem, then sedated procedures are deemed risky and are avoided.

Staging is generally based on the volume of the tumor. The St. Jude/Murphy staging system is the most widely used. Localized disease makes up Stages I and II. Stage I involves a single tumor or single anatomic node except for the mediastinum or abdomen. Stage II involves ≥ 2 nodal areas on the same side of the diaphragm, 2 extranodal tumors on the same side of the diaphragm, or a resectable primary GI tumor. Stages III and IV represent advanced disease. Stage III has involvement of both sides of the diaphragm, all mediastinal or other intrathoracic tumors, all unresectable abdominal diseases, and all paraspinal or epidural tumors. Stage IV is defined by any CNS or bone marrow involvement; it occurs in < 25% of cases.

Treatment

Treatment of NHL consists of multiagent, multiphase chemotherapy, including CNS treatment. Patients with abdominal tumors that are resected at diagnosis have an excellent prognosis with short-course, postoperative chemotherapy. Radiation therapy in NHL is usually limited to CNS disease or emergency situations (airway obstruction).

Prognosis

Most pediatric patients have a good prognosis, with > 80% survival rate overall. This varies depending on the type and stage at diagnosis. Long-term sequelae from therapy can include infertility, heart failure, and secondary cancers.

TUMORS OF THE CENTRAL NERVOUS SYSTEM (CNS)

PREVIEW | REVIEW

- Neurofibromatosis Type 1 is associated with which type of central nervous system (CNS) tumor?
- Which tumor is characteristically associated with neurofibromatosis Type 2?
- What type of tumor is seen with tuberous sclerosis?
- What type of tumor is seen in von Hippel-Lindau disease?
- Which cranial nerve finding is commonly seen in children with brain tumors?
- What clinical finding is important to look for in an infant you suspect of having a brain tumor?
- What does the "sun-setting" sign refer to?
- Differentiate between the presentations of supratentorial and infratentorial lesions.
- Describe Parinaud syndrome.
- What symptoms can occur if a CNS tumor has spread to the leptomeninges?
- What is the mainstay of therapy for most CNS tumors?
- Which age group normally is not treated with CNS radiation therapy due to increased risk of toxicity?
- What is the most common type of primary CNS tumor in children?
- Which type of astrocytoma has the most aggressive clinical behavior?
- Describe the clinical findings in cerebellar astrocytoma tumors.
- What are the most common presentations for medulloblastoma?
- If ependymoma tumors involve the 4th ventricle, what complication can occur?
- How do pineal tumors present?
- Name some of the complications from craniopharyngiomas.
- Meningiomas are more common in which patients?

OCCURRENCE

CNS tumors make up 15–20% of all childhood cancers and are the most common solid neoplasms of childhood. In most parts of the world, an intracranial mass lesion in childhood is likely to be a neoplasm. The incidence of brain tumors in all children is 3/100,000 per year. With current treatments, ~ 65% of children with brain tumors survive into adulthood.

EPIDEMIOLOGY OF BRAIN TUMORS

Occurrence

There is no difference between the sexes in the incidence of brain tumors. Caucasian children have a slightly higher incidence than African American children. Data shows that the incidence of brain tumors is increasing, but some clinical researchers attribute part of this increase to the invention of magnetic resonance imaging (MRI) and the ability to diagnose these tumors more easily.

Risk Factors

Neurofibromatosis Type 1 (discussed in the Genetics section) predisposes to CNS tumors, especially optic pathway gliomas. Other tumors include meningiomas, ependymomas, neurosarcomas of the cranial nerves, and spinal cord astrocytomas.

Neurofibromatosis Type 2 characteristically produces bilateral vestibular schwannomas. Other tumors include retinal gliomas, meningiomas, gliomas, and cranial and peripheral nerve schwannomas.

The tumor most commonly seen with **tuberous sclerosis** is a subependymal giant cell astrocytoma, which arises in the midline. Generally benign, it can grow quite large and produce pathology due to impingement on other structures.

Li-Fraumeni syndrome is a familial cancer syndrome that leads to an increased risk of gliomas, ependymomas, and choroid plexus carcinomas.

Turcot syndrome has an increased risk of glioblastoma multiforme and medulloblastoma.

Nevoid basal cell carcinoma syndrome (a.k.a. Gorlin syndrome) is associated with medulloblastomas.

von Hippel-Lindau disease increases the risk of hemangioblastomas in the cerebellum, medulla, and spinal cord.

In addition to genetic syndromes that predispose patients to CNS malignancies, **ionizing radiation** is an accepted, proven risk factor.

PRESENTATION

See Figure 25-6 for common brain tumor locations.

Children with brain tumors can vary in their presentation. Many demonstrate signs and symptoms of increased intracranial pressure, including headache (especially morning), vomiting, and irritability. Diplopia, due to 6th cranial nerve palsy, is also a fairly common sign. Other symptoms include changes in academic performance, fatigue, and personality. The "classic" brain tumor headache is a complaint of pain on awakening, which is relieved by vomiting, then lessens during the day. Frequently, though, these classic symptoms do not appear for several months. Signs and symptoms of increased intracranial pressure are a neurosurgical emergency.

Infants pose a specific problem in diagnosis because they obviously do not "complain" of headache and present nonspecific symptoms that can be confused with a common viral illness. Irritability, anorexia, and vomiting are common symptoms. Remember: The infant's cranial sutures are not fused, so a helpful diagnostic tool in an infant with these symptoms is to check head circumference or look for a bulging fontanelle.

Developmental delay and motor abnormalities are common in infants with brain tumors. Loss of developmental milestones is a worrisome feature. Impairment of upgaze and a downward deviation of the eyes ("sun-setting") can be early signs of increased intracranial pressure.

Supratentorial Lesion Presentations

Supratentorial lesions (in brain structures above the cerebellum) commonly present with headaches, weakness, and seizures. Temporal lobe lesions result in seizures with alterations in sensorium, with or without motor signs. Tumors of the supplementary motor regions can result in seizures presenting as twisting movements, posturing of the limbs, and forced tonic movements of the eyes and head. Some lesions produce generalized seizures without focality. Electroencephalography (EEG) can be helpful, but a normal EEG does not rule out a brain tumor.

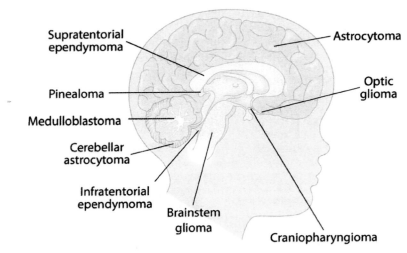

Figure 25-6: Common brain tumor locations

Tumors of the "silent area" of the cerebral cortex (the frontal and parietal lobes) rarely cause any symptoms, unless significant growth results in mass effect.

A large number of childhood tumors arise in the midline 3rd ventricle and suprasellar regions and can result in compression of visual pathway structures. It is important to attempt to elicit visual field deficits.

Parinaud syndrome is a triad of impaired upward gaze, dilated pupils with better reactivity to accommodation than to light, and retraction or conversion nystagmus with lid retraction. It is caused by compression or infiltration of the midbrain tectum, particularly with pineal tumors.

Infratentorial Lesion Presentations

Infratentorial lesions (generally of the cerebellum and below) arise in the posterior fossa and often cause problems with coordination and cranial nerve dysfunction. Tumors of the 4th ventricle present with signs of increased intracranial pressure, with or without brainstem dysfunction. Cerebellar hemisphere tumors usually present initially with lateralizing signs, such as limb dysmetria (an aspect of ataxia, with impaired ability to control the distance, power, and speed of an act), rather than increased intracranial pressure. Seizures are uncommon with posterior fossa tumors. The inability to move both eyes conjugately or to adduct an eye on attempted lateral gaze implies brainstem pathology.

Leptomeningeal Tumor Presentations

Dissemination to the leptomeninges occurs in ~ 15% of childhood CNS tumors. Symptoms include intermittent mental status changes; neck, back, or radicular pain; weakness; and bowel and/or bladder dysfunction.

DIAGNOSIS

When available, MRI has replaced CT scan as the modality of choice for diagnosis of brain tumors. Biopsy is required for histologic confirmation and to determine therapy, except for brainstem gliomas. This is usually done with tumor resection surgery; however, in instances where the tumor cannot be safely removed, stereotactic biopsy may be performed. For gliomas and germ cell tumors, the removed tissue sometimes does not correspond to the most pathologic part of the tumor and can result in a high-grade astrocytoma (worse pathology) misdiagnosed as a low-grade astrocytoma (better pathology). Tumors that cannot be safely biopsied are treated empirically based on the most likely diagnosis, given the location.

The WHO now includes molecular diagnostic criteria in addition to histology for CNS tumor classification.

Molecular classification grows increasingly complex and informative each year for brain tumors, and cancer in general. Mutations in genes or pathways are referred to as "druggable" when pharmaceuticals exist that allow oncologists to treat tumors targeted to that lesion.

TREATMENT

Surgery

Surgical resection is the mainstay of therapy for most tumors of the CNS. The main prognostic factor for a brain tumor, regardless of pathology, is complete resection. If complete resection with negative margins is not possible for a malignant tumor, then a 99% reduction in tumor burden is the goal to increase the effectiveness of radiation and chemotherapy. Preoperative corticosteroids reduce both intracranial pressure and tumor edema; steroids are tapered slowly after surgery.

Radiation Therapy

Radiation therapy is used to treat most malignant brain tumors and some benign brain tumors. One challenge remains—delivering the maximal effective dose while sparing as much normal brain tissue as possible. Several techniques, such as proton beam radiation, provide a more focused beam with less scatter and are being increasingly used in children. Due to the significant acute and long-term toxicity, radiation therapy is usually avoided in children < 3 years of age. Chemotherapy is often used to delay the use of radiation therapy until patients are older.

Chemotherapy

It is standard to use chemotherapy for medulloblastoma and high-grade astrocytoma outside of the brainstem. Agents must cross the blood-brain barrier; commonly used drugs include vincristine, cisplatin, etoposide, and cyclophosphamide. See Table 25-3 for chemotherapy agents and side effects.

Table 25-3: Major Side Effects of Common Chemotherapy Drugs	
Drug	**Side Effects**
Methotrexate	Myelosuppression, renal and hepatic toxicity
Cyclophosphamide	Hemorrhagic cystitis
Doxorubicin	Cardiomyopathy
Bleomycin	Pulmonary fibrosis
Vincristine	Peripheral neuropathy
Cisplatin	Nephrotoxicity, ototoxicity, neurotoxicity

GLIOMA

Gliomas, which can arise anywhere in the CNS, make up 50–60% of brain tumors in children and are the most common primary childhood CNS tumors. These tumors can be astrocytomas or gliomas. Prognosis for gliomas depends on the location and histologic grade.

ONCOLOGY

High-Grade Astrocytoma

Astrocytomas account for 40% of all childhood brain tumors, and 25% of these are aggressive or high grade. These tumors have an increased potential for malignancy. Glioblastoma multiforme is the most aggressive of these tumors.

Headache is the earliest and most common symptom. Vomiting, seizures, motor symptoms, and behavioral abnormalities are next most common.

MRI is best for diagnosis.

Treat surgically, but note: High-grade astrocytomas generally infiltrate the brain and cannot be completely excised. Radiation therapy may improve survival. Recently, high-dose chemotherapy and autologous, peripheral blood stem cell rescue have shown promise in adult and pediatric studies, but outcomes remain poor.

Cerebellar Astrocytoma

Cerebellar astrocytomas make up 12% of all brain tumors in children and are the most common posterior fossa tumors of childhood. They also have one of the best prognoses (> 90% 5-year survival). They peak in the 2nd decade. Most occur in the cerebellar hemisphere, but they occasionally involve the vermis.

The most common type is known as juvenile pilocytic astrocytoma, which is a slow-growing, typically well-demarcated tumor.

Symptoms with lateral cerebellar astrocytomas include clumsiness and unsteadiness of the arms and legs. Headaches and vomiting also occur. Diagnose with MRI or CT.

Treatment strategies include surgery, radiation, and chemotherapy. In children with complete resection of the tumor, radiation and chemotherapy may not be required.

Brainstem Glioma (BSG)

BSGs (i.e., those located in the midbrain, pons, and/or medulla oblongata) make up 10–20% of CNS tumors in children < 15 years of age. Peak incidence is between 5 and 8 years of age.

Focal BSGs (20% of BSGs), outside the pons, are usually low-grade astrocytomas. Symptoms depend on the location of the tumor and may have been present for months. For example, tumors of the tectum often lead to hydrocephalus, headache, nausea, and vomiting. Medullary tumors can cause cranial nerve dysfunction, dysphagia, or even apnea. Characteristic findings on MRI lead to conservative therapy. While overall survival is very good (some authors report up to 100%), many patients have disease- and treatment-related morbidity.

Diffuse intrinsic pontine glioma (80% of BSGs) have the poorest prognosis, and most children die within 2 years of diagnosis. These tumors often cause symptoms of cranial nerve dysfunction (affecting CN 6 and 7, and even CN 3 and 4), or ataxia. Remember, the more cranial nerves affected, the more likely it is that the lesion is in the brainstem. Hydrocephalus is rare. MRI is the best imaging modality and is used to determine the diagnosis without biopsy due to the substantial risk of surgery in this area. Treatment can involve radiation and/or chemotherapy, and outcomes remain very poor (< 5% long-term survival).

MEDULLOBLASTOMAS

Medulloblastomas are the most common type of malignant CNS tumor in childhood; they make up ~ 33% of all infratentorial tumors in children. Hydrocephalus is present in ~ 75% of patients at the time of diagnosis. Children with medulloblastoma typically present with morning headache, vomiting, and lethargy. Ataxia is common and involves the trunk or limbs. Most patients are symptomatic for < 3 months before the diagnosis is made. Head-tilt can occur due to 4th cranial nerve dysfunction or impending cerebellar herniation.

Surgical resection at diagnosis often results in all or most of the tumor being removed unless it has infiltrated the 4th ventricle or a cerebellar peduncle, which makes complete resection difficult. Use postoperative gadolinium-enhanced MRI to assess for leptomeningeal involvement and lumbar puncture to look for tumor cells.

Radiation after surgery is a mainstay. Chemotherapy is also frequently used in those with high-risk disease. Prognosis is poor in those with younger age, disseminated disease, brainstem infiltration, larger tumor sizes, and certain histologic and cytogenetic tumor features.

EPENDYMOMA

Ependymomas arise from the ependymal lining of the ventricular system: ~ 75% occur in the posterior fossa, with the remainder occurring in supratentorial areas. Ependymomas make up 8–10% of all primary childhood brain tumors and account for 10–15% of the posterior fossa tumors.

Symptoms depend on where the tumor occurs. If the tumor is in the 4th ventricle, CSF flow is blocked, with accompanying symptoms of nausea, vomiting, and morning headache. Diplopia typically occurs. Most patients have symptoms for 6–9 months before diagnosis. Tumors of the brainstem have more focal deficits and are diagnosed earlier.

MRI is the diagnostic tool of choice. Hydrocephalus is almost always present.

Surgery is the mainstay of therapy, and completeness of resection determines chance of cure. Postoperative radiation therapy seems to increase overall survival. Chemotherapy is not beneficial.

GERM CELL TUMORS

Germ cell tumors make up 50% of pineal tumors and 5–10% of parasellar tumors. Germinomas make up ~ 65% of germ cell tumors.

Pineal tumors can present with **Parinaud syndrome**: a triad of impaired upward gaze, dilated pupils with better reactivity to accommodation than to light, and retraction or conversion nystagmus with lid retraction. Suprasellar germinomas produce pituitary and hypothalamic dysfunction, such as growth hormone failure and diabetes insipidus. Teratomas also occur and frequently show calcium deposits.

α-Fetoprotein (AFP) and β-human chorionic gonadotropin (β-hCG) are secreted by mixed germ cell tumors—but not by other pineal tumors.

Surgical resection is difficult because most are in the pineal region. Radiotherapy is the primary mode of therapy, but chemotherapy also is effective for many tumors.

CRANIOPHARYNGIOMA

Craniopharyngiomas are benign tumors that are derived from squamous epithelial cells and arise in the suprasellar region. They make up ~ 10% of all childhood brain tumors. Although benign, craniopharyngiomas are locally invasive and can affect many structures, including the optic chiasm, carotid arteries, 3rd cranial nerve, and pituitary stalk; therefore, they are very harmful to the patient due to location.

Headaches and vomiting are typical presenting symptoms. > 50% of children with craniopharyngioma have visual changes due to optic involvement. Because of pituitary involvement, endocrinologic signs (e.g., growth failure, short stature, polydipsia) often accompany these tumors. Changes in personality or sleep patterns are also common presenting signs.

Diagnostic imaging with CT or MRI identifies the lesion. Calcifications in the suprasellar region are present in most cases. Surgery is recommended for many craniopharyngiomas, but location is frequently a problem. Radiation is usually required. Diabetes insipidus is a common complication of surgery.

MENINGIOMA

Meningiomas are rare in children except in those with **neurofibromatosis Type 2**—in which they can occur as early as 1 year of age. Meningiomas also occur in long-term survivors of other brain tumors who have received radiation therapy.

Treatment is surgical resection. Meningiomas are almost always benign.

SPINAL CORD COMPRESSION FROM A MASS

Spinal cord masses are rare in the pediatric population. They can occur secondary to conditions such as abscesses, trauma (hematoma/contusion), and developmental abnormalities. However, the most common cause of spinal cord compression from a mass is secondary to spinal cord tumors. Evidence of cord compression may be the presenting feature of a mass. Given the intricate fibers of the spinal cord, symptoms vary depending on the location of the mass and which fibers are compromised.

Most children with spinal cord tumors/masses present with back pain. Other less common symptoms include a combination of gait disturbance, weakness, scoliosis, and sphincter dysfunction. In younger children, motor regression can also be a presenting symptom. Symptoms will vary depending on the location (Table 25-4).

Table 25-4: Clinical Signs and Symptoms of Spinal Cord Masses by Spinal Level	
Spinal Cord Lesion Level	**Clinical Manifestations**
Above T10	• Symmetric weakness • Increased lower extremity deep tendon reflexes • Sensory level deficit • Up-going toes
Conus medullaris (T10 to L2)	• Symmetric weakness • Increased knee reflexes • Decreased ankle reflexes • Saddle sensory loss • Up-going or down-going toes
Cauda equina (below L2)	• Asymmetric weakness • Loss of lower extremity deep tendon reflexes • Sensory deficit • Down-going toes

In children, spinal cord tumors account for roughly 20% of tumors of the CNS and are classified according to anatomic position (Figure 25-7 on page 25-12):

- **Intramedullary tumors** arise from within the substance of the cord and grow slowly via infiltration. These are most commonly caused by low-grade astrocytoma, followed by ganglioma and ependymoma. The most common spinal cord tumors are intramedullary.
- **Extramedullary intradural tumors** are located outside of the substance of the cord but within the dura that covers the cord. These tumors are most commonly caused by neurofibromatosis, ganglioneuroma, and meningioma.
- **Extramedullary extradural tumors** are located outside of the cord and outside of the dura. They are characteristically metastatic tumors.

Diagnosis: It is important to establish the diagnosis of a spinal cord tumor as early as possible to prevent irreversible damage to the cord. MRI is the most important diagnostic test to establish a diagnosis, as well as to give a 3-dimensional representation of the mass and the extent of structures that are being compressed. In addition, a biopsy is often required to establish a diagnosis. Once a diagnosis has been established, a treatment strategy can be planned. For tumors, depending on the tumor type,

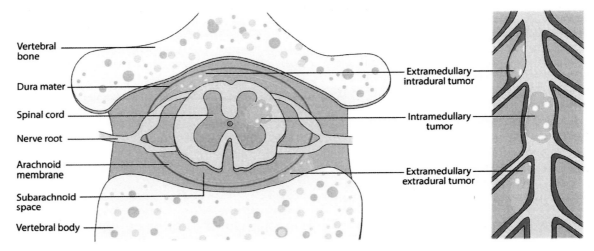

Figure 25-7: Anatomic positions of spinal cord tumors

surgical resection +/− radiation and chemotherapy may be required. Surgical resection can also be done for other mass lesions, including hematoma or abscess. Control of pain and preservation of neurologic function are important in the treatment strategies for spinal cord masses.

NEUROBLASTOMA

PREVIEW | REVIEW

- What is the most common malignancy diagnosed in infancy?

- From where do most neuroblastomas arise?

- What symptoms does vasoactive intestinal peptide cause in neuroblastoma?

- How do you diagnose neuroblastoma?

- At what age of diagnosis do children have the best prognosis in neuroblastoma?

- What is the treatment for the different neuroblastoma risk groups (low, intermediate, and high risk)?

OCCURRENCE

Neuroblastoma, the most commonly diagnosed malignancy in infancy (< 1 year of age), makes up 7–10% of all childhood cancers and is the most common abdominal malignancy. There are ~ 800 new cases per year in the U.S. It mostly occurs in the adrenal gland and presents as an abdominal mass. It is slightly more common in boys than girls. The median age of diagnosis is 22 months; 97% of neuroblastomas are diagnosed before 10 years of age.

PATHOLOGY

Neuroblastoma is characterized by small, uniform, round, blue cells under light microscopy. The malignant cells derive from neuroblasts of the postganglionic sympathetic nervous system. Molecular and genetic factors that influence diagnosis and prognosis include amplification of the *MYCN* oncogene, tumor cell DNA content (ploidy), and structural genetic changes.

PRESENTATION

40% of neuroblastomas arise in the abdomen within the adrenal medulla, and 30% originate in the nonadrenal abdomen, including paravertebral ganglia, pelvic ganglia, and the organ of Zuckerkandl (a small mass of chromaffin cells located along the aorta). About 20% occur in the paravertebral ganglia of the chest or neck. Children with localized disease can present without symptoms, but those with advanced disease present ill-appearing with systemic symptoms. The most common presentation of neuroblastoma is a nontender abdominal mass—typically retroperitoneal. Neuroblastoma in the high thoracic and cervical area can cause Horner syndrome (unilateral ptosis, miosis, and anhidrosis). Involvement of the spinal canal can occur with resulting paralysis or loss of bowel/bladder function in the lower lumbar region.

Most neuroblastomas have metastasized before diagnosis. Metastases can go to distant lymph nodes, bone, bone marrow, liver, and skin (which manifests as subcutaneous bluish nodules). In infants < 1 year of age, it is characteristic to have a small primary tumor with dissemination limited to the liver and skin. This generally has a good prognosis and is referred to as Stage 4S. For children > 1 year of age with metastatic disease, the prognosis is quite poor. Periorbital ecchymosis (raccoon eyes) due to orbital metastases must be distinguished from trauma/child abuse.

Paraneoplastic syndromes can occur but are not that common. Look for intractable secretory diarrhea and abdominal distention due to secretion of vasoactive intestinal peptide (VIP). This **VIP syndrome** may also occur with ganglioneuroblastoma or ganglioneuroma and resolves with removal of the tumor.

Opsoclonus-myoclonus-ataxia syndrome (dancing eyes–dancing feet syndrome) occurs in ~ 5% of newly diagnosed neuroblastoma patients and is characterized by rapid and chaotic eye movements, ataxia, and myoclonus. As a presenting symptom, it warrants a workup for neuroblastoma. These symptoms may resolve with removal of the tumor, but up to 80% of children can have long-term neurologic deficits.

DIAGNOSIS

Diagnosis requires biopsy with histologic evidence of neural origin of the tumor or, in the case of bone marrow diagnosis, compatible "clumps" of cells.

Because neuroblastomas are derived from neural crest cells, they take up and metabolize catecholamines. An increased level of catecholamine metabolites in the urine (homovanillic acid [HVA] and vanillylmandelic acid [VMA]) is often found at diagnosis. Urinary catecholamine excretion in neuroblastoma is useful in both diagnosis and off-therapy follow-up.

In the workup of neuroblastoma, the following tests are usually done: bilateral bone marrow aspirate and biopsy, plain radiographs, bone scan, CT, and MRI. Metaiodobenzylguanidine (MIBG) scintigraphy for evaluation of bone and soft tissue involvement is also standard for staging because the majority of neuroblastomas take up the radionuclide.

PROGNOSTIC INDICATORS

Prognosis is determined by multiple clinical and biologic factors.

Better prognosis:

- Child's age at diagnosis—the best prognosis is for patients < 18 months of age.
- Ploidy of the tumor—hyperdiploidy confers better outcome in patients < 18 months of age with metastatic disease.
- Favorable histology
- Not having MYCN amplification—MYCN amplification outweighs any other favorable characteristic, placing the patient in a high-risk category.

Poorer prognosis:

- Extent of tumor—patients with metastatic disease do very poorly.
- Unfavorable histology
- *MYCN* oncogene copy number—an increasing number of copies (amplification) correlates with poorer prognosis.
- Chromosome 11q aberration

TREATMENT

Overall, therapy is based on risk-group stratification established by the International Neuroblastoma Staging System. Risk groups are based on a combination of stage and biologic features. The lowest-risk groups are treated with surgery alone. Intermediate-risk groups receive surgery and chemotherapy. Treatment of high-risk disease includes surgery, standard chemotherapy, high-dose chemotherapy with autologous stem cell rescue, radiation, *cis*-retinoic acid, and immune-modulating therapy. Even with aggressive therapy, outcomes in high-risk children are poor.

WILMS TUMOR

PREVIEW | REVIEW

- What is the most common primary malignancy of the kidney in childhood?
- What congenital disorders and syndromes are associated with Wilms tumor?
- List the conditions in WAGR syndrome.
- What is the most common presentation for Wilms tumor?
- What is the mainstay of therapy for unilateral Wilms tumor?
- True or false? Most unilateral Wilms tumor patients receive chemotherapy.

OVERVIEW

Wilms tumor (nephroblastoma) is the most common primary malignant tumor of the kidney in childhood and, at ~ 600 new cases per year, is the 2nd most common abdominal malignancy in children (after neuroblastoma at ~ 800 new cases per year). It occurs about equally in boys and girls, with no racial differences noted. The mean age of diagnosis is 42–47 months for unilateral tumors and 30–33 months for bilateral tumors.

An important feature to remember is the association of Wilms tumor with other congenital anomalies and syndromes in up to 7% of patients.

Wilms-associated disorders:

- Genitourinary (GU) anomalies (4.4%, including cryptorchidism and hypospadias)
- Hemihyperplasia (a.k.a. hemihypertrophy; 3%)
- Sporadic aniridia (1%)

Wilms-associated syndromes:

- **WAGR syndrome**
  - **Wilms tumor**
  - **Aniridia**
  - **GU abnormalities**
  - **Reduced intellectual ability**
- Beckwith-Wiedemann syndrome (BWS)
  - Organomegaly
  - Macroglossia
  - Omphalocele
  - Hemihyperplasia
  - Wilms tumor

- Denys-Drash syndrome
  - Wilms tumor
  - Nephropathy
  - Male undervirilization

Infants with BWS or hemihyperplasia are at risk for developing Wilms tumor and other embryonal tumors such as hepatoblastoma. Screening guidelines for Wilms tumor are available.

Wilms tumor is associated with a number of genetic factors. The Wilms tumor suppression gene (*WT1*) at chromosome 11p13 and another gene at 11p15.5 have been implicated. Also, familial Wilms tumor genes have been noted.

PRESENTATION

The median age of diagnosis of Wilms tumor is around 3 years of age, with the most common sign being an asymptomatic abdominal or flank mass. These children are typically well-appearing (as opposed to those with neuroblastoma). Many masses are found incidentally on physical examination or by the parents while bathing the child or changing a diaper. Gross hematuria occurs in a small percentage. Remember to look for the common associated syndromes and anomalies: aniridia, hemihyperplasia, and GU abnormalities. Hypertension occurs in ~ 25% of patients and is due to tumor impingement of the renal artery or renal ischemia. Evaluation includes CXR, CT scan of the abdomen and chest, ultrasound, and echocardiography.

TREATMENT

For unilateral disease, nephrectomy with removal of the primary tumor is the mainstay of therapy. Assessment of tumor spread at the time of surgery is important. Most patients receive postsurgical chemotherapy.

Presurgical chemotherapy is indicated if:

- there is extensive tumor thrombus to the intrahepatic vena cava or
- there is thrombus more proximally to the right atrium or
- the primary tumor is deemed unresectable without significant surgical morbidity.

In bilateral disease (Stage 5), a renal biopsy of each kidney determines the histologic stage and appropriate chemotherapy; and, typically, bilateral parenchymal-sparing resection is performed.

The chemotherapy regimen is routinely based on staging and histologic type.

Abdominal radiation therapy is not necessary for those with Stage 1 or 2 disease and favorable histology. It is useful in Stage 3 and 4 disease. Whole-lung irradiation is a possibility for those with pulmonary metastatic lesions seen on imaging studies.

PATHOLOGY AND STAGING

Classically, Wilms tumor is a solitary growth that can occur in any part of either kidney. It is well demarcated and compresses the normal kidney parenchyma. The tumor usually is triphasic—made up of epithelial, blastemal, and stromal elements—which is favorable histology. Poor histology, or anaplasia, is found in only 10% of cases but accounts for 60% of deaths.

Stage 1 tumors are limited to a single kidney and can be completely excised. Stage 2 disease extends beyond the kidney but can still be completely excised. Patients with Stage 3 disease have residual tumor confined to the abdomen, and patients with Stage 1 or 2 disease are downgraded to Stage 3 if the surgery is complicated by tumor spillage.

Patients with Stage 4 disease have hematogenous spread, most frequently to the lung. Stage 5 disease indicates bilateral kidney involvement and occurs in only 5–10% of cases.

Histologic subtype remains the most powerful prognostic factor. Children with favorable histology tumors have > 90% survival at 2 years regardless of stage. Anaplasia is a predictor of poor outcomes.

RHABDOMYOSARCOMA

PREVIEW | REVIEW

- What is the most common malignant soft tissue sarcoma in childhood?
- What tissue/cell type is affected by rhabdomyosarcoma?
- How does rhabdomyosarcoma present?
- What is the treatment for rhabdomyosarcoma?

OCCURRENCE

Rhabdomyosarcoma is the most common soft tissue sarcoma in childhood and makes up ~ 5% of all childhood cancers. Almost 2/3 of cases are diagnosed in children ≤ 6 years of age.

PATHOLOGY

Rhabdomyosarcoma arises from the same embryonic mesenchyme as striated skeletal muscle.

There are 2 main histologic types:

1) Embryonal—found in 60–70% of cases and has a more favorable prognosis
2) Alveolar—found in 20–30% of cases, occurs more commonly in the trunk and extremities, and has the worst prognosis

PRESENTATION

The most common presentation is a mass lesion. The head and neck are the most common sites, and this includes the orbit and parameningeal sites such as the nasopharynx. The next most common site is the GU tract, followed by extremity and truncal tumors. Tumors of the orbits can cause proptosis and ophthalmoplegia. GU tumors present with a pelvic mass causing urinary frequency, urinary obstruction, or constipation. Vaginal bleeding can lead to suspicion of child abuse. In female infants, there can be a protruding polypoid "grape-like" vaginal mass (sarcoma botryoides).

DIAGNOSIS

Tissue biopsy is required for appropriate diagnosis and histologic subtype, which affects treatment and prognosis.

CT, MRI, and/or ultrasound can help delineate the extent of a mass lesion. A radionucleotide scan, such as PET, can also be done to determine extent of active disease. Proper staging workup also includes CXR, CT of chest/abdomen/pelvis, bone marrow biopsy and aspiration, and lumbar puncture (for parameningeal tumors only).

TREATMENT

Surgical excision, if possible, is paramount; however, in some cases, such as those with bladder tumors, complete resection is not acceptable because of the complications.

Chemotherapy is indicated for all children with rhabdomyosarcoma. Local control measures are imperative for disease control.

Radiation therapy is typically used and depends on the extent of tumor resection.

Prognosis is determined by stage and histology and is typically good (> 70%). Orbit is most favorable; extremities and parameningeal are unfavorable.

RETINOBLASTOMA

PREVIEW | REVIEW

- True or false? Familial cases of retinoblastoma typically occur bilaterally.
- How is retinoblastoma treated?

OCCURRENCE

Retinoblastoma occurs in 1/18,000 births in the U.S. It can be unilateral and nonhereditary (60%), unilateral and hereditary (15%), or bilateral and hereditary (25%).

The retinoblastoma gene (*RB1*) is located on the long arm of chromosome 13 and functions as a tumor suppressor gene. Malignant phenotype occurs in those with either homozygous mutation or deletion, and results in dysfunction or absence of the retinoblastoma protein. Familial cases are multifocal and bilateral.

Retinoblastoma requires 2 mutational "hits" for tumor development to occur. In the heritable form, there is one germ line *RB1* gene mutation (present in all cells in the body), with a 2nd mutation subsequently occurring in the somatic retinal cell. In the nonheritable form, both mutations must occur in the same retinal cell—which then becomes the cancer.

PATHOLOGY

Retinoblastoma can occur in any of the nucleated layers of the retina. It tends to outgrow its blood supply and becomes necrotic and calcified. Endophytic, exophytic, and extraocular extensions occur.

PRESENTATION

Classically, retinoblastoma presents with a white pupillary reflex (**leukocoria**; Figure 25-8); however, in some children, strabismus is the initial presenting complaint. Pain occurs only if secondary glaucoma is a feature.

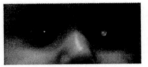
Figure 25-8: Leukocoria in a child with retinoblastoma

DIAGNOSIS

Diagnosis is best made under general anesthesia by a pediatric ophthalmologist. Orbital ultrasound, CT, and MRI are useful for determining the extent of disease. Lumbar puncture is performed for CSF cytology in patients with concern for optic nerve invasion.

TREATMENT

Treatment is aimed at cure, with preservation of vision if possible.

Unilateral disease can be treated with enucleation if there is no chance for useful vision. If feasible, small tumors can be treated with laser therapy or cryotherapy. Large tumors can be treated with chemotherapy.

Bilateral disease is initially treated with chemotherapy in an attempt to preserve vision. If responsive, then local tumor control can be attempted with laser therapy or cryotherapy as well. External beam irradiation is sometimes necessary for large, bulky tumors.

Prognosis is good for those who respond to chemotherapy or who undergo enucleation without residual tumor. Children with germ line *RB1* mutations are at very high risk for developing secondary malignancies (e.g., osteosarcoma, soft tissue sarcoma), especially if they received radiation therapy.

ONCOLOGY

BONE NEOPLASMS AND BENIGN TUMORS

PREVIEW | REVIEW

- What is the most common primary malignant bone tumor in all children? What is most common in those < 10 years of age?
- What are the classic (but nondiagnostic) x-ray findings in osteosarcoma vs. Ewing sarcoma?
- In what age group are most osteosarcomas seen?
- In what part of the bone does osteosarcoma most commonly occur?
- What are clinical clues for osteosarcoma?
- What is Ewing sarcoma?
- What chromosomal abnormality is most commonly associated with Ewing sarcoma?
- Differentiate between the clinical findings in osteosarcoma and Ewing sarcoma.
- What is an osteochondroma?
- What are the common locations for osteochondroma?
- What are the x-ray findings in osteochondroma?
- How does osteoid osteoma present?

OVERVIEW

Osteosarcoma and Ewing sarcoma are the 2 most common primary malignant bone tumors during childhood and adolescence. Osteosarcoma is more common overall; however, Ewing sarcoma is more common in children < 10 years of age. Both tumors frequently present during the 2nd decade of life. Table 25-5 lists important differences to remember about these bone tumors.

Table 25-5: Differences Between Osteosarcoma and Ewing Sarcoma		
	Osteosarcoma	**Ewing Sarcoma**
Race	All races	Mainly Caucasians
Cell Type	Spindle cell–producing osteoid	Undifferentiated; probably neural
Site	Metaphyses of long bones	Diaphyses of long bones Flat bones
Presentation	History of injury Local pain/swelling	Fever Weight loss Local pain/swelling
X-Ray Findings	Less commonly lytic "sunburst" pattern	Lytic, "onion skinning"

Benign bone tumors include osteochondroma, enchondroma, chondroblastoma, osteoid osteoma, and osteoblastoma.

OSTEOSARCOMA

Occurrence

Osteosarcoma occurs with the highest incidence during the adolescent growth spurt.

Osteosarcoma occurs at a higher rate in people with the following conditions:

- Hereditary retinoblastoma
- Li-Fraumeni syndrome
- Rothmund-Thomson syndrome (i.e., short stature, skin telangiectasias, small hands/feet, hypoplastic or absent thumbs)
- Radiation therapy for Ewing sarcoma or other malignancies

Benign conditions with malignant transformation to osteosarcoma include:

- Paget disease
- Endochondromatosis
- Multiple hereditary exostoses

Pathology

There are 4 pathologic subtypes of osteosarcoma. All show highly malignant and pleomorphic spindle cells in biopsy. Osteosarcoma usually occurs in the **metaphyseal** region of long bones and invades the medullary cavity; the diaphyseal region is involved in < 10% of cases. The 4 subtypes have no prognostic differences.

Presentation

Unilateral pain and swelling are the most common presenting findings. The most commonly affected site is around the knee (distal femur or proximal tibia), followed by the humerus. Frequently, the adolescent thinks this is a sports injury or sprain. Investigate any pain not responding to conservative therapy in a reasonable amount of time. Routine lab work is usually not helpful and is typically normal, although LDH or alkaline phosphatase can be elevated.

Clues:

- Deep bone pain
- Nighttime awakening
- Palpable mass
- X-ray showing a periosteal reaction (**Sunburst pattern** is classic but is neither common nor specific.)
- Codman triangle can also be seen on x-ray. It is a reaction seen at the junction of the mass and periosteum that is caused by the ossification of only the edge of the raised periosteum.

Diagnosis

Biopsy by an oncologic orthopedic surgeon must be performed on any lesion suspected of being a bone tumor. MRI is done before surgery to evaluate anatomy and to look for skip lesions (i.e., lesions in the bone that are not physically connected).

The most common site for metastasis is the lungs. Therefore, before biopsy, a CT of the chest and a radionuclide bone scan are performed to assess stage of disease.

Treatment

The 5-year survival rate (with chemotherapy and surgery) is 65–75% for patients with nonmetastatic osteosarcoma. Preoperative chemotherapy is standard, followed by limb salvage operations (when feasible), and further chemotherapy after surgery. The degree of tumor necrosis at the time of resection is prognostically significant. Prognosis is poor for patients with distant bone metastases and widespread lung metastases.

EWING SARCOMA

Occurrence

Ewing sarcoma is among a group of small, round-cell, undifferentiated tumors of neural crest origin. It is primarily a bone tumor but can also arise from soft tissue. A majority of patients have a t(11;22) translocation, whereas the rest have a t(21;22). Ewing sarcoma has a striking racial propensity, in that it mainly affects Caucasians.

Presentation

Clinically, these patients present with pain and swelling, similarly to those with osteosarcoma. Children with Ewing sarcoma are more likely to have systemic findings such as fever and weight loss, and they can be misdiagnosed as having osteomyelitis. Flat bones (e.g., ribs, pelvis) and the diaphyses (i.e., shaft) of the long bones are more commonly affected, as compared to the metaphyseal involvement in osteosarcoma. Paraspinal and vertebral primary tumors are also more common with Ewing sarcoma.

Suspect Ewing sarcoma in a patient with pain, swelling, and fever, with an x-ray showing a primary **lytic lesion** with a lamellated or **"onion skin"** periosteal reaction (Figure 25-9).

Diagnosis

Full workup consists of CT of the chest, abdomen, and pelvis; a bone scan; and bone marrow aspirate/biopsy from at least 2 sites. Preoperative MRI is done to assess the extent of the lesion. Confirm the diagnosis with a tissue biopsy.

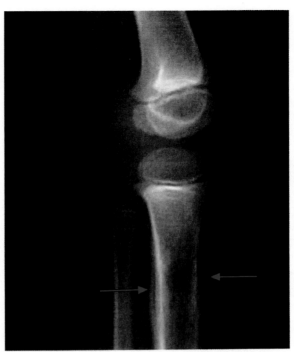

Figure 25-9: Ewing sarcoma with "onion skin" periosteal reaction

Treatment

Chemotherapy is usually given first; pain relief occurs rapidly with chemotherapy. Local control is accomplished by either complete surgical resection or radiation therapy.

Prognosis is excellent (> 75% cure rate) in those with small, nonmetastatic, distally located extremity tumors. Those with bulky pelvic tumors, metastatic disease at diagnosis, and bone marrow involvement have a poorer prognosis.

OSTEOCHONDROMA

Osteochondroma is a very common benign cartilage-forming bone tumor in children. Many cases are asymptomatic and never recognized. Most occur in the metaphysis of long bones, particularly the distal femur, proximal humerus, and proximal tibia. The lesion continues to grow until skeletal maturity.

Most are discovered between 5 and 15 years of age as a bony, nonpainful mass. On x-ray, they appear as stalks or broad-based projections from the surface of the bone. Usually, there is a cartilage "cap," which can be as thick as 1 cm. Transformation to a malignant chondrosarcoma is very rare in children but occurs in ~ 1% of adults. Typically, they are left alone unless the lesion is large enough to cause symptoms, in which case the lesion is excised.

OSTEOID OSTEOMA

Osteoid osteomas are benign tumors that usually occur in males between 5 and 20 years of age. Clinically, there is a characteristic unremitting and worsening pain (worse at night) that, in contrast to osteosarcoma, is relieved with aspirin or other nonsteroidal antiinflammatory drugs (NSAIDs; not with acetaminophen). The most common bones involved are the proximal femur and tibia. Palpation and range of motion do not worsen the pain. X-rays show a round or oval metaphyseal or diaphyseal lucency surrounded by sclerotic bone. ~ 25% cannot be seen on plain radiograph but can be seen on CT scan. Treatment is with surgical excision.

THYROID CANCER

Consider thyroid cancer in any child with a solitary thyroid nodule. A solitary mass is much more likely to be cancer in children and adolescents than it is in adults. See the Endocrinology section for more on thyroid cancer.

GONADAL NEOPLASMS

PREVIEW | REVIEW

- True or false? Few gonadal malignancies are germ cell tumors in pediatrics.

- Where are most teratomas located?

- Which patient with a teratoma is particularly predisposed to undergo malignant transformation (i.e., what age and what location)?

- Which germ cell tumor(s) has an elevated α-fetoprotein level?

OCCURRENCE

Almost all gonadal neoplasms are germ cell tumors. They represent 3% of all tumors in children. 2/3 of germ cell tumors in children are extragonadal. The peak ages for occurrence of these tumors are ~ 3 years of age and then again during adolescence. 1/3 of germ cell tumors in children are malignant, but these are mainly in older children and adolescents. Cryptorchidism is a risk factor for developing testicular cancer. Nearly all neonatal germ cell tumors are benign.

PRESENTATION

Presenting symptoms vary depending on the location of the tumor. Ovarian tumors present with a mass, abdominal pain, and distention. Ovarian torsion can occur. Testicular tumors present with a scrotal mass (with or without pain).

EVALUATION

If a testicular mass is palpated, order an ultrasound to determine if the mass is solid or not. (If it is, the next step is inguinal orchiectomy.) Never perform a needle biopsy due to the risk of seeding the biopsy tract. Evaluation of an ovarian mass begins with ultrasonography (add Doppler if ruling out torsion). A solid mass is considered to be cancer until proven otherwise. Order a CT or MRI if diagnosis is unclear from the ultrasound.

Cross-sectional imaging (CT or MRI) is used to detect metastatic disease to the lungs and retroperitoneum.

TERATOMA

Teratomas can be benign or malignant. They represent intermixed tissues that originated from pluripotent stem cells foreign to the anatomic sites in which they occur.

Sacrococcygeal teratomas are the most common congenital germ cell tumor and can be found prenatally on ultrasound or after delivery on examination.

Histologically, teratomas can be mature (composed of well-differentiated adult-type tissues) or immature (composed of embryonic tissues). Malignant elements such as a yolk sac tumor or choriocarcinoma may be present. Teratomas most commonly occur in the sacrococcyx, ovaries, testes, and anterior mediastinum. Classically, they have components from all 3 embryonic layers (endoderm, mesoderm, and ectoderm); generally, tumors presenting at a site foreign to the anatomic site are considered teratomas with ≥ 1 embryonic layers. Look for teeth and hair and other "weird stuff" (abnormal tissues) on x-ray!

In an infant with sacrococcygeal teratoma, the risk of malignant transformation increases to 50% once the infant is > 2 months of age. If malignant elements are discovered, chemotherapy is indicated.

GERMINOMA

Germinoma is a malignant germ cell tumor that can occur in the ovary (dysgerminoma) and the testes (seminoma), as well as extragonadally. The typical extragonadal presentation is intracranial and can present with hydrocephalus, headache, vomiting, or abnormal vision. It responds very well to radiation and chemotherapy. The ovarian and testicular forms respond to surgical resection and chemotherapy. Even though they are malignant, germinomas are often tumor marker (AFP and β-hCG) negative.

RARE NONGERMINOMATOUS GERM CELL TUMORS

Following are some key features of these tumors:

- Embryonal carcinoma—malignant; produces β-hCG; most commonly testicular

- Endodermal sinus (yolk sac) tumor—most common malignant germ cell tumor; produces AFP

- Choriocarcinoma—malignant; also produces β-hCG (but not AFP); often found in mixed GCT

- Gonadoblastoma—thought of as a carcinoma in situ; has low risk for metastases

- Sex cord tumors—very rare; can produce either androgens (virilizing) or estrogen; surgery is typically curative.

COLORECTAL TUMORS

Colonic tumors are discussed in more detail in the Gastroenterology section.

LIVER TUMORS

PREVIEW | REVIEW

- What are the most common liver tumors in children < 3 years of age?
- What tumor marker should be checked in all children with liver tumors?
- What is the most common primary malignant liver tumor?

OVERVIEW

Liver tumors are rare in children. Nearly 70% of liver tumors are malignant, and hepatoblastomas make up the majority of these in children < 3 years of age. Hepatocellular carcinoma increases in frequency in older children and adolescents but is still rare. Of the benign lesions, infantile hepatic hemangioma is the most common and occurs in children < 2 years of age.

Most liver tumors are painless. However, many can produce jaundice, weight loss, anorexia, and fever.

All children with a hepatic tumor need to have AFP checked.

Diagnosis is confirmed with biopsy unless infantile hepatic hemangioma or cavernous hemangioma is suspected.

HEPATOBLASTOMA

Hepatoblastoma is the most common primary malignancy of the liver in childhood. It most commonly occurs in children < 3 years of age, and there is increased risk in premature infants and patients with BWS. AFP is usually significantly elevated. It typically presents as an asymptomatic abdominal mass. Resection is recommended upfront if possible. Treatment with chemotherapy as well as additional surgery and liver transplant depend on risk group. When indicated, use multiagent chemotherapy including cisplatin (which causes a high incidence of hearing loss). Liver transplant is necessary if a complete resection is not possible after multiple rounds of chemotherapy.

HEPATOCELLULAR CARCINOMA

Hepatocellular carcinoma is the 2nd most common primary liver malignancy and the most common occurring in children > 3 years of age (usually adolescent age). Around 1/2 of patients have elevated AFP, and approximately 1/3 have cirrhosis. Hepatitis B or C infection is a risk factor. Surgical resection is the only curative option, but unfortunately, only ~ 1/3 of these tumors are resectable. Chemotherapy is not typically beneficial for these tumors.

CLUES TO DIAGNOSIS

Clues:

- A 2-year-old, born prematurely, with a liver mass and significantly elevated AFP is likely to have hepatoblastoma.
- An 8-year-old with a solitary mass and an elevated AFP most likely has hepatocellular carcinoma.
- For an adolescent female on oral contraceptives presenting with a hepatic mass, think adenoma.
- Metastatic disease to the liver in children < 2 years of age is most likely a neuroblastoma; in older children, it can be lymphoma, sarcoma, or Wilms tumor.

SUPPORTIVE CARE DURING CANCER TREATMENT

PREVIEW | REVIEW

- How do you manage fever in a patient on chemotherapy?
- What is tumor lysis syndrome?
- How is pain managed in the pediatric oncology patient?
- What is palliative care?

Advances in supportive care have improved outcomes. Key among these are prevention and management of infection and tumor lysis syndrome.

Children with fever must be emergently evaluated for bacterial sepsis and other invasive infection. Give broad-spectrum antibiotics as soon as cultures are obtained. Admit patients with severe neutropenia to the hospital for further evaluation and antibiotics. Initial therapy with an antipseudomonal β-lactam (e.g., cefepime, ceftazidime), piperacillin-tazobactam, or carbapenem is used. Vancomycin is used when additional gram-positive coverage is needed. Children are at risk for *Pneumocystis* pneumonia and are prophylactically prescribed trimethoprim/sulfamethoxazole. Some treatment protocols include prophylactic antibiotics and antifungals.

The immune system of a child receiving chemotherapy is impaired, so live viral vaccines during treatment are contraindicated.

Tumor lysis syndrome is a medical emergency and describes the metabolic complications of rapid cell lysis noted with initiation of chemotherapy or with high cellular turnover from certain tumors (e.g., AML with hyperleukocytosis, Burkitt lymphoma, T-cell ALL).

ONCOLOGY

Hyperkalemia, hyperphosphatemia, hypocalcemia, and chronic kidney disease (due to hyperuricemia) occur. Tumor lysis is expected with initial therapy. Prevention includes hyperhydration with fluids that do not contain potassium. Urate oxidase, which breaks down uric acid, is prescribed for patients with high levels of uric acid. Watch for decreased urine output as a sign of kidney damage due to tumor lysis syndrome. Tumor lysis labs include CBC, uric acid, electrolytes (especially calcium, potassium, and phosphate), and renal function.

Children frequently require transfusion support. Blood products for some oncology patients must be irradiated in order to prevent life-threatening graft-versus-host disease.

The most common pain medications in pediatrics are avoided in the oncology patient. Acetaminophen may mask fever, and NSAIDs (including ibuprofen) adversely affect platelet function as well as reduce fever. Therefore, narcotics are primarily used to control pain in oncology patients. In rare instances, the oncologist may prescribe NSAIDs when the risk/benefit profile favors their use. Gabapentin is used for neuropathic pain. Topical pain medications ("magic mouthwash") may be used for mucositis pain. Nonmedicinal means of pain management include heating pads, distraction techniques, and guided imagery. Palliative care medicine is the field dedicated to the care and support of high-risk and end-stage patients. For high-risk and end-stage pediatric oncology patients, supportive care broadens to include decisions about emergent and end-of-life care in addition to aggressive symptom control. High-risk patients and their families must carefully weigh the risks and benefits of treatment and consider their decisions in the context of their family values, ethics, and religious beliefs. For end-stage patients, the goals of care change from cure of their disease to effective comfort measures. Teams of palliative care specialists will include physicians trained in palliative medicine plus nurses, social workers, psychologists, and child life specialists for younger patients.

CANCER SURVIVORSHIP

PREVIEW | REVIEW

- What are late effects of cancer radiation treatment?
- Nephrotoxicity as a late effect is common after which chemotherapy drug?

With the advances in treatment, more and more patients are surviving cancer. Long-term follow-up is important due to the late sequelae in cancer survivorship.

Late effects of radiation therapy include hormonal dysfunction and secondary cancers occurring in the affected field. For example, growth hormone deficiency is common after cranial radiation, and infertility is common after gonadal radiation. Cranial radiation causes an increased risk for low-grade (meningioma) and high-grade (glioblastoma) tumors.

Late effects of chemotherapy depend on the specific drugs used for treatment. Secondary AML occurs at a higher rate with etoposide or cyclophosphamide. Nephrotoxicity is common, especially after cisplatin. There is increased infertility after high doses of cyclophosphamide and other alkylators. Refer to Table 25-3 on page 25-9 for more detail.

General late effects can include increased risk of obesity, liver dysfunction, and secondary cancers. There is a higher risk of heart disease when anthracyclines are given in conjunction with radiation that covers the heart.

Guidelines for long-term follow-up for survivors of childhood, adolescent, and young adult cancers are available from the Children's Oncology Group.

HISTIOCYTOSIS

PREVIEW | REVIEW

- Which cells are abnormally activated in histiocytic disorders?
- Which endocrine disease can be seen with Langerhans cell histiocytosis (LCH) involving the pituitary gland?
- Which organ systems are at high risk in LCH?

OVERVIEW

The histiocytoses are a heterogeneous group of disorders characterized by abnormal proliferation, activation, and cytokine release by cells involved in phagocytosis and antigen presentation, such as dendritic cells, monocytes, macrophages, and histiocytes.

LANGERHANS CELL HISTIOCYTOSIS (LCH)

Occurrence

LCH is the most common of the histiocytoses and occurs at an incidence of 4/1,000,000 per year. The median age at presentation is 2½ years, and the male-to-female ratio is close to 1:1.

Presentation

Lytic bone lesions of the skull are the most common presenting sign of LCH, followed by lytic lesions in the femur, ribs, vertebra, or humerus. Another common presentation is a skin rash in the diaper area or scalp (petechiae and brown scaly papules, which can resemble bad cradle cap). Patients can also present with fever, weight loss, diarrhea, diabetes insipidus (from pituitary involvement; for more information, see the Endocrinology section), and a history of draining otitis.

Pathology

On skin biopsy, LCH lesions show a large number of pathologic Langerhans cells, which are accompanied by lymphocytes, macrophages, granulocytes, eosinophils, and multinucleated giant cells. Diagnosis is confirmed by finding CD1a or CD207 (langerin) by immunohistochemistry. **Birbeck granules** are seen on electron microscopy, but this test is rarely performed.

Patients are classified as high or low risk based on specific organs involved. High-risk sites include the liver, spleen, lungs, and bone marrow. Low-risk sites include skin, bones, lymph nodes, and the pituitary gland. Treatment depends on disease characteristics.

Treatment

Treatment of disease limited to the skin may include topical steroids, surgery, phototherapy, and/or systemic chemotherapy. Indications for systemic chemotherapy include multifocal bone/multiorgan disease, painful lesions, infected lesions, and other secondary complications. Single bone lesions can undergo curettage and be observed. Low-risk patients have cure rates of > 90%, and, even if they experience a relapse, most are ultimately cured of their disease.

Patients with high-risk organ involvement can have mortality approaching 50%. The degree of response following 6 weeks of induction therapy is predictive of outcome, with rapid responders doing much better than slow responders. Advanced refractory multisystem risk disease often requires bone marrow transplantation for the best chance of long-term disease control.

THE MEDSTUDY HUB: YOUR GUIDELINES AND REVIEW ARTICLES RESOURCE

For both review articles and current pediatrics practice guidelines, visit the MedStudy Hub at

medstudy.com/hub

The Hub contains the only online consolidated list of all current guidelines focused on pediatrics. Guidelines on the Hub are easy to find, continually updated, and linked to the published source. MedStudy maintains the Hub as a service to the medical community and makes it available to anyone and everyone at no cost to users.

ONCOLOGY

FIGURE SOURCES

Figure 25-6: MedStudy illustration
Figure 25-7: MedStudy illustration
Figure 25-8: J Morley-Smith
Figure 25-9: Michael Richardson. CC BY-SA 3.0
The remaining figures are from the MedStudy archives.